The Problem of
Health Technology

The Problem of Health Technology

POLICY IMPLICATIONS FOR MODERN HEALTH CARE SYSTEMS

Pascale Lehoux

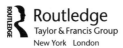
Routledge
Taylor & Francis Group
New York   London

Routledge is an imprint of the
Taylor & Francis Group, an informa business

Published in 2006 by
Routledge
Taylor & Francis Group
270 Madison Avenue
New York, NY 10016

Published in Great Britain by
Routledge
Taylor & Francis Group
2 Park Square
Milton Park, Abingdon
Oxon OX14 4RN

© 2006 by Taylor & Francis Group, LLC
Routledge is an imprint of Taylor & Francis Group

Printed in the United States of America on acid-free paper
10 9 8 7 6 5 4 3 2 1

International Standard Book Number-10: 0-415-95348-0 (Hardcover) 0-415-95349-9 (Softcover)
International Standard Book Number-13: 978-0-415-95348-1 (Hardcover) 978-0-415-95349-8 (Softcover)
Library of Congress Card Number 2005031274

Library of Congress Cataloging-in-Publication Data

Lehoux, Pascale.
    The problem of health technology : policy implications for modern health care systems / Pascale Lehoux.
       p. cm.
    Includes bibliographical references (p.) and index.
    ISBN-13: 978-0-415-95348-1 (hardback)
    ISBN-13: 978-0-415-95349-8 (pbk.)
    1. Medical informatics. 2. Medical policy. 3. Medicine--Miscellanea. I. Title.

R858.L44 2006
362.17--dc22

2005031274

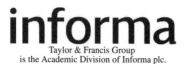

Taylor & Francis Group
is the Academic Division of Informa plc.

Visit the Taylor & Francis Web site at
http://www.taylorandfrancis.com

and the Routledge Web site at
http://www.routledge-ny.com

Contents

Acknowledgments

The somewhat audacious idea of writing a book about the social politics of health technology assessment and use first occurred to me when I was putting plans together for a sabbatical leave from the University of Montreal. At the time I optimistically believed I could, rather effortlessly, write tens of thousands of words on the subject and that they would naturally find an audience. Soon after I started to work on the project—instead of just talking about it—it became vividly clear to me that much more was involved than simply having the will to write, no matter how stubborn I am.

After convincing myself to devote my precious sabbatical year to the project, I thereupon needed to persuade an editor, who then needed to persuade her/his press, that my proposed book would not only be completed but, just as important, would sell a significant number of copies. For the latter task, I had somehow to assure serious, time-pressured people that there is, somewhere "out there," a substantial audience eager to read such a work. Because I was far from certain myself that I could convince anyone that such a specialized horde existed, I should first thank you, my reader, for devoting your time and energy to reading this book. Next, for believing in me and in the worth of this project, I extend sincere gratitude to Michael Bickerstaff, the Routledge editor who was instrumental in transforming my plans and aspirations into the three-dimensional reality you presently hold in your hands. I also gratefully acknowledge the insightful and encouraging comments and suggestions made by Routledge's peer reviewers; I hope this book merits their confidence in my work.

The Problem of Health Technology was also made possible thanks to the enthusiasm and generous support of my colleagues at the University of

Toronto, where I had the immense pleasure of spending seven months of my sabbatical. These inspiring individuals gave me invaluable support—scholarly, financial, and personal. I also found in my discussions with the mentors and fellows of the Health Care, Technology and Place (HCTP) doctoral program the intellectual stimulation that both pushed my thinking further and reminded me of what a great privilege it is to be part of a dynamic academic community. In particular, I wish to thank Patricia McKeever for sharing with me her deep respect for the natural sciences and her unsurpassed creativity in interdisciplinary research and teaching; and Peter Coyte, for his amicable, generous, and determined devotion to enriching health services and policy research. My sojourn at the University of Toronto was also greatly facilitated by Louise Lemieux-Charles, chair of the Department of Health Policy, Management and Evaluation (HPME), who provided me with office space and clerical support (without ever questioning what, exactly, I was doing!).

At my home base, the University of Montreal, I benefited from the enduring moral support of Renaldo Battista, the head of the Department of Health Administration. I extend sincere thanks also to my departmental colleagues who encouraged my aspirations and *let me focus* on writing this book. In particular, Jean-Louis Denis, with whom I have had the pleasure of conducting a great deal of research and teaching, not only sharpened my thinking but also contributed to my peace of mind during my sabbatical.

This book is informed by various research projects I led between 1998 and 2004. During that period I had the privilege of relying on several outstanding research assistants from whom I learned a great deal. Geneviève Daudelin, Myriam Hivon, and Stéphanie Tailliez were not only highly efficient and diligent but also trustworthy, insightful, and cheerful.

Several people helped to make my thoughts and prose clearer by devoting some of their precious time to reading and commenting on drafts and to advising me on the book's overall structure. During my time at the University of Toronto, a few informal discussion sessions were held around the book's prospectus and preliminary versions of two chapters. I am indebted to the helpful comments I received at those meetings from Nathalie Danjoux, Raisa Deber, Laura O'Grady, Kiran van Rijn, Jorge Silva, and Lara Varpio. For raising challenging comments—diplomatically cloaked in warm support—I wish to thank Olivier Demers-Payette, Marc Lemire, Daniel Neyland, Louise Potvin, Melanie Rock, Thomas Schlich, and the three University of Montreal research assistants I mentioned above. Near the end of the writing process, Susan Lampriere and Morgan Holmes played a pivotal role in the manuscript's final polishing.

During the preparation of this book, my feline companion, Cafeton, was my biggest fan (perhaps because he had never seen me so often at home). He slept on my desk (or rather on the thick pile of papers that carpeted its surface) and, with his purring, revealed his great enthrallment with all that I was doing. Because I am, like him, a spoiled creature, I was able to count on numerous friends and relatives who patiently listened to the obscure unfolding of the chapters and the trillion minuscule details regarding my correspondence with potential editors and publishers. However, these companions on the journey were essential in keeping me on track. Indeed, in several topics they are more deeply versed than I, and often they know how to explain those subjects much more effectively than I do. For their friendship, support, and confidence, I wish to thank Linette Cohen, Kate Frohlich, Pierro Hirsch, Pierre Patenaude, Blake Poland, Marie-Pascale Pomey, and Claude Vincent.

Introduction

Why Write and Publish a Book about Health Technology Assessment and Use?

Since the mid-1980s, health care systems in most industrialized countries have had to adapt to the continual emergence of technical innovations and the rising cost of health care services. Although the issue remains controversial, technology is often seen as the main cost-driver (Cohen and Hanft 2004). Closely connected to the evidence-based medicine movement, various initiatives to assess technologies and to introduce more rationality into decision- and policy-making have recently flourished in North America, Europe, and Australia. Health Technology Assessment (HTA) represents the most salient scientific response to such policy-related endeavors (Banta and Luce 1993 Berg, et al. 2004; T. Williams et al. 2003). Its main assumption is that the budget for health care is a closed envelope. Rational choices therefore must be made in order to sort out "good" innovations from "bad" ones and in order to select only those that yield high value for money in terms of clinical effectiveness.

While this view is partly valid, it nonetheless frames the "problem of health technology" in a way that is both too narrow and potentially misleading. When observed through the lens of HTA and through policy-makers' expectations with respect to HTA, the problem of health technology is reduced to questions of affordability and payment: Can health care systems absorb the costs of innovations? And who will pay for them? Such framing does not allow for exploring alternative policy options and leaves other pressing questions unanswered. Beyond clinical efficacy, what is the *value* of specific innovations? What impact do they have on clinical practice, population health, and social development? Why do certain innovations emerge but not others?

As the philosopher Melzer (1993, 287) suggests, technology is "the most fundamental as well as the most problematic characteristic of human existence in our age," and the "problem of technology" has become central in Western political thought. This book offers an alternative framework within which to consider health technology, thereby shedding much needed light on the social and political issues pertaining to its assessment and use.

Why Did I Write This Book?

For several observers, health technology is bliss—something that cannot be (irrationally) resisted but has to be (strategically) embraced:

> Technology has streamlined the administration of the hospital and the doctor's office, enabling more efficient and cost-effective processing and storage of patient medical and billing records. Telemedicine has advanced to the point where remote specialist consultation can take place through videoconferencing and the immediate transmission of X-ray and other images. Technology has brought noninvasive diagnostic and surgical tools to the physician's practice. And breakthroughs in medicine through computer-assisted research have reduced the half-life of medical knowledge to five or fewer years (my guess); but if there is one thing for sure, it is that technological change will continue to affect the field of medicine and will continue to accelerate. (Ellis 2000, xiii–xiv)

"Technology" sounds modern. It also evokes time. Technology must be about the *latest*. It is also supposed to be *better*. But how and when do we know that an innovation is better?

These are the daunting questions with which I have been repeatedly confronted since the mid-1990s. They combine technical and normative considerations that are usually dealt with separately—by engineers and scientists on the one hand, and by social scientists, philosophers, and ethicists on the other. Too often, however, I felt these two communities were badly equipped to understand and talk to each other. Being nonetheless interested in what both groups had to say, I learned enormously by contrasting their respective conceptual frameworks and methodological approaches to technology. Oversimplifying a long-standing debate, according to technology enthusiasts there will always be better technical solutions to social problems. According to technology opponents there will always be problems with technology because engineers and scientists do not properly understand society.

In developing my own approach, I was fortunate to be able to rely on the work of several scholars (mainly from the field of science and technology studies [STS]) whose thinking about technology has gone beyond this artificial divide and has shown that technology (including its design, production, and use) is the product of social practices (Brown and Webster 2004). In other words, humans are involved in the design of technology, and technology is involved in human practices in ways that make them mutually constitutive. As I became more familiar with STS, I realized that it should be possible to bring the technical and normative aspects together in a common framework that would make it possible to call into question why and how health innovations may or may not be *better*. I also realized, however, that such questions are not always popular within the STS community, which is often reluctant to discuss how things could be better. This reluctance may be related to the nature of the people and groups with whom STS researchers interact on a daily basis—that is, their audiences. Because, however, my "audience" is made up of health researchers, clinicians, managers, and policy-makers, I may be more concerned about ways to improve health care practices and policies. That is one reason why I decided to write this book.

Despite my pragmatic stance toward research on technology, I should warn readers that I still have not found a concise answer to the daunting question. But I trust that if they embark on the intellectual journey this book carves through various interdisciplinary perspectives, they will, at the end, be more aware of the positive and negative implications of health innovations. And perhaps, through this awareness, they will be more sensitive to innovations that are, indeed, better.

I will return to this issue in more detail later, but first I would like to consider a childhood memory that illustrates, in straightforward terms, an experience that acknowledges the superiority of a simple tool. It is taken from a work of fiction by Nicholson Baker and is about the change from milk delivered to the door in bottles to milk bought at a supermarket in cardboard containers:

> I first saw the invention in the refrigerator at my best friend Fred's house (I don't know how old I was, possibly five or six): the radiant idea that you tore apart one of the triangular eaves of the carton, pushing its flaps back, using the stiffness of its own glued seam against itself, forcing the seal inside out, without ever having to touch it, into a diamond-shaped opening which became a

> pourer, a *better* pourer than a circular bottle opening or a pitcher's mouth because you could create a very fine stream of milk very simply, letting it bend over the leading corner, something I appreciated as I was perfecting my ability to pour my own glass of milk or make my bowl of cereal—the radiant idea filled me with jealousy and satisfaction (N. Baker 1990, 42).

The experience Baker narrates is about discovering something new, something at first sight intriguing, and, more important, something that appears simple, ingenious, efficacious, beautiful, and adapted to the user's needs and abilities. In this example of use-in-context, the cardboard container is obviously superior to old glass bottles. Could that mean that technology, and more specifically *new* technology, possesses the remarkable characteristic of being able to self-evidently impose its superiority? A safe answer is "no" (as most readers would probably agree).

However, despite this commonsense appraisal, why are several new technologies introduced into the market every day in company with marketing campaigns designed to persuade users to acquire and use them? Here, the answer becomes multilayered. Although private interests shape aggressive promotional strategies, they cannot explain in and of themselves why and how the use of various technologies will (or will not) become widespread and/or sustainable (Gelijns and Rosenberg 1994).

In this book I argue that technology is profoundly human. It generates sensorial and bodily experiences that cannot be ignored even though almost all of us tend to downplay their presence. You may have lifted an eyebrow when I used the word "beautiful" to describe Baker's milk carton. This deep respect for innovation may be a legacy of my early training in industrial design, an education that first showed me how technology can be designed brilliantly. In the passage quoted above, according to the narrator the cardboard container triggered jealousy and satisfaction. Why? One preliminary response to this question might be the intense pleasure that using a certain technology generates when the action involved feels right and when one achieves the intended results (Ihde 1990). That response, of course, begs other questions: Are all technology-mediated actions that feel right in fact *really* right? Should all intended results be achieved? Trying to unpack such questions, I will argue that technology may also be gloomy, threatening, or depressing.

One thing I will never say, however, is that technology is dehumanizing. Historians know that humans have never needed massive-destruction technology to act in inhumane ways (Burke and Ornstein 1997). When observers of modern, high-tech medicine stress that technology renders health care inhuman, I instead see social practices that are inescapably mediated through technology. In certain instances, technology facilitates feelings attributed to human practices, such as closeness and responsiveness. In other instances, it supports distance and cold, machinelike rationality. Nonetheless, in both situations, humans and technology are intertwined and neither can, in itself, be declared inhuman. Judging the quality of technology-mediated actions—which is part of my inquiry about how and when a health innovation is better—requires examining the social practices that unfold in broader sociotechnical networks.

Social scientists offer several key concepts that facilitate such inquiry. They pay attention, among other things, to power relations, hierarchy, expertise-based authority, and the reproduction of social norms and routines (Lawton 2003). While conducting my research on health technology, I was struck more than once by the numerous explicit and tacit ways in which power relations pervade hospital work. Health technology is intimately linked to expertise and knowledge, and therefore is pivotal to how physicians, nurses, managers, and patients interact (Lehoux, Sicotte, et al. 2002; Lehoux, Saint-Arnaud, and Richard 2004). Recognizing that technology is human—that it is the product of human design, that it brings pleasure and pain, and that it restructures social relations in both positive and negative ways—I argue for the need to bring *intelligence* to innovations.

That is another reason why I wrote this book: I fundamentally believe that not all innovations should be put to use. Although it remains a thorny issue, I have often observed how clinicians, patients, and policymakers themselves call into question the purpose of various technologies. While some of them are more inclined to trust a quantitative, "objective," and cost-effectiveness approach to setting priorities, others raise issues that cannot be addressed appropriately through a "value for money" piecemeal approach (i.e., adding to the current health care basket of services only those innovations for which there is evidence of cost-effectiveness). For instance, reallocating health care budgets from hospital acute care to preventive community care and reducing health inequalities through integrated public policies (e.g., employment, education, transportation) requires adopting a broader perspective about what constitutes health (Evans 1984). In this book, I have attempted to offer new and potentially more fruitful points of entry for readers to reflect on and debate the relative value of technological innovations in the health care sector.

Defining Health Technology

In its early years, the U.S. Office of Technology Assessment (OTA) defined health technology as including all instruments, devices, drugs, and procedures that are used in the delivery and organization of health care services (U.S. Congress 1985, 3). This broad definition went beyond a narrow focus on high-tech devices to include technologies that were not primarily destined to provide diagnostic or therapeutic services, but that were pivotal in supporting and organizing hospital work (e.g., information systems, surgical rooms, sterilization systems). Since then, developments in information and communication technologies (ICTs) have significantly reconfigured the centrality of the hospital in modern medicine by enabling, alongside therapeutic innovations, new delivery models for health care services (e.g., ambulatory care, home care, community clinics, satellite units). It is therefore important to highlight that a technology is rarely simply a stand-alone device, but one component of larger health care delivery systems.

Furthermore, from an anthropological perspective, procedures or techniques that do not involve any apparent material support can also be conceptualized as technologies (e.g., swimming, language, hunting) (Latour and Lemonnier 1994). According to Ihde (1990), any extension of human senses, action, and cognition should be considered technologically *mediated*. That includes, for instance, the ability to see (e.g., using eyeglasses or microscope), to feel (e.g., via auscultation), to move around (e.g., on a bicycle or in wheelchair), to calculate figures (e.g., using a counting table), and to remember certain events (e.g., via photographs).

Table 0.1 provides examples of various technologies that are currently used in and around health care systems. Some of these technologies are not necessarily tools used by clinicians (e.g., health promotion technologies, occupational health technologies), but they do carry significant health implications and therefore should be included in any analysis of the value of health technology. This table reflects the types of technologies to which I mainly refer throughout this book. I discuss less often certain categories of what Brown and Webster (2004) describe as new medical technologies (NMTs), such as nanotechnology (extremely small devices that can be inserted in the body to perform various functions), cryonics (long-term preservation of body tissue and organs at temperatures below zero), cloning (duplication of biological material), regenerative medicine (use of one's cells to repair or regenerate tissues), and xenotransplantation (transplantation of tissues or organs wherein the species of the donor is different from that of the recipient). Although these innovations do contribute to shaping expectations and perceptions of health care, they are not

Table 0.1 Categories of Health Technology

Categories	Examples
Screening tests	Cytological tests, blood tests, prenatal testing, genetic testing
Diagnostic tests and imaging devices	X-rays, ultrasound, magnetic resonance imaging, computed tomography scanner
Monitoring systems	Blood glucose monitors, electrocardiograms, fetal monitoring system
Implants	Cochlear implants, left ventricular assist devices, pacemakers
Surgery and therapeutic devices	Hip replacement, tonsillectomy, laparoscopic cholecystectomy, radiation therapy
Palliative technologies	Dialysis, ventilators, parenteral nutrition
Drugs	Caplets, patches, injections, inhalers
Health promotion technologies	Vaccines, helmets, condoms, smoking cessation strategies, playgrounds and sports facilities
Occupational health technologies	Protective equipment and clothing, work safety measures, ergonomic furniture and tools, preventive measures for pregnant women
Technical aids	Wheelchairs, hearing aids, prostheses
Information technologies	Telemedicine, electronic patient records, health cards, expert systems

yet part of routine clinical practices. Chapter 2 provides a fuller description of my theoretical approach to health technology.

Aim and Approach of the Book

My scholarly journey thus far has been marked by a set of intense interdisciplinary quests in various research domains, chief among them industrial design, public health, evaluation, epistemology, sociology of science and technology, philosophy and ethics, sociology of illness, qualitative research, information technology, home care, and knowledge utilization. Each of these intellectual journeys has deepened my sense of the great extent to which research areas share epistemological and methodological concerns and of the enticing edges and territories between them that remain unexplored or insufficiently articulated. A more thorough understanding of these mutual concerns is exactly what I am looking for—the refreshing insight that comes from carefully bringing together and contrasting the border zones that each discipline or area of inquiry, over time and through hard, creative, and rigorous thinking, gradually extends a little further.

My aim in writing this book was to illuminate the main layers of scientific and policy arguments about the "problem of health technology" that are currently deployed in various industrialized countries and to show why and how they are misleading. By revisiting the clinical, commercial, and policy perspectives that dominate scientific and policy debates, I seek to develop an alternative conceptualization of health technology as it is assessed and used in industrialized health care systems.

To achieve this objective, I compare and contrast two main streams of literature that have so far evolved independently but that can, when brought together, help to identify promising areas for future research and pragmatic ways to overcome the policy challenges facing health care systems. Specifically, this book summarizes the key conceptual and methodological issues that have been examined through the work of HTA and STS scholars. While HTA embodies a rational, science-based approach to dealing with policy issues and the regulation of technology, STS focuses on the social practices that shape the processes underlying the design, adoption, and use of technology. Establishing a dialogue between these two fields appears to me to be highly warranted.

Why Read This Book?

It should be clear by now that this book is *not* about how to market technologies, to reduce resistance to change, or to manage innovation in hospitals. Rather, it is about clarifying what technology does and what humans want from it. When I was researching this subject, I sought to accentuate three key aspects. First, although this book is not an ethical analysis of how health technology should be used and regulated, it does not treat technology as an unproblematic means to an end. When the word *health* is placed in front of the word *technology*, the conjunction brings to the fore other dimensions of modernity. It raises issues such as risk, disease, death, life, and, because we are human, wonders and sorrows. Health technology is far from neutral (Ihde 1990). It moves people just as it affects lives. It creates hopes and anxieties (Callahan 1990). And it generates power and authority (Blume 1992).

Second, this book travels down intellectual paths that are often less frequently taken when experts reflect on ways to manage health technology in modern health care systems. Since the mid-1980s, the health research literature has portrayed health technology both as a tremendous opportunity to improve patients' lives and as a major threat to the financial sustainability of health care systems (Peden and Freeland 1995; Newhouse 1993). When adopting such a framework, the issue appears more or less straightforward: adopting only innovations that yield the best clinical outcomes and cost the least should help keep the health care system financially manageable. However, the trade-offs in terms of costs and outcomes are often unclear, the most salient example being when an innovation costs more *but* generates only slightly better outcomes (Johri and Lehoux 2003).

Without going into extensive detail (something better handled by health economists), measuring and valuing outcomes is an imperfect science. Furthermore, a new intervention does not necessarily replace an existing technology, although it may represent the preferred option for some patients and clinicians. As a result, restricting access to technology on the strict basis of cost-effectiveness proves much more difficult in practice than it appears in theory (Giacomini 1999; Laupacis 2002). Thus, very often the ultimate question becomes irreducibly political: Who can afford health innovations? Because there may be no limit to what wealthy societies (let alone individuals) are ready to invest in health, the cost-effectiveness approach may never fulfill its promise of increasing rationality in health technology-related decision-making. This book does not try to demonstrate why this might be the case. Rather, it relies on social science insights about the real-world use and dissemination of health technology in order to offer an alternative framing of the problem of health technology.

The third way in which this book offers a unique vista has to do with its style and format. When bringing together two relatively autonomous fields of research, one is forced to transgress conceptual and linguistic boundaries and established academic norms (Stengers 1993). Through the various research projects that I have been involved in, and because of my dual interest in social science and applied health research, I have been privileged to interact with a wide array of clinicians, decision-makers, and scholars. It took me a while to understand how to engage these various audiences, and I often had to adapt my vocabulary. Depending on the words I used and the issues I raised, my interlocutors seemed to label me as either a (anti-technology/medicine) social scientist or a (naïve/theoretically unsophisticated) applied health researcher. Beyond (or perhaps thanks to) this ambiguity in my status, I learned that each area can benefit from the other, *and this mutual learning and dialogue is what the book is largely about.*

The conceptual path I have traversed is infrequently adopted by clinicians, managers, and policy-makers, people who are generally seeking ways to adapt their practices to the rapid pace at which medical innovations are emerging. Legitimately, they may look for clinical, managerial, and financial strategies that are better exposed at state-of-the-art medical specialty conferences and in health care management and policy handbooks. Well, this book contains no strategies and no elaborate cost analyses. Neither does it rely on sophisticated sociological concepts that make "normal practices" appear more obscure than they are. I hope to have summarized the social science literature concisely so that people who are unfamiliar with the terrain will feel comfortable reading the book from beginning to end. I also hope that social scientists will not notice too many betrayals (because of course there are some; otherwise the book would not be as short as it is and would not provide recommendations), and will be both intrigued and challenged by the translation of parts of their work into the normative concerns of my quest to understand when and how certain innovations can be construed as better.

The book's main thrust is, in sum, that it is both possible and more fruitful to conceptualize the problem of health technology in a different way: by presenting health technology as necessarily embedded in broader social and political practices that can be examined, called into question, and modified through appropriate policy initiatives and organizational incentives. The upshot of such an alternative conceptualization is significant: increased influence over the types of technology that are circulated and used in health care systems.

Outline of the Book

Following this introduction (the remainder of which establishes important groundwork for all that follows), five chapters make up the main body of this book. The first chapter summarizes the development, content, and scope of HTA, stressing both its achievements and shortcomings. It also clarifies the close connection between HTA and other initiatives from the evidence-based medicine movement, such as the development and implementation of clinical practice guidelines (CPGs; Berg et al. 2004; Moreira 2005). Qualitative and quantitative data from a case study on six Canadian HTA agencies are also presented and contrasted with the international literature on HTA. Finally, the chapter explores the expectations and practices of various categories of HTA stakeholders, emphasizes the need to consolidate the academic foundations of this policy-oriented field of research, and identifies specific areas in which the input of social science work would prove useful.

Chapter 2 presents and explains key STS concepts by focusing on a question that may appear at first glance both simple and deterministic: What do technologies do? Using examples drawn from ethnographic studies (i.e., involving prolonged onsite, naturalistic observations), I argue that the value and impact of innovations can be fully understood only by considering how humans and technologies interact within the context of health care provision. By looking at what technologies do (Mol 2000), this chapter emphasizes how innovations are always embedded in complex human practices.

The third chapter moves on to explore values and expectations that are called upon to promote or to criticize the use of health technology in clinical, scientific, and policy realms. Relying on broad social science concepts, I argue that technologies, by their very design, encapsulate values and assumptions about why and how they should be used. These are often crystallized during the innovation process and may represent compromises between the views of designers, marketers, shareholders, clinicians, and patient representatives. The chapter also examines how various claims are made on behalf of patients, and stresses the need both to clarify and to try to reduce the gap between what technologies actually deliver and what people expect from them.

Next, chapter 4 addresses the institutional arrangements in which key decisions about the regulation of health technology are made. It focuses on the perspectives of influential organized groups: industry, physician associations, patient associations, and decision-makers. My approach avoids overgeneralizing and simplistic arguments, such as demonizing the role of corporate financial interests, on the one hand, and glamorizing patients' views, on the other. Rather, the chapter offers a nonnaïve, in-depth analysis of the sociopolitical tensions that shape the regulation of health technology. It also addresses the perceived value and usefulness of HTA and other types of knowledge in health technology-related policy-making.

The fifth chapter revisits the purposes and means of the evidence-based approach to health technology and makes more explicit a few of its assumptions. My objective is to lay the foundation of an alternative framework for thinking about health technology. Among other points, I argue that an increased circulation of knowledge about technology can be effective in improving the regulation of health technology only if it is accompanied by transparent deliberative processes. This chapter also outlines five overarching principles that help to refocus the discussion on the concept of desirability: explicit normativity, theoretically-informed empirical insights, reflexivity, public input, and transparency.

The book's conclusion summarizes and articulates my study's main arguments. It suggests new avenues for research and a number of policy recommendations. In a context in which the pressure exerted by health technology innovation is not likely to lessen, my concluding remarks seek to stimulate scholarly work on empirical questions that would generate original and relevant contributions to health research. This part of my book also summarizes "take-home messages" that could be integrated into policy-making practices. It then ends on a slightly provocative note by suggesting the need to add *intelligence* to innovation. This last section is intended to remind readers that any given innovation should not be seen as the only possible solution—every technology is the end result of social processes that could have led to different designs.

Revisiting the Problem

According to Campbell, normative frameworks "consist of taken-for-granted assumptions about values, attitudes, identities, and other collectively shared expectations" (Campbell 2002, 23). They lie in the background of policy debates and usually limit the range of alternatives perceived as acceptable and legitimate. Because academics contribute to the creation of normative frameworks, in the remainder of this introduction I draw attention to the ways in which health researchers and policy analysts discuss the problem of health technology in modern health care systems. In doing so, I highlight the policy implications such a framing implicitly and explicitly involves.

My analysis focuses on five characteristics of the scientific and policy debates on health technology: the relationship between values and health technology, conceptualizations of health technology, political perspectives on health, the framing of policy options, and stances toward the biomedical industry. Exploring each of these concerns is necessary for a full understanding of the sociopolitical context in which HTA has emerged (Giacomini 1999; Faulkner 1997) and why current thinking on the subject may not provide an adequate solution to the problem of health technology.

Five Characteristics of the Scientific and Policy Debates on Health Technology

1. The Relationship Between Values and Health Technology: Considering Health Technology as a Neutral Tool

Although a number of controversial health technologies and procedures have generated (and still generate) public attention and scholarly debate, health technology is most often considered neutral; that is, devoid of any axiological content. When debating medical innovations, the application of an innovation is more often at stake, rather than the innovation itself (Callahan 1990; Heitman 1998). For instance, in the case of abortion, the surgical procedure is rarely called into question, but the definition of an embryo and the time at which the procedure can be performed constitute the heart of the debate. The picture becomes more complicated when a technology to be applied changes or when an application seems hard to circumscribe. As an example of the former, regulating the use of the post-conception pill known as RU486 posed a challenge to the very definition of abortion. As an example of the latter, the use of stem cells in research became a thorny issue because the end application was still underdetermined. While it is obvious that surplus embryos generated through new reproductive technologies do not benefit from the research, the long-term potential applications of the results are very attractive for several groups (Hogle, 2000).

When technology enthusiasts hear about such ethical issues, their response is often geared to pointing out how society is stubbornly resisting technological change and is not in tune with the pace at which technology advances:

> More often than not the physician and the nurse, like most of the rest of society, are accelerating at a slower pace and learn of advanced technologies only after the fact of their deployment, leaving them with the problem of adapting quickly to new techniques and leaving the administrator with the problem of altering plans and budgets in order to acquire and install the newly available technology (Ellis 2000, xiv).

The flip side of this coin reveals that when a technology is adopted too hastily, its application can raise serious concerns (Giacomini et al. 2000). Notwithstanding the quality of the work accomplished by several ethicists, ethical tensions surrounding medical innovations are often looked at (e.g., by health care providers, managers, policy-makers, and researchers) from a utilitarian perspective: the end justifies the means. The end may be amenable to ethical analysis, but the means remain technical and, therefore, axiologically neutral (Ihde 1990).

This view perpetuates the idea that technology is "simply" a means and, as such, does not possess particular axiological qualities. Philosophers of technology, from Heidegger to Bunge, have scrutinized the various ways in which a tool might be considered value-free or not. STS scholars, following a seminal paper by Winner (1980), have also seriously debated the political and normative nature of technology (discussed further in chapter 2; see also Joerges 1999). Although none of these scholars would likely consider the debate resolved, two aspects of it strike me as being fundamentally significant for health care. First, it shows the need to revisit what we usually consider progress. According to Melzer (1993, 307), in a technological era during which avoidance of death and attainment of security predominate, life becomes "endless wanting and striving," and "the pursuit of good is replaced with the overcoming of evil." In less tantalizing terms, do innovations in health care always equate to progress? And is progress actively pursued but never really attained? The second aspect of the debate that intrigues me is the suggestion that a joint analysis of the tool (means) and its use (end) is required. As I explain in chapter 3, the ways in which health technology is applied rarely correspond closely to an initial plan, a situation that calls for a reexamination of both expected and actual purposes.

2. Conceptualizations of Health Technology: A Piecemeal Approach That Seeks to Quantify Costs and Outcomes

According to a report released by the government of Australia (Australia Productivity Commission 2005, xxvi), "Future advances, interacting with increasing demands for health services driven by income growth, the accelerating impact of population ageing, subsidized consumer prices and strong community expectations that new technologies should be accessible to all, will place increasing pressures on health systems." This view partly explains why HTA has been increasingly supported by academics and governments since the late 1970s (Banta and Perry 1997). HTA seeks to synthesize the best available evidence regarding the efficacy, safety, and costs of medical technology and, in principle, its ethical, social, and legal implications (Shemer and Schersten 1995; Cohen and Hanft 2004). Although the field has evolved since the mid-1990s and has led to original methodological and collaborative initiatives, the general approach is still to focus on one technology at a time and to produce secondary analyses of published research results that principally revolve around clinical outcomes and costs. This endeavor is definitely worthwhile; in practice, however, complex issues that are less amenable to quantitative analyses are insufficiently addressed by such a method (Lehoux, Tailliez, et al. 2004).

By adopting a piecemeal approach to technological change and by limiting issues to efficacy and costs, HTA reinforces the idea that policymakers should adopt only the most effective and affordable innovations. As Deber (1992, 135) points out, "Advocates of technology assessment have been proclaiming with increasing vehemence that we should not use technologies that are not effective. From this reasonable position comes an interesting logical fallacy, that we should use only those technologies that have been demonstrated to be effective." Although the assumption that only the most cost-effective innovations should be adopted appears to make sense, it conceals the fact that evidence of an innovation's effectiveness may not always be available because primary studies have not yet been conducted and/or published. Furthermore, HTA presumes that information about costs and effectiveness can and should drive public policy decisions (Gillick 2004).[1] As Nord (1999) indicates, members of the general public may give more weight to fairness in the allocation of scarce medical resources than to a strict maximization of health gains criteria. More globally, one is also struck by the fact that the number of new or existing technologies that deserve assessment far outstrips the human and financial capacity to perform those assessments (Deber 1992). As I show in chapter 1, there are many aspects of HTA that require further conceptualization and the use of a broader set of methods and evidence. Such work will still leave the door open for other approaches that can more broadly address technological change in health care systems.

3. Political Perspectives on Health: Conceiving of Health Care as a Market in Which Individual Demand and Ability to Pay for Technologies Should Drive the Future

Technology in health care research is often portrayed as a "force," an external factor or a variable that is powerful but unpredictable. According to Melzer (1993, 313), "When technology comes to be viewed as an independent and dangerous force, the will to control it inevitably emerges from the technological attitude itself."

Health economists have certainly contributed to a supply-and-demand conceptualization of health technology when developing a technical approach that involves, among other things, quality-of-life measurement tools and models to predict changes in health care systems. Such a technical approach may appear apolitical because it brings to the fore quantifiable benefits and the elusive notion that it is possible to maximize health gains across society. However, it underplays the extent to which broader social determinants (e.g., education, employment, discrimination, settings) affect the health of particular groups (Evans et al. 1994).

Although most industrialized countries face a similar challenge with respect to controlling health spending, one may discern particular ways of framing why health care—and health technology—is politically valuable or not.[2] Interestingly, the multiple connotations of the word "value" (ethical as well as financial) seem inextricably intertwined. In this respect, one might consider the viewpoint of Leiland Kaiser of Kaiser Consulting, who reflects on why people talk about "costs" in health care when they are considered "revenues" in other industries:

> I have never been able to figure out why we celebrate when General Motors has a good year and lament when the health care industry has a good year, particularly when the local clinic or hospital may be the largest and most important employer in the community. If we truly have high value-added health care products to offer to our aging population, why shouldn't we try to maximize revenues in the health care industry? After all, health care providers deal in the one product people cannot live without—life. Is that not worth more than 14 percent of the gross domestic product? (Kaiser 2000, x)

Beyond the contested notion (Evans 1984) that a healthy life can be considered a "product," it is indeed very difficult to estimate what a healthy life is worth. Assuming, however, that health care is a business like any other, and that medical technology leads directly to a healthy life, appears both misguided and misinformed from a public health perspective. I am certainly not saying that those working in the health care industry are ignorant. On the contrary, they know acutely that medical technology sells well. In the context of a health care system in which the individual increasingly becomes the key "consumer," it is in fact a perfectly rational way to conceive of technological change: let the demand for innovations determine the future of health care. This view, meanwhile, finds less receptive ground in countries where equity and fair access to health are seen as *public* goods that should be managed, funded, and protected by the state (Cookson and Maynard 2000; Nord 1999). But with the emergence of innovations that have equivocal purposes (e.g., body reconstruction, comfort drugs, infertility treatments), the clash between those who argue in favor of putting individual consumers and their ability to pay in "the driver's seat" (Coddington et al. 2000) and those who argue for health as a public good will escalate. With such innovations, the notion of medical necessity becomes useless, and restricting access on the basis of costs appears to some as an infringement on individual rights (Cohen and Hanft 2004). In other words, we return again to the affordability question and its political underpinnings: Will only the wealthiest have access to health care innovations?

4. The Framing of Policy Options: Explicit and Implicit Rationing by Third-party Payers

As I discussed earlier, the development of HTA and evidence-based medicine attempts to introduce rationality into policy-making. The main thrusts are that choices must be made because health care systems cannot absorb all the precious innovations that are driving up global spending on health, and that these choices should be based on scientific information about cost and effectiveness. As a reflection of this attitude, the government of Australia (Australia, Productivity Commission 2005, xxvi) noted that "improved HTA processes could help to target new technologies to patient groups likely to benefit most and improve overall cost-effectiveness of healthcare." On this understanding, HTA could help to avoid the political question of "who" should have access to innovations by reframing the issue in terms of clinical benefits: innovations should be offered to those who are likely to benefit the most from them, at a reasonable price. This is not rationing per se; it has to do with increasing rationality by setting up clear, transparent priorities (Giacomini 1999). Nonetheless, as Besharov and Dunsay Silver (1987, 521) explain, the "medical" criteria (e.g., age, comorbidity, lifestyles and health-related behaviors, caregivers' and psychosocial support) that can be used to define the relative ability of potential candidates to benefit from an intervention are entwined with socioeconomic considerations (e.g., structural inequalities associated with education and employment).

Furthermore, when HTA and other sorts of scientific studies are translated into policy-making, other mechanisms come into play. Most industrialized countries rely on a mix of third-party payers, which include the state, employers, medical insurance companies, and various other arm's-length bodies (for special groups such as veterans, disabled people, accident victims). These third-party payers usually devise coverage rules that may or may not rely on scientific evidence and clear criteria for priority-setting. Explicit and implicit rationing—limiting access to services based on the available resources—does, therefore, arise.

My chief interest in relation to health care reimbursement is how payment incentives or disincentives are perceived as bearing on the utilization of health care. According to Kuttner,

> The more patients chafe under the constraints of utilization controls, the more they demand a choice of doctors—not realizing that the various doctors affiliated with a plan have similar or identical financial incentives to constrain costs. And the more plans try to offer a choice, the further they stray from the system-wide integration, prevention, and case management that are supposed advantages of HMOs [health management organizations]. (Kuttner 1998, 1562)

Or, here again, are Kaiser's views:

> Why do I have to get sick to recover dollars in my health
> insurance?... The next time I go in for a flu shot, I am going to
> demand an MRI or maybe a bone marrow transplant. It is the
> only way to recover even a part of my investment. I have no finan-
> cial incentive to stay well. If I am healthy, I lose all my financial
> investment in my health care premiums. And while I am at it, why
> should I get treatment from the same folks who make the diagno-
> sis? (Kaiser 2000, xi)

Kaiser's provocative sentiments, like many daily conversations each of
us probably have with friends and family about health care, illuminate
dysfunctional elements in consumers' behavior that are amplified by the
way health care is paid for and rationed. His comments make a number of
crucial assumptions: to obtain more technology-based services is better
and something individuals voluntarily seek; money spent on insurance
should yield an *individual* return that takes the form of technology-based
services; and the illegitimate use of health care services threatens the health
care system's sustainability. I will not argue that these assumptions are
entirely invalid. Rather, I wish to emphasize that such assertions only contribute to framing health technology as a private, desirable good, one that
should be rationed (because of its scarcity) according to one's ability to
pay.

Here is a recent take on the desirability of technology and the idea that
individuals will need to pay[3] for it:

> In our view the growth of medical technology is accelerating and
> will continue to accelerate rapidly in the early part of the new
> millennium. Consumers will demand it and want the benefits.
> All of this will drive up health care spending, and consumers will
> be faced with the need to pay for access to the technology. We do
> not believe that any system of rationing access to demonstrably
> beneficial technology will be acceptable in the United States.
> (Coddington et al. 2000, 183)[4]

Despite the authors' rhetoric, I doubt that getting a bone marrow transplant is something I would ever actively seek (especially not to "recover
dollars in my health insurance"). I have no doubt, however, about the
symbolic effectiveness of an advertisement emphasizing that a hospital or
clinical team performs outstanding bone marrow transplants. In other
words, health technology is too easily portrayed as something desirable in

itself and, consequently, as something that should be rationed or purchased on an ability-to-pay basis. There is even some perversity in widely showing off such technological miracles and then blaming "consumers" for wanting too much of them. In chapter 3, I unpack claims made on behalf of patients (by providers, managers, and policy-makers). I also consider the extent to which patients can be conceptualized as end users of health technology and, by extension, as consumers of desirable products.

5. Stances Toward the Biomedical Industry: Downplaying the Industrial Complex Behind Innovation

The biomedical industry is both highly diversified and a major economic player: "In the early 1990s, the industry ranked among the fastest-growing US manufacturing industries, with an annual growth rate of eight percent. In 2002, industry sales totaled $71 billion in the United States alone and $169 billion worldwide" (Cohen and Hanft 2004, 65). According to Coddington et al. (2000, xiv), health care in the United States was a $1.3 trillion industry in 2000 (nearly 14% of the gross domestic product). Considering its importance in sheer financial terms, on my first exposure to HTA I was perplexed by the dodging in the literature of these large commercial and professional ramifications.[5] The intentions, strategies, and interests of the biomedical industry are too often treated as disciplinary taboos (Beck 1992); that is, as aspects everyone is aware of but that cannot be intellectually engaged.

Of course, most health research scholars are critical of private interests, the search for profits, and powerful pharmaceutical detailing strategies (Gelijns and Rosenberg 1994). As an illustration, Foote (1986, 505) questions the relationship between public funding of basic and applied research in the health sciences that "blur[s] the distinction between public interest and private behavior in several ways." Similarly, Caplan argues that "ultimately … taxpayers will be faced with the grim financial prospect of paying billions of dollars to buy back from the commercial sector a device for which they already paid" (cited in Foote 1986, 505). More recently, Hlatky (2004, 2127) criticized the industry-driven growing use of the implantable defibrillator in lower-risk patients with underlying heart disease who have never had a cardiac arrest. Aside from McKinlay (1981), who published a seminal critique showing how the evidence about the benefits of a given innovation may be highly malleable and reinforce a capitalist logic, the HTA literature has rarely offered systematic analyses of the broader industrial complex that shapes certain innovations and refrains from creating other types of products (an exception appears in the work of Gelijns; see Gelijns and Rosenberg 1994 and Halm and Gelijns 1991).

It also appeared very strange to me that HTA producers would not make recommendations or give feedback to the biomedical equipment industry about the shortcomings of the innovations they assessed. For example, why does the assessment of a technology not seek to enhance its design and application? While I admit that this question is a bit naïve, it is nevertheless true that discussing the structure and strategies of the "big bad wolf"—the private corporations developing new technology—is often both theoretically and practically avoided in the literature on health technology. As a result, the black box of health technology's constant stream of innovations is merely taken as a given (Koch 1995). While chapter 1 offers some explanations for the avoidance strategy implemented by most HTA agencies toward industry, chapter 3 discusses how various approaches to design can shape different types of technology. In order to offer new ways of dealing with the emergence of innovations in health care systems, I believe we need to address the broader industrial processes and dynamics and to take the lid off the black box of innovations (see Brown and Webster 2004).

Five Social Science Insights into Technology's Importance in Health Care

The five social issues I have summarized thus far can fruitfully be revisited from the standpoint of the social science literature on health technology.

1. The Relationships Between Values and Health Technology: The Co-production of Health Technology and Society

As indicated earlier, ethical concerns about health technology often focus on its application and rarely on its nature, form, and characteristics (i.e., what its design involves in terms of values). By assuming that tools are neutral, analyses are limited to the actual and potential effects of technology on humans. Because it is often difficult to capture all the uses an innovation will, in practice, generate, such analyses also frequently remain speculative. It is not surprising, therefore, to hear developers' and clinicians' allergic reactions to social scientists' claim that technology may not prove as beneficial as intended or even be socially acceptable. Two aspects require clarification in order to better understand what is at stake: the temporal framework that underlies any appreciation of technology benefits and the space in which values are seen as being active.

First, because innovation is closely ingrained in a progressive view of the future and because the past can always be mobilized to argue that ethical concerns are misplaced (Brown and Webster 2004; Melzer 1993), a fruitful debate on the pros and cons of any given technology appears difficult to establish. Most technology enthusiasts will indeed refer to technology opponents as being resistant to change or attached to anachronistic principles and values. A common response would be as follows: "Look,

130 years ago everyone resisted the emergence of the telephone; but now, no one would dare to not possess at least one." In other words, what might appear unacceptable at one point in time will become integrated into normal practices later. As I discuss at greater length in chapter 2, this view embodies a deterministic view of technology, whereby it penetrates society and triggers social change.

STS scholars offer another interpretation of this phenomenon that can broadly be referred to as the social shaping of technology, or the co-construction of technology and society (R. Williams and Edge 1996). This view posits that both humans and technologies evolve over time into various configurations, supporting localized uses and practices. According to Prout (1996, 203), this theory "replaces society–technology dualism with a notion of their mutual constitution and promises a way of understanding devices as participating in and performing social relations alongside human actors." Thus, there are no social effects to be analytically isolated per se. Technology is a social practice, and the processes through which sociotechnical transformations are brought about can therefore be examined both as a whole (technical and human) and in their specificities (the same tool may support various applications).

The second point I would like to stress is a corollary of the first. Ethical and social issues are generally portrayed as arising *after* a given innovation has been put to use, as if they could be divorced from the design process (Morgall 1993). Values are thus located as being active in society (or end users), not in the technologies themselves. When adopting a sociotechnical approach, however, one is forced to recognize that technology is designed in a way that constrains and shapes its users' behaviors, and that designers hold certain values about why and how an innovation will prove superior (Oudshoorn and Pinch 2003). Chapter 3 clarifies the usefulness of calling into question the rationale behind innovations.

2. Conceptualizations of Health Technology: Sociotechnical Networks That are Necessarily Enabling and Constraining at the Same Time

There are a number of reasons for broadening the analysis of the problem of health technology beyond a piecemeal approach. One is linked to the form of technological change that modern health care systems are undergoing. Instead of using independent tools, providers and patients more often than not employ components that are embedded in larger technological systems of which they may not be aware and that are not under their direct control (Tenner 1996). By "systems," I mean the endless number of technological components that are required for a single technology to be effective (e.g., power supplies, replacement parts, information systems, data archiving systems, sterilization procedures). For Casey (1998, 12), this complexity and interconnectedness can trigger significant incidents:

> Society has become highly dependent on interconnected and tightly linked technologies, technologies in which the actions of a few influence the lives of many, technologies that can bring countless benefits but can also amplify the consequences of human error in ways that were never before possible or never anticipated.

Casey goes on to tell the story of a thirty-three-year-old patient who died a few months after receiving a massive radiation overdose from a Therca-25 cancer therapy machine due to a chain of "small" human mistakes and technical bugs (lack of feedback, untested sequence of commands, a protective metal sheet that did not activate). This patient, until his premature death, maintained a wry sense of humor and at one point remarked, "Captain Kirk forgot to put the machine on stun," an unsettling comment that reflects the cultural pervasiveness of technology in the present era. This example also underscores the fact that the complexity of modern high-tech medicine cannot be downplayed. It also increases the responsibility of hospital staff and their level of skills and training, and requires the application of safety and technical maintenance procedures that may often, given the financial constraints under which hospitals operate, "slip away" in practice (Vicente 2003).

Timmermans and Berg (2003, 99) advance another reason to conceive of technology as embedded in broader sociotechnical networks: "Medicine forms an archaeology of layer upon layer of technologies, from the most mundane band-aids and pencils to sophisticated machines such as MRIs and artificial hearts, from virtually neutral infusion pumps to highly symbolic procedures and devices, such as the drug Viagra or genetic tests." In chapter 2, I build on these authors' insights to show why paying attention to "mundane tools" is key to fully understanding the effectiveness of health technology. I also argue that innovations' costs, benefits, advantages, and disadvantages should be seen as enmeshed in one another. Analytically, we often seek to balance these, to weigh the trade-offs, and to conclude that one wins over the other. I suggest, instead, that technologies are *always at the same time* enabling and constraining; forming a judgment about their value should be based on this duality.

The last reason why I believe one needs to go beyond a piecemeal approach to health technology relates to the usefulness of rethinking what is or should be the focus of health care systems. For instance, Ellis (2000, 112) stresses that his forecasts about the future of health care systems have at times been met with "accusations of hype, ignorance, and inexperience." He adds that "I must reiterate that the success or failure of any specific technological device is not the issue ... The issue is the trend or trends (to smallness, smartness, and so on) such devices represent and exemplify." Fair enough. Nevertheless, I believe that the purpose of health care systems—keeping a population healthy by deploying appropriate and effective services—should be returned to any analysis of the value of health technology (Cookson and Maynard 2000). Too many technology enthusiasts tend to accept uncritically every new innovation as is and the reallocation of resources it involves, as if technological design happens outside of society and is not open to critical examination.

3. Political Perspectives on Health: Health Technology as Part of Public Policies

Defining the proper utilization of health care services and understanding the impact of payment incentives on the provision and use of medical technology represent difficult endeavors. Perhaps those who argue in favor of a consumer-driven health care market may more easily accept the high costs of health technology. Such expense may even be seen as a marker of social status (instead of a vector of social inequalities). Coddington et al. (2000, 130) help to situate this proposition:

> From a broad perspective we know that the two most important factors that influence use of the health care system are age and income. For example, it is now an oft-quoted statistic that individuals sixty-five and over typically account for three to five times the annual health care expenditures of individuals under sixty-five. We also know that the consumption of health care services rises with income. Higher-income households typically spare no expense when it comes to obtaining the best care services, new drugs, or the benefits of the latest medical technology.

One of the things I like best in this passage is the term "oft-quoted statistic." As most of us would agree, a statistic can *mean* quite different things to different groups. Under a "social determinants of health" perspective (Evans et al. 1994), age and income are usually not used to segment a market of wealthy and desirable health care consumers; rather, they call into question the intensity of the use of medical and hospital-based services and their unequal distribution in society. For example, Gortmaker and Wise (1997) examined the relationship between infant mortality and access to health care as it differed along socioeconomic and ethnic lines. They concluded: "One of the central consequences of the increasing efficacy of health services for the newborn is an increasing burden on society to provide these services equitably. In this sense, technical progress elevates the importance of access in the determination of disparities in mortality outcome." (Gortmaker and Wise 1997, 160).

Why would the social determinants of health perspective be relevant to the problem of health technology? If one sees health technology as a public, collective good, and health as something that is influenced by factors other than health care services (e.g., education, employment, revenues), then one will likely acknowledge that what constitutes a *better* innovation may include aspects other than novelty. Let us consider why, in the first place, access to the latest health technology often stands out as the preferable option. Peters (2000) refers to the "medical arms race" to describe how competing hospitals, since the 1980s, have battled to possess the latest high-tech equipment available in their facilities. He also observes its recent issue: "The dramatic difference between the United States and our northern neighbor (and the rest of the industrialized world, for that matter) became strikingly clear; there were (and are today) more MRI machines in Detroit than in all of Canada" (Peters 2000, 195). I might be tempted to add, "So what?" (But some readers might think my Canadian fiber is too easily hurt.) More seriously, and notwithstanding the problems the Canadian health care system is facing, this reading of who won the "medical arms race" battle appears terribly shortsighted and probably pointless. The number of MRI machines is not an accurate indicator of health. It may represent to a limited extent how much having access to the latest technology is valued (and paid for) by a population, but it does not reveal a great deal about whether people are concerned that health is distributed fairly throughout their society (the number of uninsured individuals may be another useful proxy here). As I point out in chapter 4, and discuss more extensively in chapter 5, reconciling the competing objectives of technological innovation and health care systems is possible when public policies rely on transparent deliberative processes (Bohman 1996) that help to refocus the debate about health technology on its ability to contribute to a fair distribution of health care.

4. The Framing of Policy Options: Deliberative Processes and Transparent Health Policy-Making

Rationing access to health technology raises various emotional reactions. Consider Ellis's response to a question raised by Morgan: "In a world in which we can in seconds log onto a website in Tibet, is it rational to restrict the range of application of medical practice to the confines of narrow geographical areas?" Here is what Ellis had to say:

> I would add: Is it even possible to restrict it, given that the Internet knows no political or regulatory boundaries? If I hear of a Tibetan guru who (I am satisfied, after doing my own research) is a whiz at curing the malady that ails me, via fiber-optic cable from his mountaintop, what's to stop me availing myself of his services? I would be upset if the government tried. (Ellis 2000, 112)

Such emotional responses are likely to be heard when rationing access to innovations equates with denying benefits to individuals. They may also explain why certain countries engage in particular health care reforms. As Peters (2000, 196) observes, to be politically legitimate, reforms must take citizens' values and preferences into account:

> If the comparative studies of national health care systems clarified anything, it was the fact that Americans want ready access to state-of-the-art technology and services. More than anything else, what killed popular enthusiasm for a Canadian- or British-like health care system in the United States was the realization that long waiting lists (queues in the U.K.) for certain services are a fact of life in those systems, and some services simply are not available at all.

What Peters's comment does not address is the vexed issue of who knows what citizens actually want. Nor does it clarify why certain features of various systems are brought to the fore (e.g., ready access to those who can afford insurance) while others are relegated to the shadows (e.g., universal access). My point is that without proper mechanisms to seek public input and introduce accountability in public policies, debates about the regulation of health technology remain superficial and misleading. According to Abelson et al. (2003, 249), deliberative approaches "have the potential to foster a more engaged, public-spirited citizenry and early experiments suggest that the public finds these processes stimulating and informative." In chapters 4 and 5, I make it clear that decisions about health technology would benefit from a greater input of both epistemological content and civil representation.

5. Stances Toward the Biomedical Industry: Examining Why Certain Types of Innovations Emerge and Not Others

A number of years ago, I was delighted to read a book by Stuart Blume (1992) titled Insight and industry: On the dynamics of technological change in medicine. It was the first time that observations about health technology spoke to my industrial designer's background. Blume was concerned about why certain imaging devices (X-rays, CT scans, ultrasound, breast thermography) had succeeded (or not) in establishing themselves in standard clinical practice. Among other things, his study showed how interactions between radiologists and biomedical engineers affect an innovation's "career" by determining its technical characteristics, level of sophistication, and potential uses. It also emphasized the evolution of the interorganizational relationships between the state, medical insurers, technology developers, and medical specialists that tend to reinforce the desirability of diagnostic tests that require expert knowledge for their interpretation and that could, therefore, remain under their control.

There is, indeed, a very particular relationship between professional knowledge and health technology (Couture 1988; Nélisse 1996; explored in chapter 3). Health technologies are the tools through which medical experts deploy their knowledge (diagnose) and/or intervene in a given health problem (cure). One may therefore wonder what the incentives are behind medical innovation, and whether certain innovations reinforce or threaten certain medical specialties. As Ellis (2000, 139) rhetorically asks:

> What would happen to the health care industry if, tomorrow, the news reported genuine cures for cancer, diabetes, Parkinson's, Alzheimer's, and AIDS? When penicillin put pay (by and large) to tuberculosis, it certainly did not finish the health care industry. But it seems reasonable to assume that the number of careers in researching and diagnosing TB and caring for its victims dwindled rapidly, while the number of careers in the management of other diseases expanded.

Although one may stress that TB is still a problem in certain geographical areas and sociopolitically vulnerable groups, Ellis is right in pointing out the displacement of professionals that arises as a result of technological change. His analysis, though, is incomplete: "The fundamental message of the medium of technology has always been de-skilling and the replacement of humans by machines. It has happened on the farm and in the factory and is happening in the office and lab. It is clear the trend is accelerating.... The Luddites were right; only their behavior and their assessment of the pace of change were wrong." (Ellis 2000, 142) Farms and factories are not, however, comparable with hospitals. And resistance can hardly be "wrong"; it can only point out that political tensions emerge when groups do not exert an equal weight in the decisions that affect their work, lives, and futures (Bohman 1996). What is peculiar about clinical work in and around hospitals is the key role played by expertise, hierarchy, and power relations (Timmermans and Berg 2003).

It is also important to note that technological change is not a process that happens *outside* of these social processes. As mentioned earlier, technologies are designed by humans who may give priority to solving certain problems and not others, who may have a specific perception of what an innovation should accomplish or not and who may prefer to target certain types of users and not others. For instance, Udow and Seitz (2000, 224) emphasize that some current technologies may not always be fully effective in solving the medical problems for which they were designed:

> This kind of "full-blown" technology understands the underlying mechanism of a disease so that relatively inexpensive and simple things can halt it (the polio vaccine is an example of full-blown technology). At the other end of the spectrum, we could continue with "halfway" technologies—in which medical care deals with just the results of the illness without understanding its underlying mechanism.

One certainly wonders why some health care systems rely on halfway technologies that do not cure patients but maintain them in a state of dependence on medical experts. Of course, I am not suggesting that those who develop medical technologies are intentionally seeking to generate profits and create financial instability in health care while not curing anyone. Technology is not that malleable (Latour 1988), and there are true technical and epistemological challenges that may be impossible to overcome, which make halfway technologies appear to be better solutions when compared with not doing anything (e.g., dialysis). Nevertheless, it seems naïve to continue adopting halfway medical innovations without ever questioning why they were designed that way. In chapter 3, I develop this angle by conceptualizing the design processes as value-laden. And in the book's conclusion I discuss the ways in which modifying who partakes in the design process and what interests can be legitimately advanced can lead to the development of "disruptive technologies" that may cost less and be used by those with less specialized training (Christensen et al. 2000).

Summary and the Way Forward

In this introduction I have presented the main tensions that shape the scientific and policy debates about the value of health technology. I have also suggested that the affordability issue must be revisited. There are more concerns at play than cost and effectiveness, and quantifying them represents

Table 0.2 Key Issues for Understanding the Problem of Health Technology

Issue	Key points in current scientific and policy debates	Social science insights that help rethink the problem of health technology
Relationship between values and health technology	Technology is neutral; its application may be controversial	Technology embodies and reinforces values
Conceptualizations of health technology	Quantifying costs and benefits is characterized by a piecemeal approach	Knowledge and skills, as well as human and technical components, are required for innovative networks to perform effectively
Political perspectives on health	Health technology is a private good; consumers' ability to pay will drive future innovations	Health technology is a private/public good that is open to public policy interventions
Framing of policy options	Third-party payers conduct implicit and explicit rationing. Scarcity increases desirability	For health policy-making to be legitimate, public deliberations and transparency are required
Stances toward the industry	The industrial complex behind innovation is taboo; it is not to be intellectually addressed	Industry develops health technology largely according to its own logic. Why do certain innovations emerge and not others?

only a partial solution to the problem of health technology. I have also introduced several key concepts that can help broaden the analysis and, I hope, lead to a more informed framework for considering medical innovations in health care systems.

Table 0.2 summarizes the key points raised so far. It also serves as a road map for drawing links between the next three chapters and for developing the alternative framework I discuss in chapter 5.

CHAPTER 1

Health Technology Assessment: Promises and Pitfalls

The Emergence of a Policy-Oriented Field of Research

This chapter summarizes the objectives and development of Health Technology Assessment (HTA), explaining why it received strong policy support in various industrialized countries. By drawing on a multimethod case study examining the production, dissemination, and use of assessments by six Canadian HTA agencies, this chapter highlights both the achievements and the shortcomings of this policy-oriented field of research. I begin by examining the characteristics and contents of the assessments these agencies delivered over a six-year period (1995–2001) and then move on to explore the extent to which these assessments met the expectations of various HTA stakeholders.

One of my principal contentions in this chapter is that HTA is a scientific and policy movement that operates in the manner of a "regulatory science" (Jasanoff 1990), seeking to foster the institutionalization of knowledge-based changes in health care systems. This form of science has the burden of persuading a broad spectrum of stakeholders of the relevance of adopting and using technologies proven to be effective, safe, and economical. By contrasting the views of HTA producers with those of HTA stakeholders, I emphasize a number of fundamental challenges undermining the capacity of HTA to "solve the problem" of health technology. Among other things, it will become clear that there are more issues at play in evaluating health technology than cost and effectiveness. As a result, HTA and the evidence-based approach to medicine in general can offer only a partial, short-term solution to the problem of health technology. I hope it becomes clear by the end of this chapter that there is a pressing need to consolidate HTA's academic foundations by integrating concepts and findings from the field of science and technology studies (STS).

Foundations of HTA[1]

According to Cohen and Hanft (2004, 381), because medicine and technology "proliferate at a staggering pace," it "has never been more important to evaluate those innovations." On these authors' optimistic account, HTA "will become an invaluable endeavor in society, vital both to our understanding of what constitutes effective health care and to our sustained efforts to make wise and efficient use of our resources" (381).

HTA has received increasing support since the mid-1980s in many industrialized jurisdictions throughout the world. HTA development is justified by the claim that information about the efficacy, safety, and cost-effectiveness of health technologies will improve decision- and policy-making (Battista et al. 1994; Banta and Perry 1997). In principle, HTA also addresses social, legal, and ethical aspects when they are perceived as bearing on decision-making at the clinical and policy levels. According to Banta and Perry (1997, 431):

> HTA enlarges the evaluation process to encompass not only the clinical consequences, but also the economic, ethical, and other social implications of the diffusion and use of a specific procedure or technique on medical practice. Technology assessment thus takes a broad perspective and its aim is to provide facts as a basis for not only clinical decision making, but also for policy making in health care as a societal endeavor.

This "broad perspective" is the reason HTA has been defined as policy-oriented, multidisciplinary research even though, in practice, the emphasis is on epidemiology and economic analyses (Giacomini 1999; Lehoux and Blume 2000).

HTA also has close ties to other recent initiatives associated with the evidence-based medicine movement (Bero and Jadad 1997; Bero et al. 1998). One significant initiative lies in the development and implementation of clinical practice guidelines (CPGs), which are meant to make health care less variable and more reliable (Moreira 2005). Unlike HTA, CPGs focus strictly on clinical practice and systematically rely on the input of medical practitioners and clinical researchers to examine and "weigh" the strength of available evidence. When costs are considered, economists become part of the team; however, their contribution is still under debate (Berg et al. 2001; Eccles 2004; Wailoo et al. 2004). For CPGs to become legitimate tools in clinical practice, their perceived independence from governmental bodies must be established. This may explain why, although HTA agencies apply very similar methods, several of them refrain from producing CPGs. HTA bodies more generally emphasize a societal perspective and target their recommendations at health policy-makers. A brief look back at the origins of HTA should shed light on its current manifestations and concerns.

When the Office of Technology Assessment (OTA) was created in the United States in the early 1970s, technology assessment was deemed relevant mainly because of the need to know the risks, for patients, of certain novel forms of treatment and, for presumably healthy individuals, of screening tests. This early focus on safety was supported by an inescapable recognition that some innovations had been introduced too swiftly (e.g., X rays in the early twentieth century, thalidomide in the 1960s). Furthermore, the computerized tomography (CT) scanner, developed in the late 1960s, radically and rapidly affected the practice of radiology and of diagnostic medicine in general (Banta and Perry 1997, 433). The enthusiasm with which it was adopted led a number of health policy analysts to wonder about the evidentiary basis for investing such substantial resources. Creditor and Garrett (1977), among others, publicly questioned the decision-making processes of hospitals that purchased a device that, when it came onto the market in 1973, cost in excess of US\$300,000. How, many asked, could it be that such decisions were being taken on the basis of so little information regarding the scanner's benefits to patient management? As a result, in 1975 the Senate Committee on Labor and Public Welfare invited the recently established OTA to conduct a study of the kinds of justifications that ought to be required before costly new medical technologies and procedures are implemented.

Over the succeeding two decades, HTA pursued a "race against health technology diffusion" (INHATA 1997). As a result, HTA has come to be seen around the world as an essential factor in developing health policy. Not until the late 1980s, however, did the notion of effectiveness truly take shape and the methodology of randomized controlled trials become grounded in medical research (Koch 1995). In the 1990s, studies on regional variations in practices fueled the idea that clinical decisions were not based on explicit effectiveness criteria. During this period, HTA advocates promoted it as one of the best ways to prevent ineffective, unnecessary, and harmful technologies from entering health care systems (Marmor and Blustein 1994; Johri and Lehoux 2003). The cost factor was also gradually introduced and refined, along with various tools intended to make it easier to compare different therapeutic options for a given disease (cost-effectiveness) or different health programs (quality-adjusted life year [QALY], disability-adjusted life year [DALY]) (Coyle et al. 1998).[2] Finally, there arose a proliferation of initiatives relating to evidence-based clinical practices. Indeed, throughout the 1990s a call for evidence-based medicine and rational priority-setting in health care contributed to defining HTA's aims and means (Giacomini 1999). And it should be noted that today HTA still continues to undergo important developments.

In industrialized jurisdictions, HTA has taken on slightly different forms, with the former OTA often used as the organizational model. In 2005, the International Network of Agencies for Health Technology Assessment (INAHTA) comprised forty institutional members located in twenty-one countries (www.inahta.org). The structure as well as the level of financial and human resources of these agencies vary greatly. For example, in Canada between 1988 and 1993 at least five provincial agencies or formal units and one federal agency were established to conduct HTA.[3] Because health care in Canada is a provincial responsibility, and the provinces vary greatly in size and resources, each of these agencies was structured differently and has evolved within its own specific institutional context (e.g., health reforms, restructuring).

The most common types of HTA agencies include university-based research groups, arm's-length government agencies, and independent nonprofit agencies.[4] While HTA production does not appear to be affected so much by an agency's organizational model, it does seem to be shaped by the type of relationships an agency sustains with policy processes:

> There seems to be no optimal model for an assessment agency. If the agency is too close to the policy process it can lose credibility with the wider community, lack some resources of information and be unresponsive to new data and perspectives—the political agenda of the day can dominate. If the agency is too far from the policy area—as may be the case, for example, with university-based groups—assessments may run the risk of having limited impact by not taking account of the nature of the target and not meeting requirements for timing and political relevance. (Hailey 1993, 253).

Although organizational models vary, most HTA agencies focus on similar research questions and apply roughly similar methods[5] (i.e., systematic reviews of published evidence and cost analyses, sometimes supplemented by clinical and administrative data and/or analyses of ethical, social, and legal issues). Box 1.1 (adapted from Cohen and Hanft 2004, 16) lists the dimensions most often addressed in HTA, while the next section in this chapter provides a more detailed analysis of the types and contents of HTA reports.

BOX 1.1 QUESTIONS ADDRESSED IN HTA

- Economic impact: How are medical technologies changing the practice of medicine and affecting health care spending, and are they cost-effective?
- Diffusion: Are technologies diffusing too swiftly—or too slowly—into medical practice?
- Evaluation: Are technologies being evaluated appropriately?
- Ethical choice: What ethical choices (or standards) should guide the evaluation, adoption, and use of technologies whose long- and short-term effects may not be known or clearly understood?
- Organizational impact: In what ways are medical technologies influencing—and being influenced by—organizational changes in the health care marketplace?
- Access: Is access to certain technologies impeded for some population groups by financial, geographic, cultural, or other barriers?
- Societal impact: How are medical technologies affecting societal behavior and organization, including the basic demographic and institutional structures of society?
- Government role: What role (or roles) should federal, state, and other governments play in attempting to deal with these issues?

Globally, scrutiny of HTA producers' scientific achievements since the mid-1980s reveals a major drive to standardize and refine methods (e.g., grading the strength of evidence, measuring cost-effectiveness, QALYs), which my colleagues and I have labeled Phase I (Lehoux et al. 2005). This stage was consolidated by the creation in 1985 of the International Society for Technology Assessment in Health Care (ISTAHC, now Health Technology Assessment International [HTAi]), which holds annual scientific meetings and organizes professional working groups, and the launching in the same year of the *International Journal of Technology Assessment in Health Care* (Banta and Perry 1997). Phase I has yielded an enormous number of publications that have contributed to reinforcing, methodologically, the field's foundations. As Moreira (2005, 1978) aptly puts it, "Repertoires of evaluation are suited to know the world in partial, specific ways. Repertoires of evaluation also create idealized versions of the way in which different forms of knowledge entail particular form of actions." Neverthe-less, very few attempts at theorizing HTA's goals and epistemological basis were published during Phase I (Goodman 1992; Giacomini 1999). Even though this may be seen as a common feature of applied research, in the case of HTA the lack of theorization impeded its capacity to grasp the fun-damental changes through which societies that increasingly rely on tech-nological developments pass.

More recently, an issue that can be considered part of a second phase in HTA development has surfaced, underscoring the importance of concep-tualizing the mission and goal of HTA. This issue is the increasing dissem-ination and uptake of HTA products. Indeed, healthy criticism has called into question the impact of HTA on decision- and policy-making, and the active dissemination of findings was identified as a major concern as early as the mid-1990s (Battista et al. 1994; Battista et al. 1999). Since then, dis-semination and impact have become recurrent, high-profile topics at ISTAHC and HTAi conferences. Concern over dissemination has forced evaluators to reflect on and grow more familiar with the ways in which decisions and policies are made. HTA producers have had to search for their audiences and to introduce principles that have been recently pro-moted by communications and knowledge transfer experts (Bero and Jadad 1997; Lavis et al. 2002). Phase II thus represents a relatively new challenge for HTA producers, requiring conceptualization of the broader policy arena in which HTA unfolds.

The extent to which an HTA agency can bring about concrete changes in health care is affected by the policy and regulatory arena prevailing in its jurisdiction (Bos et al. 1996). Berg et al. (2004, 36) underscore the "mutual dependencies" that exist among key stakeholders, such as gov-ernments, providers, and insurers, all of whom are "fully dependent on one another for achieving their own objectives." More precisely, the regu-lation of technology and drugs, the implementation of CPGs, and the transmission of information to patients and the general public may all prove essential in determining the ultimate impact of HTA (Battista et al. 1999). In other words, if regulatory agencies and professional groups do not act upon the conclusions of HTA reports, the overall impact of HTA will probably remain limited. Hence, when appraising the "payback" from HTA (Buxton and Hanney 1996), defining who the requesters and potential users are, and drawing attention to the actions users can take and are likely to be accountable for, become pivotal. This may partly explain why the National Institute for Clinical Excellence (NICE), estab-lished in 1999 in the United Kingdom, was structurally designed to include an explicit and open stakeholder consultation process for every guidance it published, as well as general mechanisms for ensuring a certain level of accountability.

Scientific information can be seen as one of the inputs to the policy process that operates "less on the specifics of policy and more on the beliefs and assumptions that underlie it" (Lomas 1990, 526). Because beliefs about the inherently positive value of technology are often strong and widespread, regulating access to technology is a thorny issue, even when a certain innovation's effectiveness has been proven to be limited (Bastian 1998; Johri and Lehoux 2003). For instance, the geographical proximity of the most populous Canadian cities to the U.S. border makes it harder to resist technologies that are developed and promoted on the American market. A similar situation is found across European Union member states (Kent and Faulkner 2002; Faulkner 1997). Examples also exist in which the adoption of an effective technology (e.g., implantation of a left ventricular assist device as a bridge to heart transplant or a permanent solution) has been seriously compromised by both lack of resources and the economic impact of such innovations on current budgets.

For the mission of HTA agencies to be fulfilled, stakeholders that possess varying levels of economic, political, and symbolic resources must be convinced that a societal good can be attained through the application of HTA results. Implementing a knowledge-based regulation of health technology can hardly be achieved without their participation or at least passive approval. Making things more complicated, however, is the fact that in Canada and many other countries, the policy arena comprises several decision-making loci. As a result, HTA producers throughout the industrialized world have had difficulty knowing where to target their findings, while at the same time recognizing that public acceptance of the core principles supporting a given policy initiative plays an important role in the use of research findings.[6]

Phase II in HTA development consequently entails not only shaping an array of stakeholders' beliefs by providing them with scientific evidence about technology, but also understanding the regulatory mechanisms that may facilitate or impede the implementation of recommendations. From an institutional theory perspective (Edquist and Johnson 1997), HTA can be seen as a means of implementing knowledge-based change within a health care system. Such an approach implies the full development of the "sets of common habits, routines, established practices, rules and laws that regulate the relations and interactions" (Edquist and Johnson 1997, 46) between an HTA agency and the organized groups that have a stake in health issues in a given jurisdiction. Along similar lines, K. Smith (1997) argues that the innovations and changes generated by "knowledge infrastructures" are partially influenced by prevailing regulatory systems and wider sociopolitical contexts that contribute to defining public policy objectives. The "products" delivered by these infrastructures are themselves shaped by a fairly complex network of suppliers, customers, labor skills, and expertise. Indeed, the resources that can be co-opted and the rules governing this process both constrain and enhance knowledge creation. There is, therefore, a dual relationship between knowledge-producing organizations and their geographical, social, economic, cultural, and political environments.

Figure 1.1 posits that two types of HTA outputs structure the relationships between an HTA agency and its stakeholders. First, an agency disseminates HTA reports, which are concrete, tangible products that can mobilize a more or less broad scope of knowledge (e.g., efficacy, safety, cost, ethical, and legal issues). These reports seek to reduce uncertainty, or to manage conflict over the merits of medical interventions, by identifying, among other things, their costs and benefits. Second, an agency initiates processes that support the institutionalization of various HTA-derived products (e.g., CPGs, seminars, methodological guidelines, patient leaflets). The nature and breadth of these processes depend upon the overall approach to

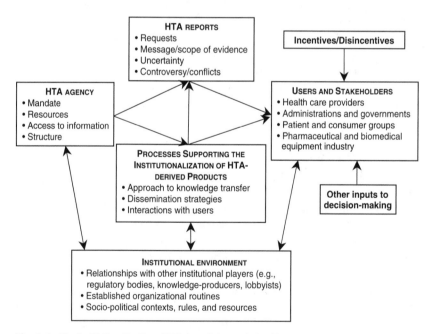

Fig. 1.1 The institutionalization of HTA-based change in health care systems
Source: Lehoux, Denis, Tailliez, et al., 2005.

knowledge transfer, the importance given to dissemination activities, and the perceived need to interact with diverse groups of stakeholders.

The HTA audience can be divided into the following four groups: health care providers, governments and administrative bodies, patients and the public, and the pharmaceutical and biomedical equipment industry. Within this framework, the first two groups can be considered direct users, while the last two can be seen more broadly as stakeholders. Within this framework, HTA agencies seek to influence, and in turn are influenced by, a specific institutional environment. This environment is characterized by the presence of regulatory bodies, lobby groups, and other knowledge producers; by the rules and routines that are established within and between these organizations; by the sociopolitical orientation of previous and present governments; and by the availability of financial and human resources. Finally, this framework recognizes that the decisions of stakeholders are shaped not only by HTA outputs but also by financial, administrative, legal, and political incentives or disincentives (Lomas 1993).

The next two sections follow this framework to examine the types of HTA products developed by six Canadian agencies as well as decision-makers' perceptions, expectations, and practices regarding the use of knowledge and HTA in technology-related decision-making.

Type and Scope of HTA Products Delivered in Canada[7]

Drawing on a study (in which I took part) of six Canadian HTA agencies, this section describes the type and scope of assessments produced over a six-year period (1995–2001), outlines the agencies' portfolios, and discusses the production challenges the agencies faced when trying to respond to increased demand. The agencies were located in the provinces of British Columbia, Alberta, Saskatchewan, Ontario (one provincial agency and one national agency), and Quebec, and they were established between 1988 and 1993. The findings presented here stem mainly from an analysis of the agencies' peer-reviewed publications, supplemented by interviews conducted with chief executive officers (CEOs) and researchers. Appendix A describes the methods used in detail.

Table 1.1 shows that decision-makers and practitioners across Canada had access to, on average, over thirty HTA products during the study period. Because the agencies differed in their annual budgets and numbers of employees, these figures should be interpreted with caution. The purpose here is not to rank agencies according to their outputs, and it is important to recognize that the populations of Ontario (11,894,000) and Quebec (7,417,000) are fairly large, compared with those of British Columbia (4,101,000), Alberta (3,059,000) and Saskatchewan (1,017,000).

Table 1.1 Number of HTA Documents Published by Six Canadian HTA Agencies (1995–2001)

	A1	A2	A3	A4	A5	A6	Total
1995–1996	0	2	3	0	4	3	12
1996–1997	4	1	12	3	6	1	27
1997–1998	6	2	19	7	7	3	44
1998–1999	1	7	11	7	8	3	37
1999–2000	7	1	7	10	6	2	33
2000–2001	7	4	9	5	5	4	34
Total	25	17	61	32	36	16	187

Note: Annual budgets for 2000–2001 ranged from CDN$600,000 to CDN$4.3 million, and staff ranged from 10 to 35 full-time-equivalent employees. *Source:* Lehoux, Tailliez, Denis, et al. 2004.

In addition, the budgets allocated to HTA by each provincial government and/or the federal government[8] varied considerably. Finally, as several CEOs stressed, all six agencies faced significant challenges in recruiting researchers who specialized in HTA.

Table 1.2 provides details of the types of products the HTA agencies delivered during the study period. While four agencies were still emphasizing the "traditional," full HTA report (representing 81% to 100% of their production), two of them diversified their products by publishing joint reports (A2: 47%; A4: 13%), a result of partnerships with key health organizations (e.g., medical associations, workers' compensation boards). Two agencies (A3: 43%; A6: 19%) also published several short documents (e.g., peer-reviewed bulletins), rapid HTAs (e.g., provisional reviews of the literature), and technical briefs (e.g., short descriptive reports focusing on an innovation's technical aspects). Overall, the bulk of HTA documents produced in Canada were full HTA reports (76%).

Among the nonpeer-reviewed documents that were excluded from detailed analysis, it is worth mentioning that three agencies did not publish newsletters during the study period, while the other three issued electronic and/or paper newsletters on a quarterly basis. The format and appearance of reports improved significantly between 1995 and 2001, a change that may have made them more reader-friendly.

Substantial variation was also observed in the number of traditional scientific outputs (e.g., scientific publications and conference presentations). Three agencies actively supported the publication of results in scientific journals (A1, A4, A5), and the majority encouraged presentations at conferences. Agency 1, which relied on several university-affiliated researchers, stood out in this regard. Overall, as most CEOs acknowledged,

Table 1.2 Types of Documents Published by Six Canadian HTA Agencies (1995–2001)

	Full HTA reports		Joint reports		Short documents		Total	
	%	n	%	n	%	n	%	n
A1	88	22	0	0	12	3	100	25
A2	53	9	47	8	0	0	100	17
A3	57	35	0	0	43	26	100	61
A4	88	28	13	4	3	1	100	32
A5	100	36	0	0	0	0	100	36
A6	81	13	0	0	19	3	100	16
Total	76	143	6	12	17	32	100	187

Note: Short documents include rapid HTAs and technical briefs.
Source: Lehoux, Tailliez, Denis, et al. 2004.

while scientific journals might not have been the most appropriate vehicles for reaching decision-makers, such publications do contribute to an agency's visibility and prestige. Indeed, establishing scientific credibility was often viewed as essential for reaching and influencing certain audiences (e.g., physicians who are involved or interested in clinical research and who value peer-reviewed publications). Given that the resources of the six agencies differed significantly, the disparity in terms of scientific outputs was not entirely surprising. This disparity nonetheless shows that conflicting legitimacies were at play—the production of traditional scientific versus user-oriented knowledge. Because the credibility of HTA is intimately linked to its scientific rigor, this tension may have affected certain agencies' ability to recruit and retain evaluators seeking to build a career according to academic standards. Several interviewees favored a balanced approach—one that encouraged peer-reviewed publications—yet did not ignore target users who did not read scientific journals.

Table 1.3 presents the types of technology the six agencies assessed. Two agencies clearly focused on health services (A1: 76%; A6: 56%), while Agency 3 focused on pharmaceuticals (74%). Four agencies were only slightly or not at all involved in assessing such drugs (A1, A4, A5, A6), perhaps because several provinces had university groups and/or governmental bodies that produced cost-effectiveness analyses of them. Diagnostic technology and screening tests did not constitute a very large proportion of HTA reports (<31%), and devices were only infrequently evaluated (<19%).[9] A limited but significant portion of the production of five agencies included essays and methodological publications. This kind of output,

Table 1.3 Types of Technology Assessed by Six Canadian HTA Agencies (1995–2001)

	Diagnosis and screening		Devices		Procedures		Drugs		Health services		Essays and research tools		Total HTA documents	
	%	n	%	n	%	n	%	n	%	n	%	n	%	n
A1	0	0	0	0	8	2	0	0	76	19	16	4	100	25
A2	24	4	0	0	12	2	29	5	12	2	24	4	100	17
A3	5	3	7	4	5	3	74	45	3	2	7	4	100	61
A4	25	8	9	3	28	9	3	1	22	7	13	4	100	32
A5	31	11	19	7	22	8	0	0	19	7	8	3	100	36
A6	31	5	0	0	6	1	6	1	56	9	0	0	100	16
Tot.	17	31	7	14	13	25	28	52	25	46	10	19	100	187

Source: Lehoux, Tailliez, Denis, et al. 2004.

which does not directly respond to users' requests, is nonetheless useful in consolidating the practice and promotion of HTA.

Excluding pharmaceuticals, most agencies presented fairly balanced portfolios. Overall, only a few focused on certain topics, several did not assess drugs, and most evaluated a number of different types of technology. The interviewees believed such practices were the result of institutional specialization arising from their specific jurisdictional contexts. As a few CEOs mentioned, a critical mass of researchers may be required before an agency engages in a new area of research. These CEOs also indicated a willingness to limit overlap between groups of knowledge producers.

Extending the analysis to examine the content of HTA reports reveals further distinctions between the agencies. As mentioned earlier, HTA is supposed to examine not only the efficacy, safety, and costs of a given health technology, but also its ethical, social, and legal issues. However, table 1.4 shows that the issues most frequently addressed were cost and effectiveness.[10] Approximately a third of the documents the agencies produced included a cost component, while the vast majority of the production

Table 1.4 Issues Addressed by Six Canadian HTA Agencies (1995–2001)

	A1		A2		A3		A4		A5		A6		Mean/tot.	
	%	n	%	n	%	n	%	n	%	n	%	n	%	n
Costs	33	8	35	6	43	26	31	10	36	13	38	6	37	69
Effectiveness	8	2	71	12	41	25	78	25	39	14	69	11	48	89
Cost-effectiveness	0	0	6	1	51	31	6	2	28	10	6	1	24	45
Quality of life	8	2	0	0	10	6	13	4	17	6	19	3	11	21
Safety	4	1	18	3	25	15	22	7	28	10	31	5	22	41
Ethical/social issues	40	10	24	4	8	5	9	3	17	6	25	4	17	32
Legal issues	0	0	6	1	2	1	0	0	8	3	0	0	3	5
Current practices	68	17	6	1	13	8	25	8	14	5	69	11	27	50
Other outcomes	60	15	29	5	33	20	47	15	56	20	38	6	43	81
Mean/total documents	100	25	100	17	100	61	100	32	100	36	100	16	100	187

Note: Because the subcategories are not mutually exclusive, the total for "n" exceeds the total number of HTA documents.
Source: Lehoux, Tailliez, Denis, et al. 2004.

of four agencies examined effectiveness (A2: 71%; A4: 78%; A6: 69%). Very few agencies, however, conducted full-fledged cost-effectiveness analyses. Only Agency 3 did so in close to half its reports. Despite the growing prevalence of chronic diseases, quality of life seldom figured as part of agencies' assessments. Safety was addressed in less than a third of their reports.

As expected, agencies did not frequently address ethical and social issues.[11] Agency 1 discusses such issues most frequently (in 40% of its reports), while Agencies 3 and 4 rarely provided such commentary. The fact that the official definition of HTA was not put into practice to its fullest extent is even more striking in the case of legal issues. According to interviews conducted with agency representatives, securing access to staff that specializes in ethical and legal issues was often problematic in a context of limited resources and immense demand. Interestingly, two agencies documented the state of current practices fairly often (A1: 68%; A6: 69%), which is compatible with the need to contextualize HTA findings for regional or provincial decision-makers. By providing information about current levels of service utilization, surgical rates, or prescription patterns, evaluators may have been aiming to better inform decision-makers about the potential gap between evidence and practice and, therefore, to support decision-making processes. Similarly, perhaps in response to specific requests, four agencies fairly frequently included other outcomes, such as findings about organizational aspects (e.g., collaboration between midwives and obstetricians, funding arrangements) or data about the impact of recent provincial policies (e.g., hospital lengths of stay, waiting lists) in their assessments.

Our research also considered the recommendations and conclusions reached in HTA documents. Except for A5 and A6, only a small proportion of HTA publications contained formal recommendations (A1: 6/25=24%; A2: 3/17=18%; A3: 6/61=10%; A4: 1/32=3%; A5: 16/36=44%; A6: 9/16=56%). This facet of their reporting is compatible with interviewees' explanations of the fragile balance between drawing conclusions about evidentiary strength and defining what should be done with findings. If the former is definitely part of evaluators' task, the latter is seen as the responsibility of decision-makers and clinicians.

The HTA outputs contained three types of conclusions: negative (24/197=13%[12]); neutral (124/187=66%); and positive (39/187=21%) (see examples in table 1.5).[12] Negative messages included reporting that a technology had not been proven effective or emphasizing the risks associated with its use. Neutral conclusions did not stipulate the actions that should be followed based on an assessment, emphasized the weakness of the evidence considered,

Table 1.5 Examples of Negative, Neutral, and Positive Conclusions Reached by Six Canadian HTA Agencies (1995–2001)

Negative conclusions	Neutral conclusions	Positive conclusions
"The trials show a very high placebo response rate. But they also show serious adverse effects for some patients." (A3) "Evidence that famciclovir provides a therapeutic advantage over the placebo for treatment of herpes zoster is scant, unreliable, incomplete, and inconclusive." (A2) "This procedure is not a medical necessity. The risks are important." (A5) "In this study we found no evidence that light level (preventive) home care actually keeps seniors alive longer or living independently longer than those not receiving the service. Our research also showed that elderly people who receive this type of home care are in fact 50 percent more likely to lose their independence or die than those not receiving the support service." (A6)	"Decisions regarding public funding of EVG technology as a replacement for open abdominal resection of AAA must await technology maturity and clinical trials results regarding specific EVG technology. The current practice of offering EVG on a compassionate basis to patients with contraindications to conventional open abdominal resection should continue under study conditions." (A2) "Survey results demonstrate wide inter-institutional variations in access to various types of stroke diagnostic services and treatments in the province. Further information is needed." (A1) "Bladder ultrasound scanning is less accurate than intermittent catheterization. Institutions using the technology should have in place suitable training procedures and validate the accuracy of the methods." (A4) "No direct evidence currently exists to suggest that mammography decreases mortality by detecting ipsilateral recurrence; however, indirect evidence suggests that clinical examination or mammography, or both, are beneficial in detecting CBC." (A3)	"For adults, asthma self-management programs are an accepted and effective approach. According to the experts, patients with insufficient control of their asthma should be the target group of highest priority during the systematic establishment of self-management programs." (A5) "Sumatriptan is efficacious and relatively safe. Furthermore, it is more efficacious than many alternative migraine drugs." (A3) "An immunization program targeted to people over 65 and HIV patients represents an effective public health program." (A5) "VF-ET is effective only for severe bilateral tubal disease." (A4)

Source: Lehoux, Tailliez, Denis, et al. 2004.

Table 1.6 Summary of the Portfolio Characteristics of Six Canadian HTA Agencies (1995–2001)

	A1	A2	A3	A4	A5	A6
Diversification of products (table 1.2)	Limited	Yes	Yes	Limited	None	Limited
Scientific outputs	Strongly supported	Weakly supported	Weakly supported	Strongly supported	Strongly supported	Not available
Agency specialization (table 1.3)	High (76% health services)	Balanced portfolio	High (74% pharmaceuticals)	Balanced portfolio	Balanced portfolio	High (56% health services)
Contextualization of findings (table 1.4)	High (68% current practices; 60% other outcomes)	Low (6%; 29%)	Low (13%; 33%)	High (25%; 47%)	High (14%; 56%)	High (69%; 38%)
Recommendations	Occasional (24%)	Occasional (18%)	Occasional (10%)	Close to none (3%)	Frequent (44%)	Frequent (56%)
Priority-setting process	Agenda is informed by the Ministry of Health No one is aware of any prioritization criteria Most HTAs are investigator-initiated	Topics suggested by several groups are given higher priority Criteria are used to plan the depth of the assessment	Input sought from several sources Priorities set through advisory committees	None; responses are provided for each and every request Criteria are used to define the depth of the assessment	Input is sought from several sources, including an advisory board Criteria are used to set priorities	The Ministry of Health submits suggestions once a year

External funding mechanisms are used	1/3 of HTAs are investigator-initiated; 2/3 are requested by the Ministry of Health and various bodies	Half of HTAs are investigator-initiated and the other half are in response to external requests	1/3 of HTAs are investigator-initiated; 1/3 are requested by stakeholders; 1/3 are requested by the Ministry of Health	Input is sought from several sources, including horizon scanning HTAs reflect the suggestions at both supply and demand ends
Position on the science vs. user-driven agenda spectrum	Scientific autonomy	Middle	Closer to scientific autonomy	Closer to user-centered services

Source: Adapted from Lehoux, Tailliez, Denis, et al. 2004.

or remained somewhat evasive, stressing that further research was needed. Positive conclusions stated that a given technology was both effective and safe or that its cost-effectiveness was reasonable.

Table 1.6 summarizes the findings I have presented so far and highlights the fact that even though all six agencies produced HTAs, they remained individual organizational entities with rather different "production lines" (see appendix B for details). Despite having similar processes, the agencies produced outputs that reflected specific interpretations of what HTA is all about and to whom HTA should be providing guidance. The agencies considered here can be situated on a spectrum that has scientific autonomy (A1) at one end and user-centered services (A4) at the other (see table 1.6). These two poles underscore a key tension inherent in the production of knowledge aimed at influencing both policy and practice: knowledge must meet scientific standards, yet also respond to the needs of its intended users.

Expectations and Practices of HTA Stakeholders in Canada

Increasing the impact of HTA on decision- and policy-making has been a significant focus since the mid-1990s. Scant attention, however, has been given to the perspective of knowledge users, and very little is known about how various groups perceive HTA's usefulness (Davies and Littlejohns 2002). This section presents findings stemming from both a self-administered survey and in-depth interviews with HTA stakeholders belonging to four groups: health care provider associations (n=223), decision-making bodies (n=105), patient associations (n=60), and the biomedical equipment and pharmaceutical industry (n=17). In all, we obtained a response rate of 27% (see appendix A for details of the study).

As Garcia-Altes et al. (2004, 307) point out, maintaining transparency and consistency in technology-related policies frequently proves challenging:

> Often, policy decisions will be made on this basis of a trade-off between the evidence available on clinical and cost-effectiveness, and several other considerations, including political pressures, availability of funding, or patient and caregiver opinion. The challenge under these circumstances is to maintain transparency and consistency of the decision making process in the face of these factors, in both the public and private sector.

Our survey asked respondents who were familiar with at least one of the six agencies how they evaluated seven of its organizational and scientific features. Table 1.7 indicates that scientific rigor (3.92 to 4.40), credibility (3.64 to 4.45), and accessibility of reports (3.94 to 4.19) were widely considered to

Table 1.7 Perceptions of Organizational and Scientific Features of Six Canadian HTA Agencies by Stakeholders

How does your organization evaluate this agency on the following aspects?	A1		A2		A3		A4		A5		A6		Total/mean	
	N	Mean	N	Mean	N	Mean	N	Mean	N	Mean	N	Mean	N	Mean
Scientific rigor	81	4.40	13	3.92	63	3.95	22	4.32	38	4.32	31	4.06	248	4.20
Credibility	82	4.45	14	3.64	67	3.91	23	4.22	38	4.24	31	4.13	255	4.17
Accessibility of its reports	79	4.06	15	4.13	68	3.94	22	4.14	37	4.03	32	4.19	253	4.05
Dissemination of its work	76	3.87	12	3.33	65	3.58	22	3.77	37	3.35	31	4.00	243	3.70
Political autonomy	68	3.90	10	3.60	53	3.51	19	3.84	31	3.68	29	3.34	210	3.67
Ability to formulate clear recommendations	77	3.66	12	3.25	59	3.20	17	3.59	36	3.81	31	3.84	232	3.56
Ability to introduce concrete changes into the health care system	69	3.10	9	2.33	52	2.83	14	2.79	35	2.91	27	3.30	206	2.97

Note: Mean scores were calculated using a five-level Likert scale: (1) very poorly; (2) poorly; (3) moderately; (4) highly; (5) very highly.

be strong assets. Respondents' views regarding the dissemination of the agencies' work were also generally positive (3.33 to 4.00). The political autonomy of certain agencies raised some concerns, however, as respondents' views were less positive (3.34 to 3.90). The table also indicates that smaller and varying proportions of respondents rated fairly highly the ability to formulate clear recommendations (3.20 to 3.84). The ability to introduce changes in health care systems was the weakest area across all six agencies (2.33 to 3.30).

Qualitative analyses of the interviews fleshed out the survey data presented above. Interviewees recognized HTA agencies as credible organizations providing rigorous studies, although some tended to challenge their political autonomy. When examining the issue more closely, a tension between scientific credibility and political autonomy surfaced. This concern appeared to be more acute in the case of HTA agencies because they must produce independent *and* usable science.

As interviewees explained, agencies' political autonomy can be challenged in two ways. First, in their assessments, agencies could give too much credit to clinical experts with vested interests in the application of the technology being assessed. Nonetheless, assessing technology requires knowledge that can hardly be entirely independent from expertise. As one interviewee remarked:

> I think it's very important to have independent bodies that validate. Now the issue is by choosing experts, you're already biased ... because the experts already have a vested interest in the application of the technology. And if you pick non-experts, the problem is they may be not biased, but they may not grasp the subtleties of the field (Physician Association 5).

It thus becomes a matter of balance, wherein agencies must both protect their political autonomy and produce irreproachable science. These tasks call for accessing specialized expertise that is not seen as blinded by or overenthusiastic about specific technological advances.

Second, as a representative of a patient association stressed, agencies may give the impression of working hand in glove with government and supporting its streamlining policies:

> In this province, it's almost a given that you're going to have some sort of government support and as I understand it, there's a bit of an arm's length relationship there, where the agencies receive their funding, but they're not run by government and I think that most

people are sort of okay with that. I think what wouldn't be okay is … if it looked like they were operating hand in glove and government was utilizing their research to make very controversial decisions that were sort of in favor of the government, to either save money or whatever, I think that would rear its head pretty fast. But I think that, generally speaking, that's not the case (Patient Association 6).

HTA producers recognize this tension. Showing autonomy requires maintaining a certain distance from government decision-makers while knowing how to meet their information needs. HTA's mandate thus embodies a paradox: to increase its use, it must fit with users' agendas; but to protect its credibility, it must appear entirely independent. Thus, the question of scientific autonomy takes on a specific coloring in the case of HTA because it remains strongly associated with its client and their ultimate purposes. If traditional university-based research has often thrived in a context where "peers" and the "quest for truth" function as convincing markers of autonomy, HTA producers' autonomy must resonate with scientific work that is both useful and used, but not by any single individual or group in any one way.

Table 1.7 shows that survey respondents were skeptical regarding the agencies' ability to introduce changes into the health care system. However, one may wonder for what role they see HTA as best suited. Table 1.8 indicates the objectives respondents believed HTA *should* pursue, and contrasts them with the objectives that respondents felt agencies *do* pursue. A strong majority of respondents believed that assessing effectiveness (3.74 to 4.71) and supporting the rational use of technology (3.62 to 4.44) were relevant objectives. A sizable majority also believed that agencies were, in fact, aiming toward those objectives (3.33 to 4.36 and 3.05 to 3.69, respectively). While the goal of improving clinical practice (3.70 to 4.44) seemed as important as supporting the rational use of technology, most respondents considered that agencies were not working sufficiently in that direction (2.75 to 3.47). In the same vein, respondents felt that health care management should be improved by HTA (3.24 to 4.07), but did not believe that the agencies were sufficiently aiming toward that goal (2.45 to 3.21). Improving policy-making was regarded as an equally important objective (3.67 to 4.02). Here again, agencies' current practices seemed to fall short (2.45 to 3.41). In summary, respondents saw two objectives as both legitimate and fulfilled to a significant extent: assessing effectiveness and contributing to the rational use of technology. Improving clinical practice, management, and policy-making were all considered crucial

Table 1.8 Objectives Respondents Believe HTA Agency Should Pursue Versus Objectives Perceived as Actually Pursued

| | A1 | | | | A2 | | | | A3 | | | | A4 | | | | A5 | | | | A6 | | | |
| | Should | | Are | | Should | | Are | | Should | | Are | | Should | | Are | | Should | | Are | | Should | | Are | |
	N	MS	N	MS	N	MS	N	MS	N	MS	N	MS	N	MS	N	MS	N	MS	N	MS	N	MS	N	MS
Evaluate the effectiveness of technology and health services	100	4.00	78	3.33	21	4.05	14	3.71	80	4.14	70	3.80	27	3.74	19	3.74	42	4.71	39	4.36	33	3.79	30	3.43
Contribute to the reduction of public spending on health care	93	2.90	67	2.66	21	2.86	11	2.55	75	2.96	53	2.70	25	2.60	14	2.14	43	3.40	32	3.03	30	3.27	27	2.81
Contribute to the rational use of technology and health services	96	3.77	69	3.14	21	4.00	14	3.07	79	3.90	62	3.13	26	3.62	19	3.05	43	4.44	36	3.69	34	3.88	29	3.24

	A1				A2				A3				A4				A5				A6			
	Should		Are		Should		Are		Should		Are		Should		Are		Should		Are		Should		Are	
	N	MS	N	MS	N	MS	N	MS	N	MS	N	MS	N	MS	N	MS	N	MS	N	MS	N	MS	N	MS
Contribute to the improvement of clinical practices	101	4.05	82	3.62	21	3.71	12	2.75	79	3.85	59	2.75	27	3.70	19	3.26	43	4.44	34	3.47	34	3.82	30	3.43
Contribute to the improvement of health care management	100	3.80	74	3.14	21	3.24	11	2.45	80	3.64	58	2.60	27	3.56	18	2.83	43	4.07	34	2.91	33	3.85	28	3.21
Contribute to the improvement of health policies	101	3.85	75	3.23	21	3.38	11	2.45	80	3.56	58	2.52	27	3.67	17	2.59	43	4.02	34	2.88	34	3.85	29	3.41

Note: Mean scores were calculated using a five-level Likert scale: (1) not at all; (2) somewhat; (3) an average amount; (4) a great deal; (5) entirely.

objectives, but respondents did not perceive agencies to be fulfilling them to a sufficient extent.

Several interviewees clarified why the agencies' role as an agent of change in their jurisdictions was limited. The following quotation describes how a lack of evidence is not necessarily the sole explanation:

> Well, there's much been written in the literature about why there's so little uptake of clinical practice guidelines and research evidence, and it has to do with why people practice the way they do ... often times, the reasons they do things the way they do them is not for lack of knowledge ... there's convenience factors, cost factors, time factors, there's administrative issues, and so that all of those things have to be understood if you're going to change behavior (Physician Association 1).

Interviewees similarly highlighted several factors that may impede agencies from playing a stronger role within health care systems. I examine each of them in detail in the following pages.

Research Agenda and Mandate

Canadian HTA agencies have developed a variety of ways to set their research priorities and to determine the topics to be assessed. As noted earlier, at one end of the spectrum a group may "inform" an agency's agenda, but most projects remain investigator-initiated; at the other end, an agency's portfolio is fashioned by a public service "pull" rather than a scientific "push." Not surprisingly, interview data show that, from a user's perspective, the public service "pull" model was far more attractive than the scientific "push" model, which was, in fact, considered to be both unpredictable and uncontrollable, as the following comments explain:

> This is specific to this agency, but may apply to some other research bodies. Most of their research agenda, year in and year out, is driven by their research scientists. So, for example, if someone comes on board and has an interest in heart disease, then they'll do more projects on heart disease. The problem with that is not that it isn't really high quality research, it's that it may or may not fit with the government's policy agenda. And so if one of the goals of health research is to influence health policy, you need to somehow keep checking to see if your research agenda fits with the government's policy agenda. And the agency hasn't normally done that (Decision-maker 1).

This preference for the "pull" model was further reflected by the fact that many users expressed a desire to see agencies embrace a broader agenda than the predominately biomedical one traditionally applied, which is closely connected to "high-tech" medicine. As one interviewee from a nurses' association pointed out, "Unfortunately, the information the agency provides is heavily focused on medical practice rather than other disciplines, and that's probably limiting in a sense for the system."

Timeliness and Turnaround Time

Timeliness is one of the most widespread and recurrent concerns regarding the usefulness of research in policy-making. Nonetheless, one may wonder whether the role of this issue is, as one respondent suggested, mainly rhetorical, aiming to shift the burden onto someone else's shoulders: "Timeliness is an overrated argument. It reflects the difficulty administrators have managing their own timelines" (Decision-maker 5). In general, users whom we interviewed recognized the paradoxical tension between the time required to produce a full HTA report and the urgency of users' needs for information while they are in the process of making decisions. Perhaps not surprisingly, for several stakeholders and producers both the causes of and the solutions to this tension resided in the opposite camp. Indeed, for many stakeholders, the time it takes to produce a full HTA report (one year, on average) was not only difficult to justify but appeared unrealistic. In order to solve this problem, they called for new methodologies, such as rapid assessments, followed by a full report when necessary. The following quotation emphasizes the pressures placed on policy-makers when an innovation is actively and publicly promoted and/or contested:

> We need to be able to respond to the substance, we need to be able to respond to the hype and we need to be able to respond to the legal issues. And it's coming at us really fast and furious, and when you're actually in the trenches and you are sort of trying to make decisions, we need more help than an 18- to 24- month technology assessment. So, maybe we need to be more skilled at searching the gray literature. We need to maybe change the methodology to reflect the reality of the very rapid development of technology and the way it's being promoted to the public … our goal is to obtain initial findings within two months. Supplementary report, if required. Eighteen months to us is next to useless. We might as well file the report in a library (Decision-maker 13).

Another respondent related a more positive scenario, discussing an HTA agency's ability to provide both rapid tech assessments and full HTA reports:

> There are the short assessments where a branch, like Claims, will have a question about a particular technology and will need an answer fairly quickly because this is related to a claim a physician is saying I did this … or if I use this technology am I going to be paid for it? So those short ones have a fairly quick turnaround and [an HTA unit] will usually do those within two or three working weeks—they're very, very quick. [The other type of report is] an in-depth analysis of a technology and for us, it allows the department, the minister to make a better informed decision, it really says what is the evidence about this technology and what kind of policy is this issue going to make (Decision-maker 3).

The timeliness argument may reflect a profound divide between HTA stakeholders and producers. The latter were often critical of, or even irritated by, decision-makers who focus on short-term, highly publicized policy issues and do not seem to care about long-term planning. These two groups may appear to hold conflicting views about how problems with the health care system should be addressed and governed.[13]

Types of Recommendations and Conclusions

The interviews we conducted showed that the question of whose responsibility it is—evaluators or policy-makers—to make recommendations is not settled. Decision-makers, in particular, called for clear recommendations and for agencies to provide not only information, but guidance as well:

> With CIHI's [Canadian Institute for Health Information] health indicators project, they sort of rate communities or districts right across Canada now, if there are elevated rates in a particular area, to help local people take action on those potential problem areas, they need to know whether the rates are statistically significant. So you can have a rate that's higher, but unless you can answer the "so what" question, like is it significantly higher?, what is there to be done? (Decision-maker 1)

The need for assessments to be more incisive—and in fact normative—was echoed by a another decision-maker:

Most often the conclusion is that "not enough work has been done, we need further research." Well, to a policy-maker, in government, that is meaningless … when you actually have to make a multi-million dollar decision, that kind of conclusion is not necessarily helpful. So we're looking for much more than an inconclusive end point to a technology assessment. We're looking for real commitment to help us move things along (Decision-maker 13).

One respondent provided an interesting comparison to clarify his expectations of HTA: "I tend to distinguish between information and intelligence and I think they're all doing a reasonably good job in providing information, but I think all of them could do a lot more to provide intelligence" (Decision-maker 1). When asked by the interviewer to explain his view, he added:

You can provide someone with sort of good facts and figures, or you can tell them what those facts and figures mean and what they should be doing with them. And so there's a sort of passive transfer of information, or a more proactive transfer of information. Then I think for the most part, they are sort of passively transferring information and saying to the users, "you decide what to do with the information," as opposed to—and that's why I use the term intelligence—saying "here's some new research findings and here's what it may mean for you and here's what we think you should be doing about it or with it."

Applicability to Local Contexts

One aspect of HTA that stakeholders deemed fairly important (and, as shown earlier, several agencies provided) was the contextualization of findings (e.g., the provision of information about the current levels of service utilization, surgical rates, prescription patterns, or dissemination of a given technology within a specific jurisdiction). Such information may be particularly helpful for stakeholders because it identifies more clearly whether there is a gap between evidence and practice, and, if one exists, what type of actions are required to reduce it (e.g., facilitating or limiting access to services and technologies). Similarly, Davies and Littlejohns (2002) observe that local priority-setting may be better informed by research that provides additional information such as health needs assessments and epidemiological analyses. The following comment by a physician association representative emphasizes users' needs for such contextualized inputs:

Because sometimes things are used without enough information, for example, there was the recent closure of some of the hospitals here in comparison to Saskatchewan, but what we really needed to know what were the size of the hospitals, what were the size of the communities, and it appears that in fact, it wasn't directly comparable, so that's when it becomes problematic...we don't have enough information about specifics, you know, how big a community, how far away were the other resources and so you can't do these comparisons (Physician Association 2).

Findings that are contextualized can also reduce the concern, noted earlier, over the perceived lack of clear recommendations. Contextualization, some interviewees claimed, provides a "local take" on concrete issues upon which users can lay the groundwork for their policy-making processes: "[A limitation comes from] an assessment that is ... high level and not really rooted in any particular community or setting, like the theoretical benefits of a particular piece of equipment or something like that. That's very helpful, but what we need to do locally here is to take that kind of information and translate it into [our local reality]" (Decision-maker 4).

Instrumental, Conceptual, and Symbolic Uses of HTA.[14]   HTA is thus integrated within planning processes and can be aligned (or not) with policy objectives currently being pursued.[15] In our research, we explored further how decision-makers, representatives of providers, and patient associations had used specific HTA reports.[16] Table 1.9 summarizes the most frequent types of use according to whether they were instrumental, conceptual, or symbolic. On Pelz's account (1978), instrumental use refers to research findings that directly shape policies and lead to action; conceptual use refers to changes in awareness, thinking, or understanding of specific issues; and symbolic use tends to justify or legitimate existing policies or positions. While there is a thin line between conceptual use and symbolic use (Weiss 1977), Pelz emphasizes the political underpinnings of the latter: "If information serves to confirm the decision-maker's own judgment of a situation, we have a conceptual use. If the evidence helps him justify his position to someone else, such as a legislative committee or a public group, the use is symbolic" (347).

Almost all decision-makers told us they used HTA reports *instrumentally*; that is, by applying findings to guide the implementation of services and programs, the withdrawal of specific health technologies, or decisions regarding staffing, coverage, and funding. Health care providers paid particular attention to reports that pointed out ineffective technologies. They

Table 1.9 The Various Forms of HTA Used by Three Types of Stakeholders

	Instrumental	Conceptual	Symbolic
Decision-makers	As a basis for coverage decisions As evidence in court Make staffing decisions As a trigger for further inquiry Eliminating services and withdrawing certain technologies in hospitals Reevaluating existing programs Implementing services and programs Funding acquisitions of technology	As a framework for debating specific issues Orienting the government Positioning of province in regard to certain services	Reinforcing decisions already made Clarifying controversy
Providers	As a basis for negotiations Identifying ineffective technologies Modifying practice standards and routine testing Organizing specific health care services on a long-term basis	As a framework for debating specific issues Formulating position statements	Justifying a position vis-à-vis the government
Patients	Lobbying health care providers Lobbying the biomedical and pharmaceutical industries	Informing members and the public Updating personal knowledge Positioning in regard to certain policies	Does not apply

Source: Hivon et al. 2005.

also explained how certain reports had informed the preparation of CPGs, the development of screening programs, and the long-term organization of certain health care services. One physician association representative noted:

> The report on mammography was a good one and was used … the government based its breast cancer screening program on

it ... from there, we were able to evaluate how much resources and equipment were needed, how many centers, staff, and so on. That's very good because we really started from the needs created by this disease and we organized the resources accordingly. It's very, very good! It took a bit of time to establish it, but it's going well now (Physician Association 5).

Patient associations also used HTA reports instrumentally.[17] For example, one interviewee explained how a radio advertisement had promoted bone densitometry testing and, as a result, their patient association received calls from consumers asking whether or not this test should, in fact, be recommended. After inquiring with two provincial agencies, the association located reports concluding there was no evidence to support the implementation of systematic bone densitometry screening programs. Subsequently, the association used the reports from both agencies to inform the public and wrote letters to both its provincial college of physicians and surgeons and to the advertising company, enclosing copies of the reports (Patient Association 4).

Decision-makers explained how they used reports *conceptually* as a framework to stimulate debate and orient government policies. For example, a report on the human genome pointed out contextual issues the government should act upon in the relatively short term, broader issues that should be discussed in the public arena, and emerging issues that would need to be managed in the future. Providers also used HTA reports conceptually as a framework for debating specific issues or for formulating position statements. Patient associations used HTA reports conceptually for slightly different purposes, mainly in order to update their knowledge, to inform their members and the public, and to refine their positions. In two cases, reports were completely counterintuitive to what patient associations had been advocating: "The [reports] were sort of saying almost the opposite of what we've been saying, so [laughter]. So we wouldn't use them for advocacy other than to probably realize that we have to speak up even louder and try to balance some of that off" (Patient Association 6). Although research results ran counter to the patient associations' thinking, they were used to anchor and to flesh out their messages.

Decision-makers used HTA reports *symbolically* to reinforce decisions already made or to clarify controversies. For instance, one interviewee discussed an HTA report on new rheumatoid arthritis drugs: "I don't think they've changed practice, because I think that people had arrived at similar decisions, but they've certainly enforced the decisions the drug plan managers have made, absolutely" (Decision-maker 2). Providers working in ethically and politically laden areas such as genetics stressed they would use reports from highly credible HTA agencies in order to lobby governments. In these cases, HTA would be deployed to give weight to their points of view. Finally, patient associations were rarely in a position to make official decisions, thereby rendering their symbolic use of information unlikely.

Organizational, Scientific, and Material Limitations in the Use of HTA
Table 1.10, which is based on interviews with the same three groups of HTA stakeholders, indicates the major perceived limitations in the use of HTA, organized into the following categories: *organizational* (i.e., limitations tied to the structure and organization of various working environments); *scientific* (i.e., limitations due to users' level of scientific literacy); and *material* (i.e., limitations related to lack of material, financial, and human resources).

One organizational issue that frequently surfaced was poor in-house communication within government, which was perceived as limiting the use of scientific advice. As a consequence, interviewees themselves recognized that HTA producers could not be held entirely responsible for low levels of uptake of their reports. They also stressed that a lack of long-term planning and decision-makers' vested interests limited the use of HTA. Perhaps not surprisingly, established routines and the prevailing distribution of authority within stakeholders' organizations were identified as major additional limitations. The complexity of health organizations was also regarded as hindering the use of HTA reports. Hospitals, for instance, involve various practitioners with different agendas and priorities, and therefore achieving consensus on technology issues is quite challenging and involves political bargaining:

> Everyone read this report that went out, I think, six months, a year ago or something like that. And since then, everyone has had their eyes on the ministry ... I called my colleagues at the ministry, I called my colleagues at the health district ... what is your position? What are you going to do with this report? Because we, at the hospital, we are interested in this technology because of our medical orientations, this technology corresponds very well to our activities. But then, well we wait, we wait. (Physician Association 5)

Another reason HTA evidence was not always used to the fullest extent lay in the scientific interpretation of HTA. All types of stakeholders mentioned the absence of skilled staff with a good understanding of the science of HTA and of clinical and administrative practices. The need for such knowledge brokers was perhaps more acutely felt in patient associations.

Table 1.10 Limitations in the Use of HTA

	Organizational	Scientific	Material
Decision-makers	Limited use of environmental scanning and lack of long-term planning Limited in-house communication restricts the circulation of information Vested interests	Lack of knowledge brokers familiar with HTA and the organization's mandate	Lack of time as well as human and financial resources for following up on recently published reports
Providers	Consultation or dialogue difficulties in practice settings Complex procedure to set priorities in hospitals providing a broad range of services Political bargaining Dependency on government decisions Lack of authority over practice settings limits their role as agents of change	Limited expertise in research hampers the application of findings to practice	Lack of time as well as human, financial, and material resources
Patients	Not described	Lack of knowledge brokers hinders the translation of research into clear messages for the organization and its membership Lack of know-how for accessing and using scientific information	Lack of time as well as human, financial, and material resources hampers access to scientific information and participation in dissemination activities

Source: Hivon et al. 2005.

Health care providers, however, also did not feel entirely comfortable with interpreting HTA findings and translating such scientific results into clinical practice. They explained that it was partly due to their limited exposure to clinical trials or to health services research in general.

A final set of limitations conveyed by interviewees belongs to *material resources*. Health care providers, decision-makers, and patient associations all mentioned that a lack of time as well as of human, material, and financial resources hindered a fuller integration of HTA into their routine. Some decision-makers recognized that, in principle, they should systematically follow up on recently released HTA reports. However, as one of them said, it may be the "eleventh priority on a top ten list."

Why would the use of HTA be so low on the priority list? Part of the explanation has to do with workload. From the patient associations' perspective, diversifying activities—no matter how promising such a change may prove—requires a strong organizational commitment accompanied by an appropriate level of resources. Indeed, representatives of patient associations stressed that small organizations often cannot afford to attend conferences or to subscribe to scientific journals.

To summarize, respondents who were familiar with HTA agencies perceived their scientific rigor and credibility in a positive light, but regarded more skeptically their political autonomy and their ability to bring about changes in health care systems. Along related lines, Berg et al. (2004, 41) note, "HTA has become an important factor in the scene—but probably more through its indirect, symbolic function of emphasizing the importance of cost-awareness than through a direct, explicit function in policy decision making."

The findings discussed above confirm such an observation, but also suggest that HTA's limited impact on decision-making cannot be construed as a failure of HTA. They suggest, instead, that the use of HTA would better be conceptualized as a shared responsibility on the part of both HTA users and producers. As one respondent observed, the effectiveness of an increased circulation of knowledge about health technology in informing policies lies in the hands of several individuals and organizations that, ultimately, are simultaneously recipients and conveyors of knowledge:

> I'm not so sure whose responsibility that is. I think in an ideal world, it is a shared responsibility. I think we play a dual role. I think we are *users and recipients* of the research and try to build that best practice thinking into our reports and our plans. But also, we can act as a *conduit* to other providers of service who often … you know, if you're working on the front line in a hospital or whatever … we can be a conduit and help in sort of the research transfer chain (Decision-maker 1).

HTA ought, therefore, to be understood as but one important source of information among others that is valued and used in making decisions and policies,[18] although several barriers and the potential lack of convergent regulatory mechanisms limit the overall role HTA can play in bringing about greater rationality in technology-related policies.

Unresolved Issues and Reasons Why HTA Should be Supplemented by Other Approaches to Health Technology

Even if, as some observers claim, the future role of HTA in health care is "indisputable" (Cohen and Hanft 2004, 381), the challenge confronting HTA is nonetheless formidable. Cohen and Hanft (2004, 375) suggest the following activities for improving current HTA policy:

> (1) development and implementation of a priority-setting system that would identify and select emerging technologies for MTE [medical technology evaluation]; (2) pooling of resources (expertise, data and funding) to support evaluation activities for selected high-priority technologies; (3) development and implementation of methodological standards for MTE; and (4) sharing and dissemination of data and information from alliance-sponsored MTE activities to support decision-making in all aspects of technology development and diffusion.[19]

Although such an approach could prove extremely useful in the short term, it might not provide sufficient guidance to overcome, in the long run, the most fundamental challenges HTA faces. Conceptualizing HTA as a "regulatory science" (Jasanoff 1990) helps to explain the paradox involved in an applied research field that seeks to establish independence while exerting a commanding influence over public policies and clinical practices. As a regulatory science, HTA must maintain a fragile balance between the spheres of science and politics. Understanding how such a balance might be achieved requires a better understanding of technology use and science-based policy-making.

The special nature of HTA—a publicly funded, independent, policy-oriented science that should be usable and used—creates four fundamental tensions. First, *denying access to health technology* is a highly contested policy option. As I underscored in my introduction, a significant premise of HTA is that it is possible and necessary to sort out good from bad innovations on the basis of their cost, efficacy, and safety. If this were always the case, HTA could perhaps be considered the most effective policy tool for solving the problem of health technology. But this, in most situations, is not the case.

As indicated in table 1.11, only when an innovation can be proven to be harmful and/or ineffective does it clearly become legitimate for a government or a third-party payer to deny access to it. Although a significant number of medical innovations may meet those criteria and thereby justify the production of HTA, table 1.11 shows that there are four other categories for which HTA can provide useful guidance but that do not entirely solve the problem of its regulation. When an innovation provides a benefit, no matter how debatable such a benefit might be, limiting its use can be seen as ethically suspect and politically challenging. Indeed, according to Berg et al. (2004, 35), the political nature of any attempt to make decisions regarding coverage of a medical innovation or of setting priorities in health care asks for a broader approach to what constitutes HTA and scientific evidence.

The second tension concerns the *nature of the decisions* that can be made. It is increasingly clear that current and future medical technology issues cannot be boiled down to a black-and-white choice between adopting and not adopting (Deber 1992). Senior policy-makers know that such a presumption[20] would be misguided:

> I think sometimes there's a tendency to over rely on HTA; it's not going to give you the yes or no answer. Policy itself doesn't consist in yes or no answers. It's a process of laying, sifting evidence and HTA is part of that, it's an important part of that, and part of the reason I think [HTA unit] is important is because their material is credible. It is seen as being objective, it's seen as being well done. So, it can be cited by the Department and the decision has credibility because of that. I think it's a mistake to say that an assessment by [HTA unit] or [HTA unit] on a pharmaceutical or a device is the sole reason or the primary reason for a decision … policy, it's really kind of mushy. [HTA] helps support the decision, but it's not the sole determinant of it. That's where I think their importance is, in supporting that policy process (Decision-maker 3).

The decisions required for a large spectrum of medical interventions are usually more sophisticated than a go/no go alternative (Giacomini et al. 2003). For a growing number of technologies, decision-making requires determining in which clinical and organizational contexts, for which patients, and with what level of professional supervision their use can be beneficial. Furthermore, the complexity of certain technologies demands not only the presence of specialized personnel (e.g., biomedical engineers, laboratory technicians, genetics counselors, or computer

Table 1.11 Five Categories of Technology and Their Associated Ethical Issues

Category/Example	Rationing Issues	Ethical Issues
Harmful and/or ineffective Electronic fetal monitoring	Limiting its use should not, in theory, pose any problems, although pressures to use it are strong because it generates both information and uncertainty	Few
Effective, but few beneficiaries In vitro fertilization	Limiting its use poses problems because it is highly beneficial from the perspective of concerned individuals	Defining disability and ability to benefit Reconciling individual and social perspectives Prioritizing outcomes vs. prioritizing the worst off
Marginally effective, many beneficiaries Dental amalgam	Limiting its use poses problems because both harms and benefits are diffuse	Trade-off: How much of a small benefit to a large group is equivalent to a large benefit to a small group?
Life-prolonging, poor quality of life Management of very-low-birth-weight infants	Limiting its use poses problems because it may run against deeply held moral intuitions	Rule of rescue requires that all that can be done, be done Institutions, clinicians, and families may have trouble bearing the responsibility for denial of care Participation of parents in decision-making may be limited
Inefficient allocation Left ventricular assist device	Limiting its use poses problems because it is effective for many individuals but unsustainable on a societal level	Marginal value of investment Opportunity cost of investment and long-term sustainability

Source: Adapted from Johri and Lehoux 2003.

specialists), but also adapted infrastructures and effective monitoring programs (e.g., a breast cancer screening program requires both equipment that is perfectly maintained and quality assurance mechanisms). As Abraham (2002, 28) emphasizes, risk assessment "cannot rely solely on a conventional model of technical science" because it involves "social and political judgments about the needs of, and acceptable risks for, patients and public health."[21]

The third tension arises because HTA's *societal purpose* that revolves around promoting rational, collective use of health technology does not automatically converge with the interests of every stakeholder. Health care does not pursue only one goal: "Other 'goals' can be more individual, such as reassurance, improvement of quality of life, the need for a last hope, and so forth. These goals are variable and context-dependent, making their explication and formalization over and above individual situations excruciatingly difficult" (Berg et al. 2004, 41). According to Tunis (2004, 2196), an important policy issue provoked by the quest for universal coverage criteria is "the pervasive and persistent discomfort with clinical decisions that are influenced by an entity other than the patient and the patient's clinician." Similarly, Wailoo et al. (2004, 536) underscore that what constitutes the "right decision" depends on one's point of view: "For individual patients the right decision is that which maximizes their well-being, and this is properly the concern of the clinician. Yet in resource constrained healthcare systems this will not always coincide with the right decisions for patients in general or society as a whole, thereby leading to some understandable tensions."[22]

In practice, HTA reports may conclude that access to technology should be either increased or decreased. Their conclusions can be translated into actions that are compatible either with cost-control initiatives (thereby reinforcing a diluted form of the societal perspective) or with facilitating the adoption of innovations (thereby potentially favoring a discretionary clinical perspective). The societal perspective is, indeed, often conflated with the issue of affordability. While health economists are routinely cast as the experts in rationalizing the use of collective resources (Eccles 2004), their view is often opposed to a clinical perspective, which would in principle give priority to patients' well-being.

Nevertheless, diminishing the role of priority-setting attempts at a societal level "shifts the burden of responsibility to individual physicians and institutions," which entails moving the locus of decision-making "outside of any sphere of public accountability and democratic control" (Berg et al. 2004, 42). This potential loss of accountability may explain why Tunis (2004, 2196) emphasizes the need to establish and maintain public trust in coverage decision processes: "Reaching agreement on the criteria that should be applied to determinations of medical necessity presupposes a level of stakeholder confidence in the process through which those criteria would be applied." Tunis (2197) also points out that the coverage process of Medicare and Medicaid in the United States is more transparent now than ever before, and that it includes appeal mechanisms and opportunities for the public to comment on draft decisions. Detailed documents that summarize scientific evidence, expert input, and other information that was considered in national coverage policies can be found on the Medicare and Medicaid Services Web site (www.cms.gov/coverage). Although such initiatives can facilitate broader access to information, they do not enable calling into question the nature of the evidence gathered and the analyses performed.[23]

The fourth key tension is associated with defining the *desirability of health technology.* HTA presumes that effectiveness and even cost-effectiveness may act as authoritative criteria for deciding whether or not a technology is valuable for society (Giacomini 1999). This belief is at the heart of its societal mission, since HTA can be influential only if it convinces a large set of players that all parties will benefit from an integrated, science-based approach to the adoption, dissemination, and use of health technology (Hailey and Crowe 1993; Jacob and McGregor 1997). Although this precept has gained widespread recognition in several countries, HTA producers still have much work to do to convince HTA stakeholders.

From a policy perspective, it may prove perfectly rational to authorize access to a given innovation on the basis that it creates economic opportunities and placates powerful providers and media-cherished patients (Weiss 1991; Cabatoff 1996). Similarly, responding to industry's concerns can be seen as rational. Tunis (2004, 2197) suggests that a fundamental challenge to developing criteria for determining which health care interventions are "reasonable and necessary" is the potential impact on industry. Because Medicare is the largest single payer of health care in the world and many private insurance companies adopt similar coverage policies, any decision Medicare makes has considerable effect on the "overall economic vitality of the pharmaceutical, biotechnology, and medical devices industries" throughout the world (Tunis 2004, 2197).

While the tensions discussed here have been poorly conceptualized and articulated in the HTA sphere, social science scholarship could bring valuable insights to the discussion. The first such insight relates to the nature of the knowledge HTA creates. Reducing the tension between context-dependent objectives and societal objectives would require a better understanding of the implications of technology use *in the real world of clinical and social practices* and a theoretically informed integration of various disciplinary perspectives. HTA's epistemic foundations are largely shaped by the postpositivist gold standard of randomized controlled trials that do not examine the context in which technology is used and that do not explore an innovation's value from users' (i.e., clinicians and patients) perspectives.

Clinical trials cannot provide information about the broader organizational and social changes that will be brought about through the diffusion of new medical technologies. Despite this lack, HTA is often promoted as an interdisciplinary inquiry that addresses a wide spectrum of issues, ranging from effectiveness to ethics. The findings presented earlier in this chapter suggest, however, that even though this may be true in principle, it is not the case in practice. There may be some obvious reasons why ethical, social, and legal issues are rarely addressed in HTA reports; for example, staff members of HTA agencies are usually trained in epidemiology and/or economics, and may feel less equipped to analyze legal, social, and ethical issues. Although HTA producers have started to address these shortcomings more earnestly (Reuzel et al. 2004; Gallo 2004; Oortwijn et al. 2004), collaboration between HTA practitioners and philosophers, anthropologists, sociologists, and jurists remains limited.

The second undertheorized area is the policy-making process and, more broadly, the institutional links and interactions between HTA producers and various stakeholders. At the present stage of HTA's institutionalization, discussions about how technology should be regulated must provide a more substantial explanation of its value to society (i.e., move beyond cost-effectiveness) and of how various stakeholders, including industry, can act together to achieve a desirable use of technology.

Although recent consultative and collaborative experiences involving representatives of patient associations and the general public have been reported in Canada and various European countries (Pivik et al. 2004; Royle and Oliver 2004), they were developed in the margins of the main thrust of HTA, often with modest resources. As one patient association representative remarked to us, such a collaboration must be reciprocally maintained and valued: "With HTA agencies, it works both ways, although more often we go to them than they come to us" (Patient Association 3). This person also provided a clear definition of how various sources of expertise can be accessed, adapted, and disseminated to the lay public:

> We have a major role in providing information about cancer to the lay public. ... The content of that information comes from a variety of sources. It may be something that is developed at our

national office … or if it's a provincial resource, then we would contact people who have expertise in that area and get their advice and input in terms of the content. So we always refer to experts as we develop our materials, because we are a lay organization, but we feel nonetheless that in that position we are the best to interpret and communicate to the lay public our focus (Patient Association 3).

For another representative of a patient association, however, informing the public was problematic. This person distrusted patients' medical intelligence, preferring to leave health care-related judgments in the hands of the experts:

The public really is not sophisticated enough to make judgment … because the patients might try, might take a variety of medications together that they shouldn't, they may mix their medications inappropriately, they might overdose, they may misuse in some way; the doctor supposedly understands interactions between chemicals and understands the patient and is able to prescribe the pill or the puffer or whatever it has to be. The patient isn't smart enough to make that judgment. So it's dangerous telling the patient about things that might not work for them, because they might start to demand it (Patient Association 1).

These two responses suggest that the people running patient associations may perceive technology-related issues in quite different ways and may, therefore, play varying roles in policy-making. As I make clear in chapter 4, this same mixed reality applies to groups of physicians, decision-makers, and industry representatives, and carries significant implications for health technology regulation. Suffice it to say at this stage that insufficiently conceptualized and timid initiatives to involve various stakeholders in the production and/or use of HTA could remain disappointing or even misguided. A stronger input from the social sciences would, therefore, help to strengthen policy-oriented research on health technology and more reflexive engagement with stakeholders (an argument I develop further in chapter 5).

CHAPTER 2

What Do Technologies Do?

An Ethnographic Understanding of Health Technology

The preceding chapter posited the emergence of Health Technology Assessment (HTA) as one of the most salient scientific responses to dealing with the problem of technological change in contemporary health care systems. Strongly rooted in clinical epidemiology and health economics, HTA has to date been preoccupied mainly with measuring health outcomes and the economic impact of innovations. Because this sort of evaluation is concerned primarily with an objective quantification of technology's effects, it has generally fallen short of providing an in-depth understanding of what technologies do in practice.

Other streams of health and social science research, however, have produced a wealth of ethnographic studies focused on the context and processes that shape human practices around health technology. In this chapter I explore and synthesize concepts that illustrate and explain, from a social science perspective, the dynamics by which health technology shapes and organizes individual and collective practices in and around various health care settings. By asking questions that go beyond the cost-effectiveness angle, I argue, social scientists offer additional points of entry and intellectual lenses that can help us define the value of innovations.

The Contribution of the Social Sciences (From Marginal to Substantive)

One reason for turning to the social sciences to understand health technology is the recognition that in the field of applied health research, insufficient scholarly attention has been given to the ways in which technology structures the delivery, utilization, and outcomes of technology-mediated health care services. As I mentioned in the introduction, health technology is often conceptualized as a black box; that is, as a given instrument that produces health effects. Nonetheless, when technologies are implemented, they deeply modify how health care providers and patients interact, and the paths of action they can and *should* take (Mechanic 2002). For instance, because the belief that information is valuable in itself is such a powerful cultural norm, when screening tests are made available, they easily become part of established practices that can hardly be opposed. Indeed, for some of the conditions tested, an appropriate treatment does not even necessarily exist. Another example is the use of electronic fetal monitoring systems that can play a significant role in medical liability suits if something goes wrong during a delivery (Johri and Lehoux 2003). Consequently, they are used extensively despite solid evidence indicating their effectiveness only in relation to high-risk pregnancies. These and numerous similar examples lead to the simple truth that health technology's use is embedded in social practices. Given this relationship, social science research can be immensely helpful (Brown and Webster 2004) in helping to shed light on the dynamics that shape the use of existing technologies and the pace at which innovations are integrated.

There are, in addition, many nonmedical variables that influence the effectiveness of health technology, including emotions, knowledge, values, beliefs, cultural practices, social interactions, organizational structures and processes, financial incentives, and regulatory frameworks (Gelijns and Rosenberg 1994; Greer et al. 2002). In short, how technology is used, perceived, and valued by providers and patients may maximize or minimize its desired effects.

Health researchers usually refer to the concept of compliance (with guidelines, in the case of physicians, or with treatment, in the case of patients) to explain some of the variations in health outcomes—a notion that appears to be empty as long as the "why" behind deviations from clinical norms cannot be answered. This concept was addressed in a brilliant study by Greer et al. (2002), a medical sociologist who, with her colleagues, examined the extent to which the interactions between physicians and women with breast cancer living in rural areas could explain why higher rates of mastectomy (versus lumpectomy) were observed in some parts of the United States. One of the elements that make Greer's study especially insightful is that the researchers did not assume a priori either that these women's rationality was deficient or that prioritizing health and bodily appearance over other life activities (e.g., taking care of the grand-children, the farm) should drive their decisions. In other words, its per-spective was strongly rooted in an academic tradition that observes and conceptualizes social practices. Its goal is not to find ways to improve phy-sicians' or patients' compliance but to explain why gaps between clinical practice guidelines (CPGs) and actual practices are observed and how they are sustained.

Such "why" and "how" questions are often best dealt with through qualitative social science studies. The adjective "qualitative" is important here because understanding rationales (why?) and processes (how?) requires exploring the viewpoints of those involved in particular practices. Such an ethnographic approach entails what anthropologists label the *emic* perspective, which encompasses listening to and analyzing what peo-ple say as well as observing what people do (Goffman 1971). Ethno-graphy's earliest roots are in social anthropology, a discipline that "traditionally focused on small-scale communities that were thought to share culturally specific beliefs and practices" (Savage 2000, 1400). According to Galanti (1999, 20), ethnography is defined by three princi-ples: "1) it is an observational method designed to get the meanings underlying people's behaviors; 2) it focuses on everyday life as events unfold naturally; and 3) its goal is to understand behavior from the point of view of those being studied." Although its defining feature for many is the use of participant observation, entailing prolonged fieldwork, it can also incorporate a mix of qualitative and quantitative methods (Savage 2000).

Despite variations from one school of thought to another, the goal of the ethnographer is not simply to give an account of these views, to assume that these views represent truth, or to talk on behalf of the research participants; it is to reorganize these perceptions and actions into a frame-work that makes the dynamics and specificities of social practices more explicit (Knorr Cetina 1999). From this perspective, changes brought about through the use of health technology can be examined more system-atically when social science concepts are mobilized. For instance, one may be interested in understanding the appropriateness of applying an informed consent procedure for a resurgent technology such as electro-convulsive therapy for vulnerable mentally ill persons (Heitman 1996). Can such people fully grasp complex information about risks and benefits when there is a fair amount of uncertainty about, and very few alternatives for, treating major depression? How can one deal with the social history that now fuels patients' rights groups? In such controversial situations, even the best evidence about effectiveness may prove to be of little help. What the social sciences can offer is a framework for making sense of the various views, claims, and actions of both anti- and pro-technology groups (Jasanoff 1990).

Another aspect that social science research can illuminate is the role of the context of health care practices and the ways various settings may influence the appropriateness and effectiveness of health technology (Andrews 2003; Kearns 1993; McKeever and Coyte 1999). Now that health care is increasingly delivered in nontraditional settings, such as home care, nursing homes, or "closer-to-patients" satellite clinics, paying attention to the variations and adaptations required to render the use of technology appropriate should help to enhance the safety and quality of such services (Lehoux, Saint-Arnaud, and Richard 2004). Indeed, when hospital-based technologies are moved to a patient's home, a number of assumptions are made with respect to what a "typical" home is, what it contains (e.g., children, pets, stairs, electricity, phone lines), and how people inhabit the space. Very often, the promises of high-tech home care conflict with the social realities and even the physical structures of patients' dwellings (McKeever 2001). Thus, an in-depth understanding of how technology can affect patients' social and private lives beyond the controlled environment of traditional health care settings may inform clinical practices undergoing health care delivery reforms.

Finally, the regulation of health technology—the policies, guidelines, and coverage criteria that are implemented to define eligibility and setting—may also benefit from a social science perspective. This potential is more acute in the case of innovations that are ethically controversial or so costly that it is impossible to introduce them into a given health care system without explicitly setting limits (Heitman 1998). For example, deciding whether left ventricular assist devices (LVAD; a battery-powered artificial heart that can be implanted in patients with heart failure as a bridge to heart transplant or as a permanent palliative technology) should be introduced in Quebec, Canada, required, in order to absorb the costs without endangering other health care services, defining the number of patients who would be permitted access to the device (AETMIS 2002). In this case, social science research highlighted the difficulty of implementing consistent priority-setting criteria from one medical team to another and, consequently, the vulnerability of a policy whose legitimacy is open to almost inevitable challenge by both the media and patients (Lehoux and Blume 2000).

BOX 2.1. REASONS FOR INTEGRATING SOCIAL SCIENCE PERSPECTIVES AND APPROACHES IN APPLIED HEALTH RESEARCH

- Technology structures the delivery, utilization, and outcomes of health care.
- Nonmedical variables influence the effectiveness of health technology (e.g., emotions, knowledge, values, beliefs, cultural practices, social interactions, organizational structures and processes, financial incentives, and regulatory frameworks).
- Providers and patients do not use, perceive, or value technology consistently; outcomes therefore vary.
- The use of health technology triggers social changes and raises ethical concerns.
- Technology modifies the settings in which health care practices take place and influences the appropriateness and effectiveness of health technology.
- Because technology modifies patients' and the general public's expectations of health and health care, its regulation requires a broader understanding of the policy arena.

Box 2.1 summarizes the points I have thus far introduced to justify why turning to the social sciences can help us to understand when and how innovations may be better. All the arguments I have offered in favor of such an integrative approach in applied health research refer to a marginal or selective[1] application of social science concepts, tools, and insights (Mykhalovskiy and Weir 2004). I suggested that relying on social science research may make it possible to introduce innovations in a more meaningful and socially appropriate way. However, to my mind, a more fundamental reason to turn to the social sciences lies in their ability *to entirely reframe what technology is and does*. This is the task on which the rest of the chapter focuses.

When compared with computers, motorbikes, water management systems, or nuclear plants, health technology plays a pivotal role in the transformation of our existence. It actively mediates life and death, health and risks, knowledge and uncertainty, and autonomy and mobility. In view of that, table 2.1 summarizes the actions that various categories of health technology support. What I want to stress is that each of these categories does different things; each thing they do carries different implications; and each is of more or less value when compared with the others. In the right-hand column I have summarized the basic assumptions embodied in each category and the issues that may possibly matter from a patient's/individual's perspective when considering a particular technology's desirability. This chapter will gradually clarify why comprehending the mediatory role

Table 2.1 Reframing What Health Technologies Do

Health technologies	Where their desirability lies	
	What they do	What these actions imply
Screening tests	Provide information that requires a confirming procedure or test (diagnostic)	Information is valuable in itself and/or it leads to a diagnosis in a timely manner
Diagnostic tests and imaging devices	Provide information about the presence/absence of disease	Information is valuable in itself and/or it leads to an appropriate and timely action vis-à-vis disease
Monitoring systems	Provide information about various vital bodily functions, psychosocial well-being, and compliance with treatments	Interpretation of the data is reliable and leads to it being acted upon in an appropriate manner; continuous surveillance does not alter identity and behavior
Implants	Restore (temporarily) bodily functions (e.g., cardiac functions, hearing)	Long-term risks, quality of life and identify alteration are acceptable to the patient
Surgery and therapeutic devices	Stop or delay the pathological process and reduce symptoms	Risks, invasiveness, and consequences are acceptable to the patient
Palliative technologies	Substitute (temporarily) natural bodily functions (e.g., breathing, nutrition, cardiac functions)	Sustaining life when quality is compromised is valuable
Drugs	Stop or delay the pathological process; reduce symptoms	Side effects and quality of life are acceptable to the patient
Health promotion technologies	Promote/discourage lifestyles and behavior; protect from or reduce harm associated with risky practices (e.g., drugs, sexuality, sports)	Alteration of practices, identity, and peer recognition are acceptable/meaningful to the individual/groups

(continued)

Table 2.2 *(continued)*

Health technologies	Where their desirability lies	
	What they do	What these actions imply
Occupational health technologies	Protect workers' health; promote/discourage work-related behavior affecting health	Overall quality of work conditions and alteration of practices, identity, and peer recognition are acceptable/meaningful to the individual/groups
Technical aids	Facilitate autonomy, mobility, and social integration	Aids are user-friendly and help overcome the social barriers associated with the disability
Information technologies	Record, archive, transmit, and provide access to administrative and clinical information	Access to and use of information respects confidentiality and brings efficiency and quality to health care

of these various health technologies and illuminating the most significant transformations they support should help us in our quest to reconsider the problem of health technology.

The Technology-in-Practice Perspective[2]

In their review of twenty-five years of scholarly work on technology and health for the journal *Sociology of Health and Illness,* Timmermans and Berg (2003) describe three general approaches to technology: *technological determinism,* which conceives of technology as a driving—and often alienating—force; *social essentialism,* which sees technology as a blank slate that is politically potentialized only through social interpretation and interaction; and *technology-in-practice,* which is concerned with more subtle technology-mediated political shifts in patients' autonomy, providers' and various experts' knowledge claims, and governments' health policies and regulations.

Technological determinism considers that technical variables alone shape innovations. A large explanatory power is thus given to technology by isolating it from the "outside" social world. According to Timmermans and Berg (2003), this type of analysis is not so much focused on explaining technology per se; rather, it seeks to construct a case either for or against a given technology. Indeed, social critics will at times refer to an idealized past or a romanticized "natural" way of doing things that has been disturbed by an inhumane technological drive, while technology fans will justify an innovation by arguing that it represents the singularly best, most logical way to accomplish a given objective. It is only rational, therefore, to embrace it (see also Akrich 1995). Scholars adopting the technological determinism perspective will often ignore or pay less attention to technologies that are seen as less controversial, while social critics will regularly be perplexed when empirical work indicates that users may be empowered by the use of certain innovations.

In the 1980s, for example, several feminist groups relied on the discourse of technological determinism to criticize the medicalization of childbirth. Certain technologies (e.g., C-section, episiotomy, induction of labor) were seen as granting (male) clinicians power over a "natural" life process and event. Conversely, critics of the medicalization thesis argued that these technologies were in fact tools that empowered women, who now could avoid some of the dangers inherent in childbirth. In both instances, technology was seen as something that emerges and evolves by itself, that generates social (positive or negative) impacts.

Largely inspired by constructivism (i.e., a research paradigm that posits reality as socially constructed), *social essentialism* views technology as profoundly malleable, something that is rendered meaningful and given shape only through cultural and social perceptions. According to Timmermans and Berg (2003), critics who adopt this perspective argue that the continued hegemony of the medical-industrial complex is maintained by interest groups. Such groups are in a position to select certain innovations over others that may threaten their privileges and power. Here again, the analysis is not focused entirely on technology; rather, it draws its explanatory power from sociological observations on power relations, compliance, illness narratives, sick roles, and the interplay among various ideologies surrounding illness and disability.

Technology is therefore posited to be a sociological catalyst that generates interactions and meanings, but that does not act, affect, or evolve (Callon 1986). As a result, the social essentialist perspective presumes that a given technology is not problematic in itself; only its socially constructed meaning and use can be examined and called into question. For instance, when patients with chronic obstructive pulmonary disease are reluctant to use a portable oxygen concentrator while visiting friends or going shopping, the bulky, noisy, and clinical-looking device is not seen as problematic. Instead, the social construction of what normalcy and autonomy represent is regarded as being at issue (Lehoux, Saint-Arnaud, and Richard 2004). This lack of attention to technology impedes analysis because social essentialism cannot conceptually address the reciprocal dynamic between technologies and humans, or what science and technology studies (STS) scholars call the co-construction of users and technology (Oudshoorn and Pinch 2003), an issue to which I will return.

Timmerman and Berg's (2003) analysis illuminates significant limitations in the technological determinism and social essentialism approaches. They suggest, instead, that the *technology-in-practice* perspective is a promising avenue for overcoming those weaknesses. In what follows, I focus on two key features of technology-in-practice that help to define how technologies mediate the construction and reproduction of lay and professional identities (Berg 1997; Pasveer 1989) as well as the normative dynamics that pervade health care practices (e.g., decision-making authority, expertise-based practices). This perspective brings us closer to a substantive integration of the social sciences into health technology analysis.

First, technology-in-practice has been inspired by ethnographic studies that examine what technologies do (i.e., what they help to accomplish in daily practice). This stream of research has clarified not only the gaps between how certain technologies were initially meant to be used and how various (often unexpected) users in practice have appropriated them (Oudshoorn and Pinch 2003); more important, perhaps, it has unpacked the concept of technology itself (Williams and Edge 1996). In defiance of the usual preoccupation with high-tech devices, scholars have shown that several mundane technologies (e.g., adhesive bandages, test kits, masks, corridors, elevators, coffee machines) contribute profoundly to the structuring and localizing of health and work practices by configuring how people interact, share information, and comply (or not) with established rules (Fagerhaugh et al. 1986; Timmermans and Berg 2003; Woolgar 1991). The recent emergence of Severe Acute Respiratory Syndrome (SARS) in Toronto, Canada, vividly illustrated how the effective detection and control of contagious cases relies primarily on the appropriate use of mundane technologies such as ear thermometers, hand-washing, and face masks (and how effective detection can fail when such basic technologies are unevenly and inconsistently applied in practice). Ethnographic studies have also underscored the ways in which technology coordinates clinical and organizational aspects of health care by forging paths of action along which a broad set of actors must travel for health care to be enacted (Berg 1997; Nélisse 1996). Furthermore, technology (and especially health technology) often generates, alongside physical alterations, profound symbolic effects on the definition of the self and identity (Lawton 2003), personhood (Kaufman 2003), and inheritance and kinship (Shostak 2003). For instance, it has been argued that diagnostic techniques do not simply reflect a patient's health—as if health were something inside one's body to be measured—but actively constitute existential meanings (Timmermans and Berg 2003). For example, a positive Prostate Screening Antigen (PSA) test result may deeply modify the self-identity of a man who may live for several years without ever noticing physical symptoms or developing cancer.

By observing what technologies do in the world, social scientists have also underlined the losses that accompany any technological expansion of human abilities (Mort et al. 2003). Commuting in a high-speed train, for example, necessitates overlooking smaller details in the use of the land that may vary from one region or town to another. Further, while a surgeon operating with endoscopic instruments can perform certain actions that would otherwise be impossible, she may notice her inability to feel the texture of various tissues through her fingers. Such losses may remain unnoticed when technology is used within the intentional and spatial boundaries of its initial script, or scenario, of use (Akrich 1995). Nevertheless, anyone attempting to use a familiar technology in a different environment will quickly be reminded of some of its specificities (e.g., attempting to use a mobile phone outside of its reception zone). There are also subtle cultural norms and routines that may render the use of technology inappropriate (or heuristically obscure) at certain times or in certain contexts (e.g., walking with an umbrella under a blue sky in a western European city). Thus, a closer examination of what happens when technologies are displaced holds the potential for making more visible some of the characteristics of their technical, spatial, and social embeddedness.

The second key feature of the technology-in-practice perspective is the recognition that technology always emerges from, and operates within, heterogeneous networks comprising various people (e.g., designers, shareholders, manufacturers, users) and technologies (e.g., mechanical or electrical components, materials, support systems, built environments) (Latour 1988, 1989). The term "sociotechnical network" emphasizes the fact that humans and technology can hardly operate without one another; power, it has been said, lies in their association (Latour 1990).

Health technologies are embedded in relationships with other tools, practices, and social groups, and it is through their location in these networks that diagnostics, treatments, or health promotion interventions are made possible in health and social care (Timmermans and Berg 2003). In addition, the emergence of a new technology always implies that designers and their corporate leaders have thought about, negotiated, and come to a certain closure regarding the "best scenario" according to which that particular innovation should be used (Bucciarelli 1994). Such observations have led some (e.g., Akrich and Latour 1992; Callon 1986; Latour 1989) to suggest applying a "sociology of translation" to conceptualize technology dissemination:

As different human actors interact with a device the alliances they form become contested, precarious, shifting and treacherous. A device is, therefore, never simply inserted or diffused into a setting but is always subject to these processes of translation during which humans interact with it, each configuring and reconfiguring the other in unpredictable and often unexpected ways (Prout 1996, 202).

More specifically, the deployment of sociotechnical networks involves delegating a fairly large number of tasks either to humans or to technology (Latour 1988). The provision of home care and ambulatory services, for instance, relies on nurses training patients and their relatives to perform tasks that have traditionally fallen under the purview of nursing staff, such as the flushing of catheters, the monitoring of clinical symptoms, and the application of emergency procedures (Lehoux, Saint-Arnaud, and Richard 2004). As I explore in more detail later, the distribution of knowledge, skills, and duties between humans, and between humans and technologies, must always be negotiated and developed (Akrich 1994).

The technology-in-practice perspective thus stresses that technology is never an isolated piece of equipment; rather, it forms a spatially unbounded and heterogeneous network in which humans and other technologies incessantly interact according to a certain distribution of skills, tasks, and responsibilities that may be contested, renegotiated, ignored, or even sabotaged. This perspective holds the potential to reconcile conflicting empirical findings concerning the partial successes and failures of medical innovations (Timmermans and Berg 2003) as well as the double-edged empowering and alienating effects they may exert on health care providers and patients. But before I examine the broader implications that sociotechnical networks bring to health care practices, I need to backtrack a bit and reexamine what health technology *is* when one adopts the technology-in-practice perspective.

Unblack-Boxing Health Technology

I have mentioned several times the need to open the black box of technology, and now I want to clarify exactly what "unblack-boxing" entails. There are at least three meanings attached to such an intellectual enquiry: (1) understanding how technology works; (2) disclosing how technology is inherently political; and (3) examining how a given technology's power lies in its association with various individuals and groups.

The first meaning is mainly epistemological, in that it emphasizes the fact that although we live in societies pervaded by technologies, each of us holds a very limited knowledge of how they all function (Tenner 1996). While some of us may acquire a significant body of knowledge about how to use certain technologies and thereby more fully exploit their potential, very often knowing how devices *work* remains secondary, if not pointless. In addition, the use of a particular technology may depend on broader technological systems that tend to disappear from the user's attention. Mitchell and Cambrosio (1997), for instance, suggest that knowledge about electricity generation and transmission is rarely necessary, even though most people in the industrialized world need to use electrically powered appliances on a daily basis: "The electricity which powers these [familiar] objects is a 'black box' for most of us; we flip a light switch or turn on the television without any understanding of the theory of physics or electricity" (222). In the health care arena, meanwhile, the idiotproof design,[3] which prevents any unskilled, unauthorized, or unequipped user from tinkering with internal mechanisms and settings is well-known to both biomedical engineers and STS scholars (Bucciarelli 1994; Oudshoorn and Pinch 2003).

Unblack-boxing's first meaning begs the question of why certain technologies are black-boxed in the first place. Black-boxing some of the technical components involved in operating a device may reflect an epistemological survival strategy, or a way to avoid information overload. The dark side of this is that users become increasingly dependent upon technicians to diagnose, repair, or prevent technical malfunctions.

Black-boxing has not, however, always been a feature of technology. Because of a widespread reliance on mechanical systems and materials that were transformed locally (e.g., leather, wood, metal), at the beginning of the Industrial Revolution many technology users could maintain and repair various tools and machines themselves (Tenner 1996). Often, these people could design new tools and, consequently, had an empirical knowledge of the tasks the tools should help perform and the context in which they would be used. In other words, users knew how to function as both designers and technicians (Oudshoorn and Pinch 2003).

By contrast, in modern health care systems, where the level of specialization of both medicine and health technology is ever-increasing, *displacement* and *fragmentation* of knowledge are ubiquitous. Black-boxing of technological components appears inescapable, since no single individual (or occupational group) possesses all the knowledge required to fully operate a technological system. This knowledge gap introduces several dependencies among various users and technicians. Even designers may be overwhelmed: "The complexity of technological systems makes it impossible to test all possible malfunctions and makes it inevitable that in actual use, some great flaws will appear that were hidden from designers" (Tenner 1996, 10). Accordingly, analyses of a given health technology would benefit from a careful examination of the various forms of knowledge that are required for its use to be safe, effective, and appropriate, and of where these epistemic sources are located and distributed.

The second meaning attached to unblack-boxing technology has a political overtone as well as an axiological character. It involves scrutinizing the ways in which a technology can act as a normative device, controlling what users may or may not do with and through it, and even sustaining exclusionary social practices. Along this line, Winner (1980) used the example of the bridges designed by the New York-based architect Robert Moses to demonstrate that specific, politicized intentions pervasively animate designers and engineers and that technology is, therefore, inherently political. According to Winner, the bridges in question were deliberately designed to be low enough so that public buses and trucks could not access the islands. As a consequence, people of lower socioeconomic status (including African Americans, many of whom used public transport) were excluded.

Though hotly debated, Winner's analysis is still used as a learning case in the STS community[4] and points toward the decisions that are made during the design process and that are, by definition, embedded in social, economic, and political ideologies (Pinch and Bijker 1987). Recognizing such embeddedness enables the axiological unblack-boxing of technology by disclosing the norms that are active in the design phase. Following Woolgar (1991, 59), unpacking how technology designers "configure the users" by "defining the identity of putative users, and setting constraints upon their likely future actions," can help make more explicit why certain groups of users are targeted, what assumptions are made on their behalf (e.g., regarding preferences, needs, behaviors), and the range of forbidden and authorized actions. This process can lay the foundations for a broader sociopolitical analysis that seeks to identify power dynamics around the design and use of health technology and its impact on vulnerable groups (Brown and Webster 2004).

The third meaning attached to the unblack-boxing of technology draws heavily on Latour's (1989) proposition that the power of technologies lies in their *association* with various humans, the alliances those humans forge over time, and the trials they endure. Although this view focuses on the strategic and political dynamics that fuel innovation processes, it is devoid of any axiological connotation, since Latour's concern is not to judge whether certain innovations are better or worse, desirable or despicable. For him, black-boxing is unavoidable; it happens over time and through scientific and political struggles in order to bring controversies to a close, to authoritatively select certain technological scenarios over others, and to enable various groups to pursue their projects once a few key social and technical solutions have been black-boxed along the innovation path.

The crucial element of Latour's theory is its determined quest to regard both social and technical entities as potential objects of black-boxing. Joerges (1999) has adopted and elaborated on Latour's perspective. For him, it seems clear that

> the power represented in built and other technical devices is not to be found in the formal attributes of these things themselves. Only their authorization, their legitimate representation, gives shape to the definitive effects they may have ... in particular, built spaces always represent control rights. They belong to someone and not to others, they can legitimately be used by some and not by others. Variable control rights over built spaces constrain what can pass in and around these spaces. Only rarely and in the most trivial senses can one show that such constraints are coupled to building form. In this view, it is the processes by which authorizations are built, maintained, contested and changed which are at issue in any social study of built spaces and technology. (424)

In other words, technology's coercive power cannot be explained solely through recourse to designers' intentions. Unblack-boxing must go beyond disclosing political interests thought to be inherent in their design. On this view, it is only through understanding associations between social and technical entities that the powerful persuasiveness of sociotechnical networks can be appreciated. If humans did not forge alliances with and around specific technologies, the power of those technologies would be limited or nil. An instructive case in point is the example of a surveillance camera system that is promoted as being able to reduce crime rates in public spaces and lead to arrests (Neyland 2004). Although some passersby might feel the system exerts some kind of power over their behavior, it is mainly because of their belief that humans will act upon the images gathered. For public video surveillance to gain social legitimacy, several social groups must act together, aiming toward a more or less consensual goal and realigning some of their competing interests. In this perspective, the fluent functioning of an innovative network is nothing but a *joint performance* of human and technological entities involved in its maintenance and use (Akrich and Latour 1992).

This third view of technology's black-boxing stresses that certain social entities formulate authorizations and define how they should be distributed across social and/or technical entities and enforced. This process of granting and enforcing authorizations is far from predictable and can be contested at any moment, especially if a black-boxing process has not been entirely secured. It should be kept in mind, however, that black-boxing may be so effective that no one will dare to challenge what has been agreed upon in the past and everyone will accept the constraints of sociotechnical networks as absolutes (Bijker 1987). Callon (1987), for instance, has shown that certain associations between economic, technical, social, and political entities acquire irreversibility; in other words, they are institutionalized as established practices.

Unblack-boxing, meanwhile, is a powerful means to analytically and retrospectively reopen scientific, technical, and sociopolitical controversies that have paved the way for the evolution of an innovation. In particular, health technology's unblack-boxing enables scrutiny of the epistemological and axiological assumptions that are embedded in an innovation's design and that define by whom and how it should be used. It also provides insights about the social and technical struggles that shape innovative processes as much as the deployment of innovations.

But why would health technology analysts be interested in the unblack-boxing process? The answer lies in the fact that such an examination makes more explicit the competing and/or converging claims of medical experts, biomedical engineers, shareholders, policy-makers, and patient representatives about the value of medical technology, and brings the social and technical factors to the analytic forefront (Brown and Webster 2004). Unblack-boxing avoids the shortcomings of technological determinism and social essentialism, and it seeks to understand more incisively the role of health technology in daily practices.

Adding Verbs to Health Technologies

This chapter's title asks an apparently simple question: "What do technologies do?" I first tried to anchor this question conceptually by situating it among various approaches to technology, stressing the need to examine what technologies do "in practice." Then I started to unpack the question by defining why and how technology must be unblack-boxed in order to understand its normative features as well as the role of knowledge in its design and use. I will now weave another layer of theoretical insights into this question. "Adding verbs" to health technologies should help complete our analysis of what they do by defining more clearly the active relationships between technologies and humans in the context of daily practices.

A scholar who has examined blood sugar measurement devices recently argued that "medical technology serving to acquire knowledge tends to do more than passively registering facts" (Mol 2000, 9). When people measure their blood sugar levels and discuss the meaning of their variations over time with medical specialists, the measuring "is not only a matter of getting to *know* something. It also implies something is *done*" (10). The measurement device alters the subjectivity of a patient's physical sensations by (un)validating their relationships to an objectively measured health state, which may increase one's physical self-awareness. Technology, therefore, *does something* by modifying its users' identities, perceptions, knowledge, and range of actions. Furthermore, technology does something by constituting epistemic objects (i.e., entities that can be problematized as knowledge over time and trials; Knorr Cetina 1999) that alter the potential paths of, and perceived need for, action.

This sense of what technology does, alludes to a broader notion that is quite controversial among STS scholars and social scientists: the idea that technology has *agency*, that it performs actions and produces sociotechnical practices (Latour 1988; Mol 2002). Stressing the productive character of technology requires clarifying the power relationships associated with it. A Foucaultian analysis, for instance, would conceive of various technologies "as producers of new types of humans, and new types of relationships" (Vos and Willems 2000, 3).

Instead of dealing directly with the concept of agency, however, my interest is in illustratating how, empirically, health technology is always both enabling and constraining in any individual or collective action, an important aspect to consider when one tries to set a value on innovations. As Mol (2002, 32) remarks, "It is possible to say that in practices objects are *enacted*. This suggests that activities take place—but leaves the actors vague. It also suggests that in the act, and only then and there, something *is*—being enacted." Mol's wording aptly conveys what the ethnographer of health technology observes in daily health-related routines.

A useful (albeit erroneously perceived as outdated by some) key to conceptualizing what technologies do and how practices are enacted is found in phenomenology. This approach, developed by such landmark philosophers as Husserl, Heidegger, Sartre, and Merleau-Ponty, centers "on analysis of the phenomena which flood man's awareness" (Reese 1980). According to Ihde (1990), a philosopher of technology, "life-world"—our sense of being in the world—is inescapably technologically mediated; there is no human action that is not in one way or another filtered, supported, or extended through technological means. From the very moment our reliable alarm clocks wake us up in the morning until we put our children to bed at night with the reading of a story, a multitude of tools, techniques, and devices have been mobilized.

As I mentioned in my introduction, Ihde (1990) defines technology as any extension of the human senses, cognition, and action. Technology may be used to increase our vision and our ability to measure distance or move around. Under certain conditions technology can even shape all these dimensions of experience at the same time. For example, electromagnetic field measurement devices (dosimeters) may "constitute a form of vision, a way of seeing the space around us in profoundly altered forms, as numerical displays, graphs and plots" (Mitchell and Cambrosio 1997, 251), which may be used, under commercial pressures, to map zones in one's house considered to be potentially unhealthy. Furthermore, as technology can hardly be isolated from what individuals see, feel, think, and do, someone who uses technology can be regarded as a dynamic, technologically mediated entity. For instance, when a person rides a bicycle, she becomes a "biker" (i.e., a person embodied in a technology that provides mobility). The fact that we have coined names to define those human–technology hybrids (e.g., airplane pilot, deer hunter, commuter) is not insignificant. As Merleau-Ponty (1962, 143) says of a situation in which the distinction between the human and the technological blurs experientially:

> The blind man's stick has ceased to be an object for him and is no longer perceived for itself; its point has become an area of sensitivity, extending the scope and active radius of touch and providing a parallel to sight … the position of things is immediately given through the extent of the reach which carries him to it, which comprises, besides the arm's reach, the stick's range of action.

Drawing on Merleau-Ponty, Ihde (1990) suggests that humans relate to technology in two ways. Technology may act as a *transparent mediator* between one's self and the world, enabling a smooth engagement of the individual in a world made accessible by technology. A woman wearing a pair of glasses to read her newspaper, or a surgeon cutting skin with a scalpel may illustrate this type of fluid and empowering interaction (see table 2.2). For Ihde, it is through such technological embodiment that humans experience the world as if technology did not exist. In contrast, technology may also act as an *opaque interference* between one's self and the world, obfuscating the relationships between individuals, technologies, and the world. Such relationships are opaque because both the world and a technology become experiential obstacles calling for interpretation. Driving a

Table 2.3 Two Ways in Which Humans Relate to Technology

Type of relation	Embodiment relation	Hermeneutic relation
Phenomenological structure	[Human-Technology]–World	Human–[Technology-World]
User's experience	A user becomes a technologically mediated entity	Technology disrupts a user's experience of the world
Examples	Bicycle ridden on a smooth road, wheelchair traveling in a friendly environment, well-adjusted glasses, scalpel used in a simple procedure by a skilled surgeon	Subway system in a foreign country, thermometer with an unknown scale, dysfunctional monitoring system
Role of technology in experiencing the life-world	Transparent mediator	Experiential obstacle calling for interpretation

wheelchair in an unfriendly environment or estimating the level of fetal distress through a dysfunctional electronic monitor illustrates this type of awkward and thwarting interaction. Ihde calls such an interaction a hermeneutical relationship because a person no longer directly experiences the world; technology is now visibly and disruptively part of the experience, and this disruption calls for that individual's attention.

As table 2.2 indicates, the ways in which humans experience the world is affected by the knowledge required to handle the situations at hand (e.g., reading a map in a foreign public transit system) and by the context in which technology is used (e.g., the results of a monitoring system that is regularly dysfunctional are interpreted differently by various clinical teams) (Mol 2002). It is important to recognize that these two types of relations can occur both sequentially and simultaneously. For instance, when a person in a wheelchair maneuvers her way from her house onto a bus and thence to a public library, she is likely to experience both embodiment and hermeneutic relations (McKeever et al. 2003). It is also possible to imagine that a particular combination of the characteristics of knowledge and context may lead to a situation wherein the experiential obstacles do not totally disrupt a user's activity. For instance, when installing and using a new version of software, a user will expect that its core functions will remain similar while its new features may appear a little obscure for a short while. This implies that the user is both embodied in a technologically mediated activity and estranged from some of its aspects.

The phenomenological conceptualization of technology does not provide an answer to whether or not technology has agency, but it brings to the fore the experiential texture of the relationships through which technology does something. It can also emphasize the processes through which a "domestication of technology" occurs. Drawing on Serres (2001), for whom domestication involves the "reciprocal breeding of humans and animals" (Lehtonen 2003, 363), Lehtonen suggests that domestication of new technologies "entails a state of becoming affected" and unfolds according to "a learning process whereby things and people reciprocally influence each other" (364). In his qualitative study on the consumption of digital technologies in everyday life, this author observes that

> the technological sphere seems to have an autonomy of its own, and the interviewees feel strongly that they are *subjected* to it. At the same time, they strive to create and maintain a critical distance from it, to retain a degree of control. Their attitude is simultaneously one of enthusiasm and reserve. On the one hand, the informants express interests in seeing new devices and trying them out and they eagerly show competence in being able to recognize novelties. One the other hand, they see waiting as a rational—even virtuous—way of behaving. Moreover, virtue has to do with responsibility, the ability to control oneself and to resist the temptation to purchase new things at whim. (368)

Phenomenological sensitivity also seems particularly useful for analyzing how technology enhances or interferes with the experience of patients, their relatives, and their professional caregivers when health care or health promotion interventions are deployed in various settings. In a recent study (in which I took part) on the use of high-tech home care by acute and chronic patients, we observed that several devices and broader technological systems shaped how patients coped with technology in the context of both their private and their social lives (Lehoux, Saint-Arnaud, and Richard 2004). In accord with this finding, a phenomenological perspective encourages one to conceive of technology as an extension of one's range of potential action, gaze, knowledge, and power; and an enigma, an obstacle, the trigger of an unanticipated accident, and an unknown intermediary between one's self and the world.

Awareness of technology's phenomenological dimension makes it conceptually awkward (if not futile) to try to disentangle whether a technology generates *either* positive *or* negative effects, since it is likely to do both, depending on the knowledge mobilized and the context in which it is used. For instance, medical technologies, after they have been demonstrated to be safe and generally effective, are disseminated across a variety of settings and used by freshly trained practitioners with new categories of patients (McKeever and Coyte 1999). These real-world implementations may lead to more or less optimal treatments because several key variables (especially knowledge and clinical context) are modified along the way. Such modifications may render the use of health technology hermeneutically instable.

To my mind, we need to reconcile these two types of dynamic relations (embodiment and hermeneutical) and conceptually integrate the tenet that technology is simultaneously enabling and constraining, reassuring and threatening, empowering and alienating (Tenner 1996). Anyone familiar with alarm systems can recognize how they create feelings of anxiety alongside feelings of safety. Tenner (1996, 7) goes further and draws attention to the "revenge effect" of an increasing reliance on technology: "The electronic gear that lets people work at home doesn't necessarily free them from the office; urgent network messages and faxes may arrive at all hours, tying them more closely to business than before."

Once combined, medical expertise and health technology often create as many certainties as uncertainties by constituting knowledge that amounts to a probabilistic interpretation of disease prognosis (Lock et al. 2000). Thus, a dualistic interpretation of what technologies do may be helpful in more globally valuing innovations and critically examining what they are supposed to do for us. Figure 2.1 offers a crude overview of the various perceptions and actions health technology may mediate in the context of routinized health care practices. I have introduced an intentionally incomplete list of verbs that reflect the dualistic nature of what technologies do. Encompassing those actions I have also provided broad spheres of ontology and praxis that pinpoint the specificities of health technology. Such a schematic rendering is a first step toward integrating into my analysis the normative dimensions that are both parts and extensions of health innovations.

Most important, figure 2.1 brings to the fore the principle that technology is not neutral; rather, technology acts on, transforms, modifies, and reinforces human perceptions and actions. For instance, it is pivotal in the very act of defining what is life and what is death. Kaufman (2003, 2250), who has studied the technologically produced border zone between life and death in palliative care units for comatose patients, remarks that "the various kinds of *uncommon personhoods* residing in hidden medical spaces and the ongoing anxieties and debates they elicit invite us to consider the proposition that we may never understand certain states of being or how

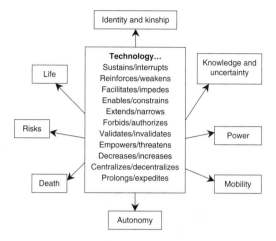

Fig. 2.1 The dual performative potential of health technologies

best to respond to them." Indeed, although major efforts have been invested in defining objective, technologically measured criteria for deciding whether (brain) death has occurred, upon closer examination conflicting knowledge claims seem to be at play in the daily activities of medical specialists, nurses, and family members surrounding these patients.

The use of health technologies also modifies individual and collective identities. For instance, genetic technologies are transforming the current definition of inheritance and kinship, which goes well beyond the individual to encompass past and future family members (Shostak 2003). Similarly, studies in the sociology of illness and disability have revealed the extent to which chronic patients and disabled persons may struggle in redefining their identities, overcoming social and material barriers that constrain their mobility and finding creative solutions to enhance their autonomy (Lawton and Gabe 2003). For example, refusing the medicalized definition of deafness as a "disease to be fixed," several associations for the deaf across western Europe protested vigorously against the use of cochlear implants (an implantable device initially used to restore some auditory function in late-deafened adults) in young children (Blume 1997). Some in the deaf community perceived the promotion of these devices as a form of eugenics by societies that could not understand cultural minorities who rely on, and express themselves through, their own means of communication. Adding another twist to the narrative is the fact that a deaf person who uses a cochlear implant may decide to switch it off if she wants to withdraw from the hearing world and, instead, communicate in sign language with other members of the deaf community. Thus, beyond a categorical definition of the sense of self, individuals may prefer to use technology in a way that fits, momentarily or for longer periods, with their multiple, localized identities.

More broadly, health technology is central to organizing, coordinating, and locating health care trajectories. As a result, technology contributes to shaping the temporal and spatial dimensions that underlie health care practices. For instance, the results of screening and diagnostic tests and the availability of various treatments often put "patients on a diagnostic and treatment trajectory from which they have difficulty extricating themselves" (Mechanic 2002, 464). Dialysis presents a vivid example of this situation. The cleansing of blood through hospital-based dialysis imposes a particular time–space grid (treatments can last for up to four hours, three times a week, for the rest of a dialysis patient's life) to which patients may more or less strictly adhere, but which clearly is not optional (unless one accepts facing almost certain death as an option). This temporal and physical constraint explains why certain patients prefer nocturnal, at-home peritoneal dialysis—it frees up their time during the day and may facilitate keeping a full-time job (Lehoux, Saint-Arnaud, and Richard 2004).

As this phenomenologically inflected discussion has illustrated, adding verbs to health technology introduces the *dualistic performative* dimension of medical innovations into the analysis. At the same time, it keeps the social and technical entities together by foregrounding what one does with/to the other. As I will show in chapter 4, keeping them together increases analytical acuity when one asks for whom and in what conditions an innovation should or does prove better. A phenomenological sensitivity toward the everyday use of health technology also enables articulating the significance of *possessing* knowledge about health technology's deployment that the most common types of health technologies bring to the division of clinical tasks.

Redistribution of Skills and Knowledge Among Technologies and Humans

In the introduction I alluded briefly to the notion that throughout history, innovations have had an impact on work, often leading to a deskilling of occupational groups by replacing humans or rendering some of their skills obsolete. I also emphasized that health care represents a special case in this regard because of the expertise-based hierarchy that prevails and the ensuing power relations—enforced through, among other things, professional corporations—over who is (or is not) allowed to perform certain tasks (Freidson 1975). Furthermore, medical specialization has been fostered mainly through the development of powerful and sophisticated technologies that do not strictly replace humans; rather, they often magnify and extend the role of the expertise people embody. For example, since World War I radiology has thrived as a specialty through the emergence of various imaging devices that have advanced the art of radiologists' diagnostic abilities (Blume 1992). The emergence of interventional radiology, which in some cases infringes on the clinical territories of other medical specialties, also benefited from the development of new technologies (e.g., angiography).

Instead of examining them in isolation, it is thus more accurate to explore the reciprocal relationship between medical innovations and clinical expertise. According to Abbott (1988), who produced seminal work in the area of the sociology of professions, maintaining control over the abstract, noncommodifiable knowledge required to perform tasks is key to maintaining a professional group's authority over its work jurisdiction (see figure 2.2.). For Abbott, the "system of professions" is an ecology wherein various existing and emerging groups compete to defend or redraw epistemological and praxis boundaries around their work tasks. In this process, developing new tools that cannot be appropriated by other groups and delegating "procedural" tasks to subordinate groups are strategic moves. Extending Abbott's analysis, medicine can be seen as maintaining its dominant status by constantly developing new knowledge and technologies that render physicians essential, while other health care providers (e.g., nurses, occupational therapists, nutritionists, social workers) are generally relegated to the role of highly skilled "technicians." Abbott's thesis may also help to explain why many nurses (especially in Canada) are vigorously engaged in researching and theorizing why "caregiving" is a pivotal and unique expertise-based skill (Witz 1992).

This general overarching trend that shapes technology-intensive medical care and professional epistemological turf battles can also be examined at a micro level; for instance, during the design and implementation of innovations and new health care delivery models (Prout 1996). Earlier in this chapter I stressed that the development of sociotechnical networks requires distributing skills, tasks, and knowledge among human and technical entities. This distribution process implies defining which tasks can be delegated to a machine and/or to a human, as well as what knowledge and skills a user will or will not have to master to operate the device safely and effectively.

Of course, not all tasks can be delegated to a machine, or at least not entirely. According to Collins and Kush (1998, 119), there are three kinds of machines: *proxies* that "can replace us by doing what we already

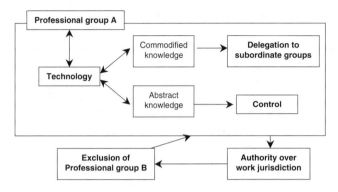

Fig. 2.2 Technology in the evolution of knowledge-based health care professions[5,6]

do" (e.g., thermostat, calculator); *tools* that "can amplify our ability to do what we can already do" (e.g., hammer, word processor); and *novelties* that "do types of things that we could never do without them" (e.g., bridge, freezer, laser). *Proxies* include, for example, health technologies that are designed to reduce the tedious (e.g., cognitive, physical, clerical) tasks that are performed by physicians, nurses, or lab technicians. In the early 1980s, computerized medical records were strongly promoted, backed by the claim that they would reduce the need for clerical staff (and cut personnel costs). Empirical research later showed that "paperless" clinical records came at a high price (if they came at all), creating in turn the need for staff specialized in the management and use of information technology (IT) (Berg 1997; Sicotte et al. 1998). The introduction of proxies may henceforth merely translate into a shift in human resources, not a direct substitution. Medical innovations that fall under the *tools* and *novelties* categories are those that generally trigger scientific and professional controversy. In the case of tools, the levels of skill and knowledge their users possess are key variables in the quality, safety, and effectiveness of health care. The feasibility and effectiveness of novelties must first be clinically tested and researched.

The type of delegation made possible by these three types of machines is intimately associated with knowledge. It is widely known that health technologies may, in certain situations, replace humans, be they professional or lay users. Most of the time, however, people will use health technologies to perform a number of tasks, including gathering the pathophysiological information needed to create medical knowledge (Mol 2002). Some knowledge, however, is *embodied* in a given health technology, not produced by it. Consider, for instance, a monitoring system that records, graphically represents, and sets out various actions (e.g., alarm system, feedback to a call center), depending on decisional algorithms that clinicians and biophysicists have previously defined. All automation mechanisms reflect the embodiment of such codified knowledge (Vicente 2003). Knowledge that cannot be codified usually is expertise or experiential knowledge embodied in humans (e.g., localized, practice-based, and vernacular forms of knowing).

Over time, relationships between knowledge, technologies, and users change and the type of delegation may be deeply transformed. One might consider, for example, childbirth. Although there are sharp variations among different countries and cultures, the role of midwives and their ability to use technologies and health care resources has often fueled significant debate. Looking at the history of this occupational group, Daly and Willis (1989) observed that the use of forceps by midwives in the early 1900s was strongly opposed by obstetricians. Interestingly, the most persuasive claims that midwives are currently forging in Canada relate to the *avoidance* of technology, the nonmedicalization of a *natural* life event, and the superiority of holistic and woman-centered care. Unpacking such claims reveals that midwifery is fashioning another globalizing technology around its work, one that requires pregnant women to adhere to a different, nonmedical, yet pervasive ideology of what constitutes a *good* birth (Armstrong 1983; see also Sullivan 2003). As another example, Remennick and Shtarkshall (1997) observe that for physicians who had been trained in the former Soviet Union and then had emigrated to Israel, mastery of technology became a contentious issue. For these physicians, "the attitude often expressed was that the advantage of Israeli medicine is mainly instrumental, while some important clinical skills 'have deteriorated' as a result of physicians' dependence on modern technology" (197). The deficiencies of Soviet physicians were perceived as situational, superficial, and improvable by training, while "the drawbacks of Israelis were seen as something more essential," related to a fragmentation of the classical body of clinical skills (197). As these two examples attest, fully understanding the processes by which technology generates deskilling and reskilling necessitates examining the knowledge claims and persuasiveness of its professional users. Once tools and novelties in health care have been intimately coupled with a defined set of expertise and skills, it may become increasingly difficult to renegotiate the established distribution of knowledge, skills, and tasks.

Figure 2.3 illustrates three types of delegation that can occur in health care practices. Each requires that a knowledge component be possessed by an already trained user, acquired by a less trained or lay user, or automated in a new technology. This figure also introduces two concepts that

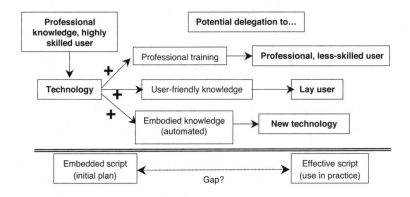

Fig. 2.3 Delegation of skills and knowledge in order to perform tasks

emphasize the tensions involved in negotiating and establishing a new delegation of tasks and skills (i.e., a script) when health care delivery models or technologies are being designed and implemented. A script is a type of scenario that defines how an innovation should be deployed and used (Akrich 1994). The term "script" is useful because such a scenario does not simply involve an abstract theoretical plan, but relies on tangible, technical, and procedural components that orient and/or forbid action. For instance, rules of access to a patient medical record system grant various categories of providers and clerical staff different possibilities of accessing and modifying clinical and administrative data. This is an *embedded* script; that is, one that conforms to the initial definition of how an innovation is supposed to work. It is therefore closely linked to the views and hypotheses of its engineers, promoters, and implementers (Kling 1991; Lehoux et al. 1999).

An *effective* script defines the way users employ a new device, how they reorganize their tasks and routines, or how they circumvent the embedded script (Akrich 1994). For instance, a study in which I took part found that nurses and physicians were creative in finding ways to bypass the established rules of access to a computerized medical records system that was seen as too cumbersome or time-consuming (e.g., by sliding in a personal ID card, by keying in a password) (Lehoux et al. 1999). In addition, the bedside terminal that was initially perceived as enabling a close contact between nurses and their patients was rarely used to enter data. Instead, nurses preferred their old, yet comparatively more efficient, routine of gathering all the clinical information in a notebook during their rounds, and then taking time later to sit down, sip coffee, and fill out all their patients' charts at once. These nurses reallocated their tasks and time in a manner that made sense to them but that was not seen as an option by the system designers. As a result, the objective of recording and accessing "real-time" data was not entirely achieved.

When an embedded script is difficult to outsmart, however, users may have to adopt new routines that may be at odds with how they perceive their roles or identities, resulting in a sense of alienation or passive acceptance (Prasad 1993). In chapter 3, I explore more deeply the implications of the gap between embedded and effective scripts and how it results from a more or less tacit strategy to change clinical practice and behavior *through* new technology.

The professional tensions I touched upon above are as much political as they are epistemological/clinical (Knorr Cetina 1999). That is to say, if clear rules need to be drawn up in formal medical/legal frameworks, and therefore into technology design, it is also true that interpretatively flexible rules are often enacted in local contexts. Indeed, several studies (Berg 1997; Dodier 1995; Fagerhaugh et al. 1986; Mol and Law 1994) have shown the extent to which physicians and nurses are less reluctant to circumvent established rules and to accept practices that, while they deviate from the rules, are seen as legitimate (when quality is maintained) and convenient (when lack of resources is at play). Conversely, the use of certain innovations may be shaped by factors falling well beyond the clinical domain: "Emergency physicians are sensitive to the fact that their treatment decisions may be susceptible to litigation on the part of patients, both for failure to use a medication in cases where there are bad outcomes, and for failure to warn patients of the risks of treatment" (Mather et al. 2004, 57). Hence, in certain contexts, which technologies become strict standards of care "might ultimately have more to do with decisions made in legal courts than with those made in clinical settings" (Mather et al. 2004, 57). Figures 2.2 and 2.3 thus remind us that medical innovations emerge and evolve within a professionally driven context, wherein significant ideological, deontological, and legal tensions accompany the development and diffusion of sociotechnical networks. They also underline the dual role of technology in the creation and commodification of knowledge.

What Do Health Technologies Do for Humans?

In the introduction, I suggested that a critical examination of health technology could not avoid asking fundamental questions about the value of innovations. I challenged the view that assumes that innovation equals progress. Ellis, a technology trends pundit, takes a rather different view of the matter:

> Progress is progress, right? It's what happens when things advance, get better. Not at all. It's a "noxious, culturally embedded, untestable, non-operational, intractable idea that must be replaced if we wish to understand the patterns of history" according to Stephen Jay Gould. Whew! Fortunately, for our sanity, Dr. Gould is expressing no more than his opinion, and it can mercifully be ignored. (Ellis 2000, 251)

Personally, I would choose *not* to ignore Gould, for doing so would involve ignoring a sizable amount of empirical research conducted by applied health researchers as well as social scientists. For these scholars, progress is not always achieved through technology and, if progress is achieved, it is not done exclusively through technology.

One sure thing is that health technology deeply transforms how humans live, struggle, thrive, and die (Brown and Webster 2004)—and all of this happens in the social world of which we are a part (Stengers 1993). By recognizing that humans and technologies are coproduced, STS scholars stress that humans can no longer be seen as solely natural, but only understood in their varying degrees of simultaneously artificial and natural hybridity (Haraway 1991). As Mitchell and Cambrosio (1997, 222) suggest, there is no point in despairingly concluding that humans have been "denatured." Rather, recognizing that a "particular production of nature" is occurring should generate fresh insights into the study of the impact of new and emerging health technologies. The philosopher Melzer, whom I quoted earlier in this book, opines: "Our whole understanding of the 'problem of technology' was itself formulated from the standpoint of man's quest to master all the conditions of his existence" (Melzer, 1993, 318). Getting rid of this quest for control appears intricate.

Any attempt to formulate fundamental questions about the desirability of a medical innovation appears largely doomed to failure, at least if one is looking for a systematic and coherent philosophical approach. My objectives, however, are more modest and pragmatic. I want to find out whether it is possible to avoid falling into the trap of a schizophrenic discourse about the problem of health technology. On the one hand, this discourse embraces the desirability of innovation; on the other hand, it reiterates the need to control costs and therefore restrict access to innovations. Aiming to open up an alternative, more fruitful intellectual path, in this chapter I have laid out an analytical template that draws on the social sciences to unpack what innovations do in order to understand their value. I also have argued that examining technologies without paying attention to the certainties and uncertainties they reveal, and to the skills and knowledge required to use them appropriately, appears fundamentally misleading. Furthermore, several medical innovations are not so much geared to intervene directly in a health problem as they are to seek to produce information about its likely presence and evolution, insight that may contribute primarily to increasing medical knowledge. This very particular effect of health technology poses significant challenges for evaluators (Cohen and Hanft 2004). Could the most tangible outcome of a technology (e.g., positron emission tomography [PET scan], prenatal genetic test) be strictly confined to providing information to patients and contributing to research? And how much of our collective resources should such innovations use up? In the case of genetic tests, consideration of resources also begs the question of who, exactly, will benefit from the information, especially when no treatments are available in the short term. The issue of who benefits is one reason why Shostak stresses the need to reflect further upon the desirability of various foreseeable scenarios that lie ahead: "The introduction of genetic and genomic technologies into the field of public health opens up a range of possible futures that will not be determined by the technologies themselves but by how they and the knowledge they both produce and reify are used" (Shostak 2003, 2329).

Existing technologies, when disseminated broadly across large geographical areas, also raise ethical issues that might not have been anticipated at the outset. A vivid example is given by the use of prenatal screening to facilitate "family balancing" (Malpani et al. 2002) (e.g., the selective abortion of female fetuses). Of course, I am now walking on shaky moral and cross-cultural ground. Who am I to judge whether a government or culture should or should not exert direct control over its population demographics when facing huge economic and political problems? I nonetheless believe that I, as several others should, pursue explorations along such normatively treacherous paths. Otherwise, I might just as well forsake my "intellectual citizenship" (LaCapra 1997) and mind my own business. When technologies are used for equivocal purposes, or when their usage is steered by political and commercial abuse, the desirability of medical innovations requires, to my mind, a pragmatic response. We should not be afraid to create space for dialogues, no matter how demanding and thorny they may be. In chapter 5 I offer some guidance on this issue by summarizing principles and experiences associated with public deliberation and increasing the accountability of policy-making.

In this chapter I have tried to convey a number of thoughts about the potential contribution of social sciences to the policy problem posed by health technology. I have argued for the usefulness of an ethnographic turn in HTA, stressing the meaningfulness of in-depth investigations as well as the importance of conceiving of technologies as pivotal mediators in the construction and reproduction of patient and professional identities and in the organization of health care. I also have underlined the fact that entire generations are now born in a technological society, with significant technological expectations yet with little knowledge about how technology works. In my discussion on the unblack-boxing of technology, I have suggested that in the early phases of design, "interpretive flexibility" (Pinch and Bijker 1987) around innovations may reinforce the privileges of the groups that possess authority over those stages and that are in a better position to bring controversies to a close (Latour 1989). Further, the use of technology becomes an "obligatory passage point" (Latour 1989) only when economic, social, and political arguments are perceived as persuasive and when a particular innovative path converges with various groups' interests. I have stressed the insights one may gain by considering that patients, health care providers, and health technologies are mutually coproduced and that this coproduction regularly challenges the definition of patients' health and well-being (Oudshoorn and Pinch 2003).

It is possible at this stage that readers may feel that in the STS conceptualization, innovations that are supposed to be *better* may simply be conceived of as *different*; in other words, they generate a set of advantages and disadvantages not necessarily superior to previous options. However, as I suggest in chapter 4, health care is comprised of competing and conflicting objectives, not all of which are worth pursuing. The next chapter picks up on these questions by reflecting on what humans want from technologies. That consideration sets the stage for an examination of the normative dimensions of health technology, which become more apparent when considering the gap between what health technologies are supposed to be doing—their embedded scripts—and what they actually do—their effective scripts (Lehoux et al. 1999). As I ask (and begin to answer) in chapter 3, how much of that change is welcome? And by whom?

CHAPTER 3

What Do Humans Want and for Whom?

A Sociopolitical Understanding of Health Technology Design and Use

Man is a creation of desire, not a creation of need.

—Gaston Bachelard

In the preceding chapter I introduced several key concepts from science and technology studies (STS) and other social science fields of inquiry that can help to clarify how health technology transforms and affects health care practices. I highlighted the various ways in which technology becomes active in, and part of, the social fabric that constitutes everyday life in health care settings. My discussion also stressed the need to examine the distribution of knowledge, skills, and duties involved in health technology's use, suggesting that this distribution relies on a normative understanding of what physicians, nurses, and patients (and their friends and families) can and should do with and through technology. Finally, I introduced the idea that the desirability of health technologies lies in what they disclose, perform, help bring about, or settle, and I argued that most of these actions have both positive and (unavoidable) negative effects.

In this chapter I explore the extent to which the things technologies do are consistent with what humans expect from them. In order to distill such a broad issue to a manageable size, I examine several independent bodies of literature, switching between health research and technology design perspectives. I begin by clarifying the role of various categories of humans in health technology design, dissemination, and use (e.g., designers, manufacturers, clinicians, patients' advocates, policy-makers, managers). To accomplish this, I ask "who" wants something out of technology? Answering this deceptively simple question enables me to expand on a key point raised in the introduction to this book: technology embodies values as well as intentions (Brown and Webster 2004). Expanding on that insight, I also stress the need to clarify *whose* values and intentions are reflected and encapsulated in various technologies. Relying on the work of political scientists, ethicists, and sociologists, I then explore the relationships between desires, wants, needs, intentions, and values. Following that, I review the literature relevant to the theory and principles of design, emphasizing the goals of "responsible" or appropriate design and the role of users in the design process. This review is intended, in part, to refocus our attention on the way designers both explicitly and implicitly define how innovations in health care can constitute an improvement and lead to progress. Finally, I return to the perspective of health researchers to ask whether designers' definitions are compatible with those of providers and patients, and whether they further the objectives of various health care systems.

These interconnected pathways of inquiry will, I hope, deepen understanding of what humans want from technology by highlighting that, while some groups obviously want things for themselves, they also often desire things *for others*. Indeed, technology is often a vehicle for shaping others' perceptions, needs, values, and practices. Examining the processes by which certain groups can exert influence on what individuals and other groups will or might want, and will or might have access to, can help illuminate the social and political specificities of health technology. In particular, such an exploration should make more explicit why the question of health technology's affordability is deceiving unless one unpacks the way its desirability is enacted.

Who Wants Something Out of Health Technology?

The answer to this question is not as straightforward as it might at first seem. In health care, technological advances are often viewed as intrinsically beneficial and, therefore, as not requiring an explanation of the motives that have led to their existence or the reasons that have rendered their use desirable. The question "Who wants something out of health technology?" could, according to this interpretation, be discarded as too obvious because the answer is "everyone!"

In this chapter I try to show that not everyone expects the same thing out of technology, not everyone can satisfactorily voice her concern in the design process, and not everyone's wishes can be and are fulfilled by those who design health care innovations. In addition, by creating technology in particular ways, designers and the organizations for which they work impose and encourage certain behaviors upon/by others (Garrety and Badham 2004). As a consequence, technology acts normatively on health care systems, clinicians' practices, and patients' lives (Murray et al. 2003). This normative drive, Grunwald (2004, 177) argues, must be called into question:

> The idea of shaping technology … is inherently correlated with normativity. If one wants to shape technology, one of the inevitable questions coming up is: To which ends and objectives should technology be shaped? What are the goals to be approached by technology, and how can we organize the processes to determine those goals?

Given these multiple considerations, it is clear that determining "who" wants something out of health technology is far from a benign activity. Trying to answer the question, however, underscores the sociopolitical dynamics that contribute to making certain innovations more likely to come into existence than others.

At the outset, it should be acknowledged that design is an intentional endeavor, one that seeks to articulate means and ends as well as to give shape to interventions in the world (Gauthier 1999). The conception of any intervention starts with the assumption that the current ways of doing things are neither optimal nor satisfactory. The first step in design usually involves "problem-setting" (i.e., defining the problematic situation at hand that requires improvement). New interventions are thus, by definition, normative, because they bring together various means to correct, improve, or support *better* practices and actions. Articulating a problem accurately may call for a large spectrum of knowledge, including not only technical understanding of the properties of the technological means to be employed, but also practical awareness about those who will use the eventual problem-solving innovation in order to perform certain tasks (Bucciarelli 1994). Acquiring and articulating these various bodies of knowledge requires, among other things, decoding and reinterpreting intentions: What do users want? How can this new tool fulfill their wishes? Because a perfect translation between wants and technical performance is rarely realized (at least unambiguously), intentions, desires, needs, aims, and expectations are all subject to negotiation.

In this chapter, therefore, I devote several sections to clarifying what designers are aiming at when they develop new technologies. I also spend considerable time defining how users might intervene in the design process. As I show, any design process evolves according to numerous decisions, some of which are largely technologically constrained while others are fundamentally value laden. Each decision pushes the design process in a certain direction, one that may ultimately prove more or less in tune with initial explicit intentions. Before examining further what normative decisions the design of health technology may entail, however, I need to clarify where those values come from and who, exactly, may express or dictate them.

Figure 3.1 posits "designers" as the central group of actors through whom society's desires and expectations about health care are translated into concrete technologies that users can apply. Of course, the three categories—society, designers, and users—must be unpacked and more clearly defined, since this figure obscures the many different subcategories of people who intervene directly or indirectly in the design process. The "society" box appears in this figure to remind us that although technology design involves micro-level social processes aimed at problem-solving, it is also shaped by broader societal trends, opportunities, and perceived needs. These broader trends are influenced by the changing demographics, economics, and politics prevalent in jurisdictions that develop and consume health technology. However, these societal trends do not act as discrete, deterministic forces. Rather, they are partially constructed and interpreted by various experts (e.g., market analysts, economists, political scientists, scientists) and acted upon by people who have an interest in the marketing of health technology (e.g., shareholders, policy-makers, patient groups, physicians). Through their actions, these two groups forcefully contribute

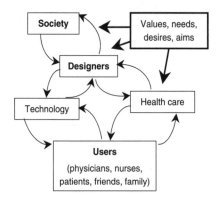

Fig. 3.1 The social and normative embeddedness of health technology design

to making these trends "real" (Blume 1992). For instance, the growing elderly population, which is thought to be more educated and wealthier than parallel cohorts in previous generations, has been shaped over the past two or three decades into a sizable market for health technology (e.g., home monitoring, alert systems, new drugs). Accordingly, the desires, values, and expectations of this demographic group have contributed to the evolution of existing health technologies and the creation of new ones. The fact that this group is well represented in decision-making bodies and institutions that shape research and development (R&D) and health policies, may have facilitated this process.

Technology designers are influenced by these societal changes. In figure 3.1, the "Designers" box represents the expansive array of people who intervene more directly in the emergence of a given innovation (e.g., engineers, physicists, biochemists, technicians, chief executive officers [CEOs], shareholders, marketing specialists). Such people may interact with scientists in public institutions such as universities, research centers, and laboratories in order to derive concrete applications from new knowledge; most, however, operate in private firms (Bucciarelli 1994). Some of their staff members (mainly representatives) will also interact frequently with clinicians, which may help them to understand the constraints under which clinical work is performed and some of this cohort's values and needs. Furthermore, a number of companies that develop health technology hire clinical staff to consolidate their internal knowledge about health care. Nevertheless, the extent to which health technology designers are perceived as being truly knowledgeable about health care practices is a matter of considerable debate. The potential gap between designers' and users' worldviews and perceptions of health care is even more salient in countries that have a publicly funded health care system. Telemedicine projects that have been driven by strong private incentives, for example, have not been well received in hospitals, which traditionally envision health care as a public good. In other words, the values that drive health care delivery may clash with ones that are operative in the private-sector enterprises that create health technology.

Finally, the "Users" box is also heterogeneous, comprising clinical experts such as physicians and nurses, but also lay users such as patients and their friends and families. Indeed, in the case of ambulatory and home care, patients are increasingly being asked to become more active users of health technology (Kaye and Davitt 1995; Coyte and Young 1997). Private companies are also resorting more often to direct-to-consumer marketing strategies in order to convince large patient groups to acquire and use health technologies that are sold in community pharmacies or via the

Internet (e.g., hypertension monitoring, glucose meters, paternity tests). During the R&D process, these firms may run a few focus groups with patients (or employees acting as proxies) in order to map their perceptions and needs and to fine-tune their marketing strategies (Akrich 1994). Meeting physicians' and nurses' expectations and needs also requires that elaborate mechanisms be woven into the R&D process (e.g., advisory committees, prototype testing, preclinical trials). Sometimes clinicians themselves come up with an innovative idea and seek out partners to develop and manufacture a new device. In this case, a clinician possesses specialized knowledge required to develop an innovation that should meet its users' needs and expectations. Later on in this chapter, however, I explore the reality that for each prospective innovation it still remains to be determined how many users must be consulted in order to know exactly what the "average" user's needs are.

As I have outlined in this section, health technology design is an intentional process that lies at the confluence of public and private sectors' value-laden endeavors. It involves articulating needs and expectations regarding appropriate and useful interventions in health care and agreeing on compromises that are able to rally a large and heterogeneous group of actors who have various, sometimes competing, stakes. Therefore, no technological innovation can be seen as an unproblematic response to a demand, let alone a given (health) need. In order to better understand the role of health technology in health care systems, it is necessary to explore the full spectrum of the normative issues embodied in innovations.

A Note About Needs, Values, Desires, and Intentions, and How They Become Part of Health Technology

Notwithstanding the pervasiveness of the broader institutional and market structures I sketched above, every industrial designer is trained to identify users' needs and to conceive of a technical solution that can meet those needs as smoothly and closely as possible. Along that creative problem-solving path and through work experience, designers often realize that needs are far from discrete entities. Rather, they are usually enmeshed with perceptions, desires, and values, as well as influenced by other technologies. As Siu (2003, 73) notes, "Even users themselves often do not know how to articulate their dynamic, temporal, and subjective feelings on a designed object, and the needs, hopes, and fantasies of their everyday lives." In addition, the need for a technology is constructed over time and through social and cultural practices.[1] In this regard, "defining a 'need' refers to a practical process that continues all through a technology's career in use" (Lehtonen 2003, 371).

Market opportunities and constraints likewise significantly shape the types of solutions designed, which may or may not fulfill all identified needs. It is misleading, therefore, to assume that health technologies are created mainly to fulfill explicit needs. I prefer to see them as social vehicles of values, aspirations, desires, and intentions. What renders discussion about the desirability and value of health technology (i.e., the reasons people want it) more sensitive compared with discussions about the desirability and value of other industrial design products is the relationship with health. Before exploring how values and desires become part of health technology, however, a brief overview of the work of bioethicists and political scientists is in order to provide us with general concepts about values specific to health and health care.

"The exact relationship between preferences, principles and values is the object of intensive discussion in parts of the philosophical literature" (Hasman 2003, 43). According to Hasman, the tendency is for economists to examine preferences, for political scientists to consider political incentives and public opinion, and for ethicists to explore principles and values. Despite this disciplinary variation, a large range of researchers, practitioners, and policy-makers commonly refer and have recourse to values. As Giacomini et al. (2004, 16) show, the appeal to values has been pervasive in Canadian health policy reforms of the past few decades: "Most policy analysts would agree that values influence policy goals, decisions, and conduct," and ideologies, interests, principles, and goals "figure prominently in explanatory models of the health policy making process." However, when examining up to thirty-six major policy documents published between 1990 and 1999, these researchers concluded that "health reformers do not share a precise or consistent understanding of what values are" (19). Values, they found, were not explicitly defined or always justified as more or less important in relation to one another. For instance, policy-makers assumed that all Canadians shared a belief in the fundamental right to universal health services. Other supposed values included health states, equity, access, economic viability, caring, inclusiveness, individual responsibility or rights, pride, dignity, identity, and quality.

Giacomini et al. (2004) also observed the extent to which appealing to values reveals different ontological assumptions about their very nature. They organized the values mentioned in the policy documents under five general ontological categories: (1) goodness (e.g., quality, effectiveness); (2) physical entities (e.g., health system, programs); (3) principles (e.g., efficiency, equity, responsibilities); (4) specific goals (e.g., prevention, access); and (5) attitudes and feelings (e.g., compassion, well-being, respect). This diversity is not in itself problematic. It likely reflects the multidimensionality of a public health care system that revolves around fighting disease and alleviating suffering through technological means and clinical practices viewed as public services that should be universally accessible. Nonetheless, one may still wonder how health technology contributes to, rather than conflicts with, values.

As I mentioned in the introduction, technology has traditionally been conceived of as a neutral entity—only an application and the consequences of that process may (possibly) trigger an ethical dilemma. This view has increasingly come under attack by social scientists and bioethicists. Indeed, a number of bioethicists are now arguing in favor of *empirical ethics research*, a form of inquiry that seeks to transcend time-honored disciplinary divisions. According to Molewijk et al. (2004, 70), the cooperation between bioethicists and social scientists "is traditionally based on the assumption that they are representatives of two *essentially* distinct scientific disciplines, with bioethicists representing the prescriptive sciences, and social scientists the descriptive sciences." In the same vein, Reiter-Theil (2004, 18) points out that ethicists actively avoid committing naturalistic fallacies such as deriving value judgments from facts or concluding an "ought" from an "is." This avoidance explains their reluctance to engage in empirical research. The result, she observes, is "a striking gap or deficit in the epistemological discourse in bioethics or medical ethics: it seems that no reference is made to empirical research, neither at the methodological, nor at the epistemological level" (19).

For Molewijk et al. (2004, 71), there are three different ways of using empirical data in bioethics: (1) applying a moral theory to empirical results in order to evaluate an action or policy (e.g., knowing the consequences in order to judge the appropriateness of someone's behavior); (2) assessing the empirical validity of the assumptions of a moral theory or principle (e.g., examining the cognitive requirements behind informed consent); and (3) generating insights into social practices that help improve moral theory (e.g., reappraising the notion of kinship in the context of new reproductive technologies). In illustration of the third approach, these authors examined the production of an evidence-based decision-support brochure for abdominal aortic aneurysm. They concluded that "different choices in the process of producing and presenting facts appeared to lead to different moral consequences, in particular regarding patient autonomy" (73). For instance, showing in graph form (i.e., giving the distribution curve, not just the mean value) the average life expectancy of patients who have undergone the surgical procedure, instead of just presenting the numbers, may affect the way a reader assesses her own life expectancy as well as the extent to which she feels reassured by the facts presented. Furthermore, the brochure is not a stand-alone tool. As one of the surgeons interviewed in their study stated, "I do not present all risk information as numbers. I manipulate the presentation of the information in the way I assess it. I almost always succeed in convincing the patient. I change the way I present the information if I think that the patient unjustly hesitates with respect to a certain treatment" (83).

Given the reality that information is not as neutral as one may wish, and given that risks may be over- or underestimated by various individuals, a surgeon may want, according to her clinical appraisal, to "correct" the picture for a patient and ensure that she is making the right decision. Nonetheless, the above quotation shows that informed consent is an ethical principle that deserves careful rethinking and improvement if it is ever to achieve its purposes in practice. Molewijk et al. (2004, 87) conclude, "It is likely that actual patient autonomy in the decision-making process is more strongly determined by the implicit normativity in information than by physicians' and patients' conscious and rational moral argumentation with respect to patient autonomy." More generally, they also emphasize how "awareness of the implicit normativity *within* facts and technologies creates a broader scope than traditional empirical research in bioethics and raises interesting theoretical, methodological and normative questions for future empirical research" (70). This statement reflects the perspective I have adopted in this book: technologies are normative devices, and judgments about their desirability must therefore be anchored by a disclosure of their implicit and explicit normativity.

Along the same line of thought, Berg et al. (2001, 79) stress that clinical practice guidelines (CPGs) and cost-effectiveness analyses (CEAs) embody normative issues in two ways: in the implicit and explicit assumptions that are used to develop them (e.g., preferred situations, logical next steps) and in the translations that must be made when a concrete medical situation is represented in a formal model (e.g., cutoff point, number of alternatives and branches, types of costs to include) (79). Creating CPGs and CEAs requires the collaboration of researchers familiar with conducting economic analyses and systematic reviews of randomized controlled trials (RCTs) as well as clinicians familiar with treatment options, patients' characteristics, and probable outcomes.

For Berg et al. (2001), the major problems besetting these tools are the invisibility of the assumptions and norms that are black-boxed into CPGs and CEAs and the fluidity of medical decision-making, which tends to be tailored to individual patients and to evolve over time and events. When interviewing researchers and medical specialists who had collaborated in creating guidelines, Berg et al. observed significant disagreement about the role of costs in clinical decision-making:

> A cardiologist: I want to have a longer and better life for a patient. That should be the starting point, I think, no matter what it costs. … Although you can't set age-limits officially, it constantly happens in practice. So although I might say to you that I always put quality and length of life first, I have become affected by the system that we have to live with, that has been enforced upon us, or that we have accepted. There are constraints that we have to live with. And that you implement in your everyday actions and thoughts. So to answer your question: of course you consider costs, consciously or maybe even subconsciously. I mean, you're not just going to send a 60-year-old for transplantation, because you know that will be turned down. (90)

> A researcher: We only deliver data: if someone has a high blood pressure, of this or this level, then that costs me so much and these are the benefits when you intervene in this way. You decide. Our experience is that 40,000 guilders per gained life year is often drawn as the limit for cost-effectiveness, generally speaking. But we don't make any recommendations about this limit, we're just calculating … that wouldn't be our task, wouldn't it? We only deliver data. (91)

The cardiologist quoted above is quite direct about the implicit rationing that appears to be reinforced through policies and institutional pressures, of which CPGs and CEAs are part. Interestingly, rationing partly contradicts his own ethical stance (not worrying about costs); however, it is also partly compatible with a clinical aim (when maximizing longer and better life, it becomes reasonable not to recommend costly invasive treatments to older patients). Here, then, values are seen to be of different sorts, but they do not entirely negate each other. The quoted researcher, on the other hand, is keen to avoid stepping into value-loaded terrain, leaving such decisions to clinicians and the proper authorities.

The fact that this researcher considers "delivering data" to be a value-free endeavor, however, is more perplexing. To deliver data, one must first identify and select the indicators and outcomes measures that will be relevant to decision-making. This involves translations between the worlds of research and clinical practice. As an example of such translation, Berg et al. (2001) observed that "effectiveness" meant different things for researchers and clinicians. The latter were more inclined to set reasonable, individual objectives for each patient as indicators that treatment had been successful. The former, meanwhile, wanted to obtain a clear-cut value that could be used to determine, across RCTs, whether or not an intervention was, on average, successful. According to Berg et al., these different orientations are not so much linked to the respective values of researchers and clinicians, but rather to the fact that their tools are created for different purposes and under different constraints: "Many of the differences in normative choices we encountered, in fact, resulted not so much from the normative differences between the researchers and the specialists, but were due to the features of the tools they handled, and the pragmatic choices they had to make in doing so" (94).

Priority-setting analysis is another important area of study that has emphasized the role of values in guiding health care decision-making. At the crux of such analysis is the fundamental axiom that choices must be made because not every service is affordable. As Hasman (2003, 42) remarks: "Scarcity is an established structural problem in health care, where demand for services in many cases outstrips resources available for provision." When cast at the societal level, priority-setting has a distinct connotation in the field of bioethics, emphasizing "social justice, fairness, equity, legitimacy and entitlement" (42). These elements refer to ethical principles that invoke a sense of solidarity among citizens. These ethical principles also stipulate that decisions regarding the allocation of scarce resources should be based on fair, transparent, and nondiscriminatory criteria that entitle each and every person with a particular health need to receive appropriate health care services.

There remain intense discussions among bioethicists, clinicians, political scientists, economists, and policy-makers about the framework required to identify, justify, and organize a clear set of priorities. For instance, Martin et al. (2002) conducted a qualitative study on the priority-setting processes of two provincial-level committees—one in cardiac care and the other in cancer care—located in Ontario, Canada. Their objective was to examine the extent to which the "accountability-for-reasonableness" framework developed by Daniels and Sabin (1997, 1998) was meaningful to decision-makers. This framework posits that fairness is achieved when four conditions are satisfied:

Rationales for priority-setting decisions must be publicly accessible (*publicity condition*).

These rationales must be considered by fair-minded people to be relevant to priority-setting in that context (*relevance condition*).

There must be an avenue for appealing these decisions and their rationales (*appeals condition*).

There must be some means, either voluntary or regulatory, of ensuring that the first three conditions are met (*enforcement condition*) (Martin et al. 2002, 280).

By conducting in-depth interviews with twenty-one committee members, Martin et al. (2002) identified eleven specific elements of fairness that either confirmed or expanded the accountability-for-reasonableness framework (see table 3.1). The committee members stressed the procedural aspects (gathering multiple perspectives, reaching consensus, avoiding conflicts of interest, appeals mechanisms) that injected into their deliberations a broad and shared sense of impartiality and fairness. For instance, one member stressed the fairness of the process by highlighting the need to deal up front with potential conflicts of interest:

> It was fair because I think [the chair] did a very good job in making sure pros and cons were brought to the table. Although he is at the forefront of the use of [technology], he was also cautious and he wasn't overzealous in his approach. So I think that the way that he was able to give enough airtime to all of the issues ensured that the process was fair. (284)

Committee members also pinpointed features of their group work (e.g., leadership of the committee chair, transparency, understanding of scientific

Table 3.1 Accountability for Reasonableness and Fairness According to Decision-Makers

Conditions for accountability for reasonableness	Elements of fairness according to decision-makers
Publicity	External transparency
Relevance	Multiple perspectives
	External consultation
	Consensus
	Honesty
	Identification of potential conflicts of interest
Appeals	Appeals mechanisms
Enforcement	Leadership
	Internal transparency
	Understanding
	Opportunity to express views
	Agenda-setting

Source: Martin, Giacomini, and Singer 2002.

issues and of various views, agenda setting) that reinforced the impact of their deliberations and consensuses on priority-setting in the areas of cardiac care and cancer care. Not surprisingly, mastery of scientific content and terminology was seen as a key feature of the deliberations, one that helped ensure consistency from one decision to another:

> I think part of [the chair's] job is to make sure that everybody understands a reasonable amount of the content of the discussion. The specialists can drift off ... it's sometimes important for [the chair] to bring people back a little bit and ensure that the statements made about a specific drug or specific condition are rephrased in terms that everyone understands, and also, but probably more importantly, that they're rephrasing in the same kind of terminology that was used when we discussed the previous drug or the previous condition. (285)

Based on the insights they gathered during the interviews, Martin et al. (2002) concluded that the accountability-for-reasonableness framework was meaningful to those responsible for making decisions and that gathering their views helped enhance it. Nevertheless, such a framework appears slightly less satisfactory when one is interested in judging the fairness of decisions. For Martin et al. (287), "fairness is a goal of priority-setting. It has been recognized that health care institutions wishing to achieve fair priority setting must follow a fair process. Moreover, by focusing explicitly on fair process, health care institutions can enhance public confidence in particular priority setting decisions." This last point is especially significant in light of the belief that public policies should appear legitimate to those who contribute financially to the provision of health care (i.e., citizens as taxpayers), to those for whom public solidarity matters (i.e., citizens as civic members), and to those who may eventually need access to services (i.e., citizens as potential patients). However, an argument for applying this framework still begs the question of whether fair processes lead to fair decisions and outcomes. Further, does a general sense of fairness in a process necessarily equate with fair outcomes? And what happens if several committees formulate conflicting priorities despite having followed fair processes?

Furthermore, although the notions of fairness, social justice and equity have gained increasing recognition in health research, the issue of *whose* values and rationales should underpin the priorities remains controversial. Should patients'? The general public's? Clinical experts'? Patients are often seen as legitimate sources of values and preferences because the health care system is supposed to meet their needs; however, their lack of neutrality on the issue appears problematic to some (Hasman 2003). This is why several critics argue in favor of surveying the general public, a process that could potentially elicit preferences that would encompass a broader spectrum of potential values and needs and inject more reasonableness (i.e., impartiality and consideration of resource scarcity) into priorities (Abelson et al. 2003). Clinicians are also often seen as knowledgeable sources for deriving priorities, although here again their neutrality and ability to think in terms of a societal perspective are questioned (Hasman 2003).

Understanding the respective merits and shortcomings of these views as they pertain to defining the value of health technology is a hugely important endeavor if one wants to fully comprehend the nuances of decision-making in the health care sphere. In what follows, I therefore consider these issues in greater detail and suggest that perhaps we need to rethink how actual clinical decisions are made in practice. I also believe we must recognize that individual, clinical, managerial, economic, commercial, and social perspectives are concurrently active and contribute to forging values and expectations about health technology.

I began chapter 2 with a table summarizing the functions different categories of health technology fulfill, as well as the main assumptions underlying the desirability of those functions (table 2.2). This table emphasizes the variety of reasons why health technologies become part of the normative framework of public health and modern medicine. Their normative stature includes the relationships between technologies as well as the goals and values that are actively pursued and tacitly embodied in health practices and policies (Hasman 2003).

Health technologies are supposed to help meet a diverse range of (valuable) aims. But are they all equal, or are some of them more important than others? Should resources be allocated preferentially to technologies that fulfill the most important needs? Or should every technology be assessed according to its ability to meet its specific aim(s)? Box 3.1 helps to clarify and respond to these salient questions by summarizing the various ways in which health technology contributes to reaching specific goals and enacting certain actions or states of being deemed to be valuable.

Comparing the value of technologies across the main areas of public health (e.g., prevention, cure, end-of-life treatments, occupational health) is certainly a thorny enterprise. Before drawing conclusions, it might help to know the respective budgets allocated to each area. In several health care systems, for instance, a large component of costs is concentrated on end-of-life interventions. Alternatively, we may want to examine the burden of illness across social groups and, according to a principle of

BOX 3.1 GOALS AND VALUES THAT HEALTH TECHNOLOGY HELPS REACH

- Knowing about the absence or presence of a disease and its evolution (e.g., screening and diagnostic tests, imaging devices)
- Surveillance of health behaviors and states (e.g., monitoring systems)
- Intervening in the body or in pathological processes while coping with risks and side effects (e.g., implants, surgery, therapeutic devices, drugs)
- Extension of life duration in the context of possible diminished quality of life (e.g., palliative technologies)
- Risk reduction and protection (e.g., health promotion and prevention, occupational health technologies)
- Autonomy and mobility (e.g., technical aids, home care)
- Access and use of administrative and clinical information; efficiency, and quality assurance (e.g., information technology)

redistributive justice, more fairly redistribute resources or inject new ones. Such issues have been raised by academics in recent decades, and they are increasingly becoming a concern for the public, most vividly during election campaigns (Giacomini et al. 2004; Sang 2004). At the very least, dealing with such issues requires examining current resource allocations, the distribution of the burden of illness (health needs), the relative values of different areas for interventions, and the technologies best suited to alleviate the burden of the sick and improve their quality of life, as well as to prevent injury and disease in the healthy.

Although I cannot offer entirely satisfying short-term recommendations about ways to settle these debates, this book may be able to shed light on the fundamental processes that have paved the way so far. It may also help us to consider how we might more creatively reframe the choices that lie ahead. At this stage, my most important observation is that health technologies embody values and act normatively on health care practices. Needs, desires, values, and intentions all become blurred in the design of health technologies. Accordingly, one may want to exert more influence on the types of technologies that enter the health care system in the first place. In addition, it seems necessary to recognize that current practices are largely shaped by needs, desires, values and intentions that are co-constructed by clinicians and patients (Oudshoorn and Pinch 2003). Normativity shapes the ways physicians define patients' eligibility for treatments, level of potential compliance, tolerance of side effects, lifestyle, ability to benefit from interventions, resistance to pain, and expressions of anxiety and fear (Murray et al. 2003). Patients may also hold values that affect their perceptions of scientific knowledge, handicaps, corporeal interventions, outcomes, quality of life, and costs (Heitman 1998). There are also conflicting theories about health and disease processes that may increase the difficulty of choosing one approach over another (e.g., surgical treatment versus drugs, physical activity versus social support). Thus, by recognizing that both technologies and human practices are normative, we may be in a better position to assess the relative legitimacy of various clinical options. Such assessment will require clarifying whether current norms are individually as well as collectively appropriate, and whether it is possible to avoid normative actions that are undesirable. Before embarking on such a journey, however, I want to explore how technology designers conceive of their role as creators of normative devices. This will offer another lens through which we can examine the ways technology and humans jointly affect the world.

Design Theories: From Technical Fixes to Social Action

Some readers might wonder why I am positioning design as such an important issue, one significant enough to justify devoting several pages to it in a book dealing primarily with the impact of health technology on modern health care systems. As I mentioned briefly in the introduction, my initial academic training in industrial design has shaped the way I examine the entire problem of health technology. But is that sufficient reason to delve into the literature on design theory? In the following pages I hope to prove that it is. To further my scholarly project, I have selected a number of issues from the literature on design theory that I believe hold great promise in helping us to better understand the fact that designers—and everyone else who deals with technology—aim to change society *through* technology.

Industrial design is a fairly recent academic discipline whose emergence is closely linked to the rapid expansion and commercialization, since at least the beginning of the twentieth century, of the capacity to transform natural resources into manufactured goods. When compared with engineering, training in industrial design is less focused on amassing technical skills and more interested in drawing from art history, aesthetics, ergonomics, and the study of human–machine interfaces and human factors (Petre 2004). Industrial designers work in a large range of private and public areas, designing objects as various as domestic appliances, motorcycles, playground equipment, medical devices, safety accessories, and office furniture. Due to growing concerns about pollution, environmental degradation, the overconsumption of fossil fuels, the spread of consumerist culture, and the deskilling of workers by machines and automated systems since the late 1970s, designers of all stripes have had to revisit their core mission. One recurrent criticism continues to be that technology designers are blinded by their quest for "technical fixes," which, some critics contend, they naïvely believe can solve all the environmental, economic, and sociopolitical problems that previous technologies, and a capitalist socioeconomic drive, have created (Cross 2004).

Among other things, advocates of socially responsible design "argue that consumerist market structures provide lucrative incentives for designing the ephemeral, the gimmicky and the superfluous. By catering to economically powerful groups, market-led design practices create ever more products while leaving many basic needs unaddressed" (Nieusma 2004, 21). This is in spite of the recognition—resulting from reflections on technology transfer to Third World countries in the late 1970s—that "developing appropriate technologies require[s] accounting for the needs of others by paying careful attention to the use context of that technology, as well as to local perspectives on the problem to be solved" (13). Similarly, some have pointed to the ironic fact that while industrial societies have grown more diverse, manufactured products and a consumer society have fueled a standardization of objects and, by extension, of users (Cross 2004; Martin 2002). For Tatum (2004, 75), "what is required for the designer is a vigorous awareness that the way the world is put together for them—that is, their *reality*—is by no means objective or unvaryingly shared among sane and rational people. Much of the disciplinary education, certainly in engineering fields, runs contrary to that message, instead reinforcing singular images of reality."

This last point should be expanded upon because it conveys another vital principle. Design involves both problem-setting and problem-solving; therefore, the epistemological standpoint from which one defines the nature of a problem—its scope, roots, and relation to various individuals and groups—is a key departure point in any creative and normative endeavor. In what paradigm (e.g., positivism, constructivism, critical theory) does the understanding of a problem lie? How is knowledge about a problem constituted and gathered? Whose views about a problem are considered? A designer's epistemological stance also influences the scope and nature of the solutions she envisions. For Bucciarelli (1994, 71), and in the eyes of the teams of specialists who contribute to almost any technology-oriented design process, the object of design "is a constructed and contested object in the sense that more than one explanation of its behavior, more than one account, or harder still more than one analysis of its behavior is possible, meaningful." Not surprisingly, the technological solution that will, at the end of a process, be realized is not the only solution that could have been selected. Consider the examples Tatum (2004, 70) provides:

Possibilities for the design of single artifacts are much more open that we ordinarily imagine. A refrigerator designed for use in a traditional setting may, for example, be radically different from one designed for use in a home with its own independent renewable electric power supplies. Variability in electric power availability in the latter case, along with concerns about electricity storage and the higher cost of power from photovoltaic and other renewable sources, may suggest thicker insulation, separate compressors for refrigerator and freezer compartments—even a "built-in" configuration sharing insulation with the building's exterior walls, and moving the condenser (heat-dissipating coils of the refrigerator) outdoors to reduce energy use in winter months when less solar energy is available. The design of machinery to slaughter and prepare chickens for market is likely to be radically different in the small-farm context of "community supported agriculture" than it is in the mass production plans more common today. And the design of a vehicle for local grocery shopping by low-income single parents may not resemble the highway-capable "car" that now is almost the only option available.

In other words, just because most of the objects now surrounding us are familiar and because most of the machines we use in our daily activities fit our environments and habits fairly logically, does not mean they *must* be the way they are.

I am certain that readers who are sensitive to objects and technological systems have already spent some time imagining how various technologies in their lives and homes could be different, or have even created their own tailor-made solutions or tools. The same under-determination toward an end product animates the work of designers and engineers. As Bucciarelli (1994, 187) notes, "the object is not one thing to all participants. Each individual's perspective and interests are rooted in his or her special expertise and responsibilities. Designing is a process of bringing coherence to these perspectives and interests, fixing them in the artifact. Participants work to bring their efforts into harmony through negotiation. "

The lesson for students of health technology is, therefore, that health care systems do not revolve around technological platforms and devices that are the exclusive technical means to deliver, organize, and manage health care services, no matter how widespread and customary their use might be.[2]

Scholars of industrial design know very well that technological solutions are shaped by a variety of socio-political forces and reinforce a wide range of socio-political projects. Starting from this recognition, debates about the ethics of the roles of designers and engineers—debates that still divide these professional groups (Martin 2002)—significantly influence the evolution of industrialized societies. These debates have proven productive in the sense that several important reflections about design's theoretical foundations and socio-political implications have recently been advanced. According to Nieusma (2004, 13), for instance, several "alternative design" communities are currently active, including universal design, participatory design, ecological design, feminist design and socially responsible design. The aim of these new design discourses is to

> understand how unequal power relations are embodied in, and result from, mainstream design practices and products. Alternative design scholars analyze how technologies and other designed artifacts are implicated in larger social problems, such as rampant consumerism, sexism, ecological abuse, lack of user participation and autonomy, and restricted access to built environments, among others.

These alternative design communities have raised important questions about key features of technological innovations, such as diversity (universal design), disagreement (participatory design), uncertainty (ecological design), governing mentalities (feminist design), and agency (socially responsible design).

Universal design theorists go further than merely advocating for adaptations and arrangements that render public buildings accessible to disabled persons. They argue that spaces and objects can be designed to be usable by a broad range of people, whatever the abilities and needs of various sub-groups. However, according to Siu (2003, 65), "quite a large number of designers still expect and believe that they are able to predict users' ways of operating, predetermine users' likes and dislikes, and then produce appropriate designs. ... The most discouraging thing to designers is that users' needs and wants continuously change." Participatory design is a response to such fluctuations, in that it "is a tool for arbitrating disagreement over which objectives to pursue." As Nieusma puts it, "instead of ignoring the fact that conflicting interests underlie many important design decisions, participatory designers attempt to leverage such differences to arrive at outcomes suitable to diverse interests" (2004, 16–17). Meanwhile ecological designers such as Todd are seeking to develop technology that can work *with* environmental forces and incorporate flexibility and biological compatibility (www.oceanarks.org). For instance, natural organisms can be used to process wastewater in a series of "human-designed but self-managing micro-ecosystems" (Nieusma 2004, 18). Feminist designers, for their part, are concerned about gender-based power relations that are reinforced and reproduced through technology, a focus that aligns with Cockburn and Omrod's observation that "'technology is gendered. We collectively gender it, of course; but, in turn, it individually genders us'" (quoted in Nieusma 2004, 20). Various objects we use often (e.g., children's toys, cars, purses and attaché cases, baby strollers) or occasionally (e.g., speaker's podiums that are too high for many women, "tie" microphones, lawn mowers) are made in ways that reinforce power-inflected gendered identities. However, the possibility of designing technologies that would shift or level gender-based power relations remains elusive, mainly because they may not modify the underlying values that created various inequalities in the first place.

A concern with differential power relations might explain why some scholars of industrial design are more ambitious in their quest for socially responsible approaches. According to Gauthier (1999, 40), one of the design field's major difficulties is that it is not "sufficiently oriented toward the elaboration of hypotheses on the usage of objects. At best, such hypotheses sometimes are borrowed from marketing or from ergonomics which, moreover, are not interested in uses per se but rather in the needs and identity of types of users." Design theory requires, for this critic, a more elaborate understanding of what is at play between persons and things. This is in tune with Siu's (2003, 66) observation; "it is the participation of the individual user that gives a design its meaning." In other words, a design has no *real* existence until it is used. In order to comprehend this existential participation, Siu recommends in-depth analysis and observation of users' environments and actions. For Gauthier (1999, 42), meanwhile, socio-political issues should be examined more systematically as "objects entail changes on the social level because they represent a kind of confirmation of the primacy of certain interests or, to use the terms of Boltanski and Thévenot, because they establish the grandeur of different actors." Gauthier's view is deeply rooted in a sociological understanding of the normativity of technologies that emphasizes the social embeddedness of objects:

> Usages are inscribed in specific cultures, in habits, in manners, and in historical traditions. They contribute to the mutual recognition and reconciliation of persons and, thus, to the maintenance of the social bond. Therefore, we consider the object to be a stakeholder of the common good, not because of its value or utility, but by the actions that it serves, materializes, and transmits. (47)

Accordingly, design projects should rely on ethical deliberations that can produce "conditions that are favorable to the universal or common good"

(Gauthier 1999, 41). It is important to break away from the assumption that these conditions reside in the value of certain objects (their performance and effectiveness) because this view tends to cast the design process as an endeavor that pursues, first and foremost, the goal of "valorizing objects in the eyes of individuals" who have a stake in them (Gauthier 1999, 41).

Critical scrutiny of design's ethical dimension is exactly what I have in mind when I stress that the desirability of health technology is often constructed out of the very attempt to decipher its affordability and to rationalize, through health technology assessment (HTA), its dissemination and use. By exploring the literature on design theory, my goal has been to elucidate the creative and normative processes that shape technologies, but that cannot be divorced from the broader socio-political dynamics that permeate the values we attach to technologies and our reasons for wanting them. Accomplishing this goal entails asking and answering several questions: Is the quest for socially responsible design and, by extension, socially responsible health technology, reasonable? Is it feasible? And would such a quest yield better technologies? I concur with Nieusma (2004, 22) that, "given the pervasiveness of consumerist market structures shaping design," it is likely that hoping for alternative practices that "result in more than trivial resistance" *appears* farfetched at best. But when one scrutinizes the types of changes gradually taking place in various societies, one may well conclude that socially responsible design is already happening, even if not at the level and scope, or even in the direction, its theorists would like to see. Changing power relations is, after all, not a straightforward or rapid task.

Recognizing that technologies take part in social struggles is, however, key to a fresh new way of assessing which problems they are supposed to be solving and for whom. For instance, Margolin and Margolin (2002) suggest that designers collaborate with allied health professionals around socially relevant projects in order to work in "institutional frameworks that are somewhat insulated from market priorities" (quoted in Nieusma 2004, 22). Although one could argue that modern health care is certainly not insulated from private interests, it nevertheless does nourish a culture that seeks to increase quality of life, to respond to suffering, and to address social inequalities in health. Finally, I would also ask why, even if socially responsible health technology might at times fall short of its promises, one would *not* support it? As Tatum (2004, 76) notes, "every design serves certain interests, certain objectives, to the relative disadvantage of other real or possible interests and objectives. Ignoring this fact is no less a moral or value-based position than attending to the matter explicitly." Between normatively questionable ignorance and ethically informed restricted power, I prefer the latter.

The Role of Users in Technology Design

Alongside industrialization, an important phenomenon occurred that made designing technology more convoluted: labor specialization. As a result, a vast array of technologies is currently conceived for a wide variety of purposes, which are intimately linked to users' specific tasks and occupational duties (Lock, Young and Cambrosio 2000). According to Norman (1989, 156), "there is a big difference between the expertise required to be a designer and that required to be a user. In their work, designers often become expert with the *device* they are designing. Users are often expert at the *task* they are trying to perform with the device." In health care, such differential specialization often adds to the complexity of a designer's work because she is not an end user of the device and is unfamiliar with the complicated tasks performed by health care providers using the technology. Furthermore,

> design, by its very nature, is an uncertain and creative process. In every design task there is an opportunity for creative work, for venturing into the unknown with a variation untried before, and for challenging a constraint or assumption, pushing to see if it really matters. Uncertainty in one sense allows participants to exercise their creativity. But uncertainty in another sense ensures that there will always be unforeseen outcomes (Bucciarelli 1994, 123).

In addition to that germane uncertainty, how do designers interpret and define users' needs? Do patients, physicians, and nurses represent the same type of user? How do designers come to understand a user's practices and relationship with a medical device? And finally, how are patients' needs, tasks, and social/work environments taken into account by designers?

Oudshoorn and Pinch (2003) describe in detail various social science approaches that have shed valuable light on the relationship between designers and users. In what follows, drawing on their analysis I focus on three approaches that have particular relevance to health technology. First, the social construction of technology (SCOT) approach has revisited the role and contribution of social groups and early users in the design phase. Some two decades ago, SCOT theorists rejected the view of users as passive consumers of technology by empirically investigating the role of "relevant social groups" in the emergence and design of innovations (Pinch and Bijker 1987). By relying on historical analyses, the SCOT approach emphasizes how different groups of users can contribute to transforming the meaning of a nascent technology (when still interpretatively flexible) and thereby carve out certain evolutionary paths. Despite an early phase during which innovations are open to the influence of potential users, Pinch and Bijker (1987) have shown that, over time, the shape and purpose of a new technology is more or less stabilized, a situation that leads to a predominant or established use. In the case of medical technology, finding new uses or expanding the types of patients that are clinically eligible for certain treatments may be seen as problematic because of increased utilization and costs (Gelijns and Rosenberg 1994). Although manufacturers and physicians often drive such new uses, some technologies may also acquire an additional meaning through interaction with groups that were not initially seen as main end-users. Ultrasound, for instance, which was initially meant to provide obstetricians with information about fetal development, has now become a way to reinforce bonding between future parents and their babies (Oudshoorn and Pinch 2003). As a result, parents have themselves become technology users.

Who, then, decides who the users of a given technology are (or will be)? And which uses should be deemed legitimate? According to Oudshoorn and Pinch (2003), one limitation of the SCOT approach has been its neglect of groups that do not play a visibly active role in the genesis of technology. This neglect stems from the fact that entrepreneurs and designers do not perceive these groups as relevant. Such situations have lead scholars to insist that vulnerable groups and people indirectly affected by the diffusion of technology be conceptualized as *implicated* actors (Clarke, 1998). This warning seems particularly relevant to health care research, because in that milieu experts are usually those people who hold the authority and power to intervene in technological development and who claim to know what is best for patients and, by extension, society (Rip, Misa and Schot 1995).

The second approach, feminist studies, has taken more seriously the negative consequences of technology on women and the recurrent absence of women as a social group in historical accounts of technological development (Odshoorn and Pinch 2003). In fact, technology was and still is perceived to be largely a male domain (Cockburn 1983). Nevertheless, an important body of feminist literature has examined how technology affects women in the workplace (Wyer 2001). Some feminist studies have also criticized the fact that the consequences of technology on women have frequently been underestimated and that technology has often reinforced gender-based inequalities (Cowan 1983).[3] In addition, several scholars have shown how the introduction of medical technology not only assumes that women's traditional responsibility for familial caregiving and the good health of their children are the result of a "natural inclination," but also increases women's personal and social burdens. Leslie (1989), for instance, exposed how the World Health Organization's policy for improving children's health in developing countries was disconnected from the reality mothers faced because it assumed they could easily reallocate their time and mobilize the necessary resources to apply treatments such as oral rehydration therapy or to seek preventive services such as child growth monitoring. In a similar vein, literature on home care has shown that caring for a technology-dependent child negatively affects a mother's revenue, career, and mobility (McKeever et al. 2003).

Woolgar (1991) paved the way for a third approach, opening up a new set of empirical questions by stressing how the design process entails "configuring" users, that is, shaping and constraining their actions. In an early stage, designers engage in brainstorming and problem-setting activities that involve "defining the identity of putative users, and setting constraints upon their likely future actions" (Woolgar 1991, 59). Although prototypes may be tested with actual users, large companies often ask employees to act as potential users in order to save time and money (Oudshoorn and Pinch 2003). According to Akrich (1995), designers assess users' needs by applying *explicit* techniques based on expertise and qualifications in specific areas (e.g., market studies, tests with limited groups of consumers, feedback from early adopters), and *implicit* techniques based on appraisals made on behalf of users. Akrich's empirical work revealed further that both techniques may be used in tandem: during the design phase, hypothetical scenarios can be developed and representatives of potential users consulted to "validate" whether designers' assumptions about users' needs and ways of interacting with a new technology are probable and whether additional features should be built into it to avoid unwanted behaviors.

In a research on the design and implementation of a computerized medical record system, my colleagues and I observed a telling example of the disconnect that can arise between designers' plans and users' practices (Lehoux, Sicotte and Denis 1999). During the development phase, a major design activity involved defining the level of access to patient data for various groups of professionals (e.g., physicians, nurses, archivists, pharmacists). This activity was carried out by a providers' committee, which formalized rules for data entry and modification that turned out to be at odds with practices established in several clinical wards. As Akrich (1995) notes, sometimes users simply ignore how to fully exploit the technical potential of a new device and, therefore, cannot articulate their "need" for it. In addition, designers rarely, if ever, walk in users' shoes. How, therefore, could they avoid projecting preconceived ideas regarding users' preferences and behaviors? Following the same line of thought, in another study my colleagues and I explored the "theory of use" behind telemedicine (Lehoux

Sicotte Denis et al. 2002). We found that telemedicine falls short of understanding how medical specialists, when they discuss patient cases at a distance, actually appraise the validity of clinical information provided by referring physicians.

Taken as a whole, the social science literature highlights the fact that several different groups play an active role in the emergence of innovations. Designers themselves might even be considered "amateur sociologists" (Callon 1989); that is, people who redesign society according to their vision of the tasks that should be delegated to humans and technologies, and of which economic, political, cultural, and social assumptions should be accepted as convincing claims by shareholders, politicians, tax payers, and other interested parties. Making health technologies desirable thus involves more than merely responding to users' needs. It begs the question of who exactly are the end-users of health technology—clinicians or patients?

Do Clinicians Know What They Want Out of Technology? And Is Such Knowledge Needed?

Asking such questions may to some appear unseemly. Nonetheless, the high-tech health care environment in which we find ourselves, and that seems to be increasingly financially unsustainable, can be seen as the result of physicians' intensifying expectations (beginning in the early 1980s) of the means through which health care services are organized and delivered. As an illustration, Blume's (1992) work on the development of medical imaging devices from the late 1970s to the early 1990s has shown that obtaining a high-quality tri-dimensional image was strongly requested by medical specialists who were not satisfied with having to make sense out of numerical data. While the emergence of computer science facilitated the process, major R&D efforts also had to be redirected to meet these users' expectations.

Physicians are, of course, not the only players involved in health technology design and use. Their specific role, however, must be examined to get a full picture of the role users play in the process of technological innovation. Such analysis is especially important given current constrained fiscal realities. As Chervenak and McCullough (2001, 875) note, physicians are now operating in an increasingly depleted financial environment and "management styles that have been successful in the past, in an era of economic abundance in health care, are at risk of becoming prescriptions for failure today in an era of quality and cost control." Despite economic constraints, Chervenak and McCullough (2001) believe unequivocally that physicians should play a pivotal role in the delivery of medical diagnostic services and treatments. They argue that the "physician as the moral fiduciary of the patient" should be seen as the core concept of medical ethics and should lead to enhanced professionalism in health care organizations. For them, "the physician's ability to meet fiduciary obligations to patients is adversely affected by decisions to ration resources that do not take those fiduciary obligations into account" (Chervenak and McCullough 2001, 876).

Physicians' "moral fiduciary" role relies on four virtues: self-effacement (i.e., clinical judgment must not be affected by differences between physician and patient, such as class, gender, or ethnicity); self-sacrifice (i.e., physicians should accept reasonable risks to their health, income, and job security in meeting patients' needs); compassion (i.e., physicians should be aware of a patient's pain, suffering, and distress, and seek to ameliorate them); and integrity (i.e., physicians should practice according to intellectual, scientific, and moral standards of excellence) (Chervenak and McCullough 2001, 876). These authors also stress four vices that threaten medical practice: unwarranted bias, primacy of self-interest, hard-heartedness, and corruption.

This view of physicians' moral responsibilities is not only too starkly dichotomous to be of any help in clarifying empirically what actually happens in clinical practice, it is also at odds with the numerous social movements that have criticized the paternalistic model that has prevailed in medicine since at least the turn of the twentieth century. Furthermore, many physicians themselves would hardly adhere to such a role. Physicians often invite patients, their family members, and their friends to participate actively in decision-making, and they frequently ask authorities to issue guidelines and policies that provide clear rationales on which to ground their clinical and social duties. Strong evidence of physicians' deep involvement and investment in patient care appeared in a recent multimethod study with physicians in Germany about the ethical challenges they face in caring for dying patients (Reiter-Theil 2004). End-of-life care emerged as a pressing issue for those physicians. The various specialists and generalists surveyed reported having difficulty with the following eight issues: decision-making about foregoing life-sustaining treatment; communicating with the relatives of a dying patient; providing conditions for dying with dignity; informing a patient about an unfavorable diagnosis or prognosis; respecting a patient's wishes; providing adequate pain control; having doctor-patient conversations about dying; and dealing with living wills. When physicians were asked how well they considered themselves prepared to care for dying patients, 50 percent said they felt "insecure," 15 percent replied "not adequately prepared," and only 35 percent claimed they were "adequately prepared" (Reiter-Theil 2004, 23).

When interviewing intensive care nurses and physicians (health care professionals who are generally more sensitive to ethical issues), Reiter-Theil (2004, 26) noted that ethical considerations are a part of their everyday clinical work: "For most of the team members, ethics here seems to be a matter of personal sensitivity, integrity and conscience, rather than knowledge and skills." Intensive care nurses and physicians offered some treatments that they believed, erroneously, were illegal, but nevertheless provided because they were personally convinced that it was the right thing to do (Beck 2002, cited in Reiter-Theil 2004, 26). Reiter-Theil (2004, 25) also observed that these clinicians were often confounding ethical and legal terminology as "they were not able to distinguish reliably between 'passive,' 'indirect' (active) or 'direct active' aid in dying and confounded these with each other as well as with other legally relevant constructs such as 'neglect'." Reiter-Theil (2004, 26) therefore recommends that ethics experts should not simply teach clinicians the "correct" use of the terms; rather, they argue that "ethics, guidelines and law should be informed and further developed from the perspective that terminologies have to serve practical problem-solving—not the other way around."

Extending the analysis beyond what physicians think to include their social interactions with patients, Neves (2004) suggests an anthropological view of the concept of informed consent. For him, "consent is the expression of proximity, communication and interaction" (Neves 2004, 97) and promotes encounters among people:

> It is in that encounter, that can be achieved through dialogue or silence, through gesture or glance, or through some cultural ritual, that each person is recognized in itself, in his/her unique originality (subjectivity), and not considered homogeneously and undifferentiated (objectified) among the others. Therefore, "consent," through the respect for the difference that it testifies, is necessary and effective in maintaining the human character of relationships among individuals in extreme situations of deep vulnerability, to guarantee the ethical nature of those relationships, that is, "a non-violent relationship"—in the words of the philosopher Emmanuel Lévinas.

In light of these ethical considerations, revisiting the role of the physician in the use of health technology should involve articulating that role in the context of clinical work and their various professional and personal support networks. Some of that communication may remain implicit, and will likely always involve a degree of translation back and forth between varying interpretive schemes. In this mutual interpretive process, expectations may be projected onto others, without ever being entirely validated. For instance, in our evaluative research on the design and implementation of "closer-to-patient" satellite and mobile dialysis units in Quebec, Canada, my colleagues and I observed the extent to which several professional and lay claims contributed to the shaping of new dialysis service delivery models (Lehoux Daudelin Pineault et al. 2004). Nephrologists, nurses, managers, medical internists, civil servants, and patients' representatives all voiced their concerns, expectations, desires, and intentions. The fact that some of these claims complemented each other, while others were in conflict, is not in itself surprising. But acknowledging that some claims were made *on behalf* of others, no matter what those other individuals and groups really thought about the issues in question, opens a new avenue to examine why certain innovations emerge. Most nephrologists, for example, strongly approved of having closer-to-patient services. The appropriateness of dialysis itself was not debated: "So, the solution is that patients be dialyzed in their own environment; that's a basic health service" (Nephrologist 2M). For another nephrologist, the service that was currently offered in remote regions—home-based peritoneal dialysis—was second-class:

> Nephrologist 1M: I believe that patients are entitled to [closer-to-home services]. In [region], you know what happened to patients? Well, they were forced to go on home peritoneal dialysis. So they were at a disadvantage right from the start.
>
> Interviewer: Yes. So they were at a disadvantage because … .
>
> Nephrologist 1M: Well, you know, it's not me who said this; it's the patients … .
>
> Interviewer: This is what they are saying?
>
> Nephrologist 1M: This is what they say. And you know, patients who didn't want peritoneal were forced to be on it. I'm not saying that it's not as good, but we live in a free country and it's the patient who chooses after we've given him all the facts. So those patients were at a disadvantage.

Although Nephrologist 1M denied making the claim that home-based peritoneal dialysis was a second-class service, he nonetheless signified that it was not a desirable option by using words such as "forced" and "disadvantage." He also later added that costs and preferences were associated with the decentralization of services: "People want to stay home. When we started dialysis 30 years ago, it cost a lot; improving it has cost a lot; and now regionalizing it costs even more." This observation is interesting because it highlights how dialysis has become increasingly expensive over time, and how it has also come to be viewed as a necessity to which patients are entitled. This last point, however, is controversial among clinicians, as illustrated by a medical internist's view:

> The nephrologist thought it was terrible that their hospital was so poorly equipped while 10-12 patients were treated like pashas in dialysis, and when the indication for some of them appeared doubtful since they would have died three years ago. And they were kept and kept on dialysis … . That's easy to say when it's not you who has to tell them that they're going to die. But we felt that some of them would have died from their conditions if they hadn't had renal failure (Medical Internist 1S).

Here again, defining exactly whose view is expressed is complicated. First, the medical internist referred to "the nephrologist," then used the catch-all "we" after characterizing patients as "pashas" and then evoked the not-yet-dead-patients. To make interpretation even more complicated, I will add another voice. When discussing the issue of treatment cessation, several nephrologists stressed how difficult such a situation is because it involves several people in addition to a patient: "Sometimes it's hard. Families don't want this, and some physicians find it difficult and time-consuming. So we end up doing all of them. But sooner or later relatives understand that it doesn't make sense anymore" (Nephrologist 1M). The desirability of dialysis is therefore also assessed by people who are not direct users and it fluctuates across time.

In our research (Lehoux Daudelin Pineault et al. 2004), we discovered that the idea that, at some point in time, dialysis becomes less meaningful was a recurrent theme. There was also a shared, though tacit, recognition of the fact that dialysis is often inappropriate or of limited use. This widespread awareness was tightly coupled to the fact that there is an ever-growing population of patients, as older and sicker individuals are increasingly offered dialysis on a regular basis. To this point, one medical internist said,

> we now have diabetics on dialysis, plus all the elderly who have renal failure because of advanced kidney-related vascular disease and people over eighty who are waiting for renal transplant. Where are we going to draw the line? That's a social question, but I have a hard time with transplanting the elderly when there are kids going to school hungry (Medical Internist 1S).

In light of these ethical and socio-political quandaries, it would be misleading to assume that all physicians are comfortable acting as patient trustees. Equally misleading would be the idea that they do not struggle with ethical dilemmas and do not care about resource allocation. Although the brief excerpts from the above-mentioned study do not do justice to the great difficulty inherent in determining whether dialysis is a desirable therapy, they do illustrate the fact that several groups' wishes and concerns are (re)interpreted and rationalized into several layers of claims that appear, ultimately, to be deeply enmeshed. Trying to distinguish who says what and on behalf of whom, let alone to ascertain whether the claims made are valid, is extremely challenging.

The design of technological innovations as well as clinical practice involves precisely these sorts of thorny decision-making processes. In order to avoid such messiness, should technology researchers focus strictly on the view that matters most; for instance, that of dialyzed patients? But what about nurses who manage and attend dialysis units on a daily basis? And what about citizens who, through their taxes, pay for life long treatments that seem to know no limits?

Should Patients Be Considered End Users of Health Technology?

To help settle some of the controversies surrounding the merits of health technologies, I would like now to turn attention to the view of the patient. Sullivan (2003) argues that the growing interest in the patient's perspective is the result of convergent trends in health and social science research. There is, indeed, a mounting appreciation among health researchers of the ways patients' values affect their experience of acute and chronic health states (Wensing and Elwyn 2003). Although clinicians are often concerned about patient compliance, they underestimate the individual, social, cultural, and political dimensions at the root of this problem (Pierret 2003). Among other things, medical sociologists have shown that shifting familial and social relationships shape patients' perceptions and coping strategies (Lawton 2003). Some of these strategies may, in addition, run contrary to patient's adoption of the sick role. Lowton and Gabe (2003), for instance, observed that adults with cystic fibrosis who were not expected to live for long found various ways to downplay the importance of their illness and to compare themselves favorably to "normal, healthy" people. Accordingly, Sullivan (2003, 1602) stresses that patient-centered medicine is gradually seeking to integrate the "perceiver of ill health as well as the ill body" into a more complete object of study. But, he cautions, "outcomes research is as yet undecided if [the object of study] will be the patient's health or the patient's life. Each step in this direction brings medicine closer to pursuing 'what really matters to patients' and also brings greater scientific, ethical, and social complexity" (1602).

In order to define the ways health technology matters to patients, we need to address three issues: the extent to which patients must use health technology; designers' and researchers' abilities to determine how patients appraise the value of health technology; and the limitations of resorting to the patient's view as a panacea for improving health care.

First, although physicians usually remain responsible for prescribing them, there are a number of key interventions in which patients can be seen as the end-users of health technology; in particular, screening and diagnostic tests, prescription drugs, high-tech home care, implants, preventive devices and safety equipment, and technical aids. Despite the fact that these interventions may be designed and offered with the best intentions, patients do not always require or even desire them. For instance, with the large number of prenatal tests that are now available and often part of the clinical "routine," many pregnant women are faced with results they may not have asked for and about which they receive little information (Paravic et al. 1999). Drawing on such an awareness, Kenen (1996) examined how "at-risk" labeling is closely associated with the "gift" of knowing, which may not be always welcomed. She concludes that providers' invitation to know, which is offered through various screening and diagnostic technologies, is problematic when the line between prevention and overuse is not clear: "this technologically oriented invitation presented by some health care professionals to their clients is predicated on the belief that knowledge is intrinsically good, enabling clients to make informed decisions. Therefore, the possession of knowledge is equated with empowerment" (Kenen 1996, 1546).

The presumption that technology and its associated epistemic objects are empowering is difficult to ascertain empirically. Scott et al. (2005, 1875) conducted interviews with fifty-eight users of a cancer genetics service in the United Kingdom and found that some participants were less pleased than one might have expected with the "good" news of not being at risk. Conversely, "those who were categorized as "high risk" seemed to be quite content with the way in which the genetics service had configured their status. Indeed, the "fortunate" outcome of receiving a high-risk estimate appeared to create feelings of safety, reassurance and trust in the power of medical knowledge."

Understanding the context in which knowledge, its corresponding labeling, and its accompanying services may not always be empowering to patients, is necessary. Furthermore, the very existence of a particular innovation may not be the direct result of a users' demand. A good example of this is the diffusion of the cochlear implant that has met with unanticipated resistance by associations representing the hearing impaired, an issue I briefly visited in chapter 2. Some argue that medical doctors and technology innovators are imposing on deaf people unacceptable definitions of their "impairment" and why it should be fixed (Blume 1997; Lehoux and Blume 2000). These groups refuse to become "patients" and, therefore, users. Moreover, if users are resolutely a heterogeneous category shaped, in part, by designers, it must be acknowledged that they can also be manipulated by business entrepreneurs. Blume (1997) has shown, for instance, that successful stories of deaf children who received an implant have often been used to gain public acceptance. In addition, when health technologies are moved away from hospitals and into patients' homes, the technical and symbolic characteristics of medical devices become more salient because patients must learn how to operate them safely and confidently.[4] The extent to which patients are voluntary, informed, and supported (or empowered) users of health technology must, therefore, be critically examined.

Second, researching and articulating how patients themselves appraise the relative merits and shortcomings of various health technologies is not an easy task. Some clinical care areas raise major challenges when researchers attempt to gather patients' views (Sinding 2003). For example, after examining seventy patient cases in oncology (where the shift from curative to palliative is fraught with ethical issues), Reiter-Theil (2004, 25) observed that "in more than half of the cases," patients had not been informed of, or involved in the process of end-of-life decision-making. By extension, attempting to define the value of end-of-life treatments for patients requires research methods that are sensitive to patients and their social networks, and that can foster a collaborative partnership with clinicians who care for those patients.

Returning to the dialysis study discussed earlier (Lehoux Daudelin Pineault et al. 2004), my colleagues and I observed that despite marked discontent among the patients, the question of the appropriateness of dialysis was, across all informant groups, rather like a Pandora's box: not to be opened under any circumstances. During interviews, patients overtly referred to other patients who had died and to older and sicker patients who could not hope for a renal transplant. As one patient telling by put it, "it must be depressing for them. … I don't know. I don't know how they deal with it. We don't really talk about it. When you know the person has serious health problems and is going to die, you just don't talk about it" (Patient BS1).[5]

It is difficult to define what a *successful* technological intervention entails when the anticipated outcomes are delayed and not as clear as one might wish. Shedding light on this challenge, Menkes et al. (2005) employed a mixed method design to explore the views of twelve patients who underwent stereotactic radiosurgery (SRS) in New Zealand. SRS is used for treating brain tumors and vascular malformations and it involves a full-day procedure that entails fixing a metal helmet on a patient's head with bone screws and using computerized tomography (with or without angiography) followed by focused irradiation. The authors commented on the long period of uncertainty that follows this imposing procedure:

> Although the SRS procedure represents the endpoint of waiting and journeying for treatment, it only dissects the period of "time out" described by participants. Most return home after this "pilgrimage" understanding that they are still impaired and at risk of further catastrophic ill health, typically from AVM [arteriovenous malformations] bleeds which are still common in the months after SRS. Although anxiously hoping the treatment will prove successful, patients must wait up to three years for this to be confirmed. (2571)

From a methodological standpoint, research on the patient's view also begs the question of how to define the groups whose views are to be investigated. Is it possible to obtain an "average" opinion? And can such a thing even exist? Although some designers may seek to gather the views of potential users during the problem-setting phase, there will always be variation within user groups. When designing a building that was meant to be universally accessible, Luck (2003) observed numerous differences among the views of a range of informants. Among other things, these touched on whether the opinion of a hearing person working with hearing-impaired people be considered significant and on what happens if such an opinion contradicts the views of hearing-impaired people? Reflecting on his experience, Luck (2003, 529) concluded that such variation illustrates "the problem of 'presumptive' designing (assuming knowledge of a user group), and also the fact that people's preferences within a user-group are neither predictable nor constant." Luck (2003, 533) also stressed that beyond the problem of finding the right spokespersons, there is the difficulty of ascertaining to what extent designers and users truly understand each other, as "dialogue and the exchange of concepts between designer and user can be limited by the use of common terminology." This caution certainly also applies to researchers and their informants. Examining the patient's view thus requires a thorough problematization of the variables (e.g., sex, gender, socioeconomic status, physical and mental health) and dynamics that structure a range of informants' perceptions, as well as an understanding of how temporal dimensions may contribute to the evolution of coping strategies and preferences regarding technological interventions.

Finally, it is far from clear that focusing on the patient's view, although a potentially extremely valuable endeavor, can solve all the controversies related to the appropriateness of health care services. Sullivan (2003, 1595) stresses that there is a "radical realignment between the objective and subjective elements of clinical medical science." This realignment poses an epistemological challenge because researchers must examine how patients value their health *in the broader context of their lives.* In my opinion, this brings us closer to an area of enquiry that may not even be legitimate for health researchers: Who are we to examine anyone's attitudes toward their own life? Are the common theoretical and methodological health research frameworks appropriate for dealing with such a topic? I would rather be cautious and emphasize that there are limitations to keep in mind when embarking on a quest to discover the patient's view. Conducting such research in an epistemologically coherent way would require, at the very least, that researchers master the theories and implications of such research (e.g., understanding the biographical construction of the self across a myriad of personal, age-related, cultural and other variables).

That being the case, there remain important lessons to be drawn from researching the patient's views regarding specific aspects of technology-mediated health care. In the dialysis study, my colleagues and I noticed that patients' quality of life was deeply structured by the time-space dimensions imposed by dialysis itself (i.e., being hooked up to the machine for up to four hours, three times a week). For some patients, dialysis was compared to "doing time" in prison. For many, reducing the distance of their trips to the clinic represented a gain, but this gain remained more or less marginal considering the large amount of time spent hooked up to the dialysis machines. Several patients made regular attempts to reduce this duration by 15, 10, or even 5 minutes. One medical internist helped clarify this tactic: "I think they're tired of being here. Every minute counts from the moment they arrive, and they can't tolerate any delays" (Medical Internist 1S). Because of the reduction in time lost traveling from their home to the clinic, only a few patients we encountered were able to engage in new activities and this depended upon whether their treatments were scheduled for the morning or the afternoon. From a patient's perspective, therefore, the quality of dialysis services could have been improved by reorganizing the schedule of those services. Such schedules, however, are usually under enormous organizational constraints because the clinical staff must try to maximize machine use while accommodating physicians' and nurses' varying shifts. On the purely technological side, meanwhile, I could not help wondering why dialysis machines, which have been around since the 1960s and have become increasingly more sophisticated with respect to data monitoring and alarm systems, have not evolved to reflect what appears to matter most to patients.

The patient's view is clearly a relevant angle from which to appraise the value of innovations. Nonetheless, it must be articulated within a framework that can illuminate the clinical experience as a socially enacted practice, and therefore it must include the influence of interactions with clinicians, family members, friends, and other members of society (Lawton 2003). Such a framework should also be sensitive to the technical dimensions of health care and to the processes through which the design and use of health technology reinforces values and intentions that may be neither entirely explicit nor necessarily held by those who are considered to be the original possessors of those values and preferences.

A Few Design Challenges Specific to Health Technology; or, What is User-friendliness?

Three things should be clear by now: patients are neither the only nor primary social group for which technology is designed, patients' perspectives may be ignored or manipulated during the design process, and designers, even if they want to understand and fulfill all the needs of clinicians and patients, may not be able to. Thus, one cannot hope to solve the problem of health technology in modern health care systems solely by emphasizing user-centered design. That being said, it should also be clear that part of the appropriate response to the financial and ethical challenges facing health care lies in the improved design of health technology. In this section, therefore, I discuss in detail how designers seek to make health technology as user-friendly as possible and thereby reduce barriers to its use and improve its safety and effectiveness (Vicente 2003).

According to the *Longman dictionary of the English language* (1984), the term "user-friendly" characterizes an object (often a computer system) as "easy to operate or understand; not needing special training." This term has gained a prominent place in the lexicon of industrialized, English-speaking jurisdictions over the past twenty years.[6] Its prevalence is largely the result of the growth of information technology and research on human computer interface (HCI), along with the recognition of the need to design interfaces that users can rapidly understand. In general, the human-machine interface is seen as key to enabling a smooth fit between users, tasks, and technology (Lun, 1995; Norman, 1989). The principle of user-friendliness thus tries to bridge the current marked gap between the world of designers and the world of users.

The French word that encapsulates best the concept of user-friendliness is *convivialité*. This term's primary meaning (derived from *convive,* a guest sharing a meal) designates positive social interactions and, by extension, hospitable environments. Several decades ago, Illich (1973, 21) distinguished "convivial" tools from "industrial" tools: [7]

> [Convivial tools are] those which give each person who uses them the greatest opportunity to enrich the environment with the fruits of his or her vision. Industrial tools deny this possibility to those who use them and they allow their designers to determine the meaning and expectations of others. Most tools today cannot be used in a convivial fashion.[8]

Interestingly, the idea that technology should generate or sustain users' autonomy seems central in contemporary user-friendly-design discourses. Less clear, however, is the extent to which technology should sustain a collective ethics, and to what extent users' autonomy should concurrently be limited. In effect, by creating technology that generates autonomy, designers will perforce constrain users' behavior and range of action. In their research on voice recognition tools, for instance, Wooffitt and MacDermid (1995) observed that interactive speech systems are designed in a way that confines the range of human behaviors. Due to inherent technical hurdles, a user must behave as much as possible like the system she is using (e.g., speaking slowly and pausing distinctly between words); otherwise, the technology will be ineffective. Turning the issue on its head, technology will prove to be fully user-friendly only if users learn how to be *technology-friendly.*[9] Examining how users become attached to objects (as opposed to strictly examining decisions to adopt or not new digital devices), Lehtonen (2003) suggests that when users put new devices on trial they are testing themselves as well: Can they master a new device's technical components? Can they learn to use it swiftly and effectively? Lehtonen (2003, 377) concludes that "the more actively one is attached to one's technology, the more controlling and restraining—but also potentializing—will be its effects on one's life."

In order to assess the level of user-friendliness of HCIs, Lun (1995) suggest we must pay attention to two components: user acceptance—the extent to which a user favors using a given information technology; and user competence—the abilities required to use it effectively. These two components interact with each other: the more technically complex a technology is, the more elaborate the user training required. Lun also posits three principles for designing user-friendly HCIs: the human-machine interaction is pivotal; this interaction evolves through use; and the user should be the key informant. Methodologically speaking, these principles imply that designers should directly observe how a technology is used, compile users' perspectives, and identify users' learning curves for appropriating the technology.

One may wonder whether the use of HCIs or technologies meant to support leisure activities or work tasks is similar to the use of health technologies, including those that sustain life and on which patients depend. Observers of high-tech home care have already stressed that certain health technologies are, by their very design, *un*friendly (Parent and Anderson 2000). Nevertheless, very little is known about the characteristics that facilitate or impede the use of medical devices and whether health care providers and patients perceive them as user-friendly or not.

The work of scholars who have studied technical aids for the disabled and the elderly brings another dimension to the definition of user-friendliness. If one conceptualizes disability as a social phenomenon, then technical aids' user-friendliness must be gauged with respect to their ability to assist users in moving freely in their social environments (McKeever et al. 2003). From this perspective, autonomy and mobility become pre-eminent considerations, as does the impact of a given technology on users' social identities. Pippin and Fernie (1997) conducted focus groups and interviews with the elderly in order to explore their acceptance of dependence, experience of social stigma, recognition of personal physical loss, appearance of technical aids, autonomy, and perceptions of options. Their work reveals that technology users must cope not only with specific devices but also, more importantly, with the limitations they themselves experience (e.g., architectural barriers, deteriorating physical condition) and with becoming the object of others' gaze as soon as they enter environments outside the private sphere.

Accordingly, user-friendliness must also be understood as a function of the type of settings in which users maneuver and that affect how they succeed in (re)constructing their identities as technology users. Social science research on patients learning how to cope with chronic illnesses and life-sustaining technology has yielded similar results, highlighting the way each patient tends to go through a personal trajectory (Sinding 2003) or to engage in "biographical work" aimed at giving meaning to a constellation of unfolding events (Lawton 2003). The context in which technology is used is likely to alter these identity reconstructions. Although hospitals allow patients to adopt the sick role rather straightforwardly, the home setting may force them to be more active and optimistic (Kaye and Davitt 1995). Family members, friends, and other caregivers may also be affected by the use of health technology. They might, for example, be asked to give technical and moral assistance and, in certain cases, providing assistance implies inflicting pain and discomfort through the application of technology (Kaye and Davitt 1995).

The literature on the use of medical technology and technical aids thus highlights dimensions the HCI literature cannot explore to any great extent. It also shows how a disability or a disease may interfere with a user identifying herself as a technology user. As figure 3.2 shows, health technology's user-friendliness results from a combination of technical (e.g., shape, functionality, complexity) and human (e.g., self-image, autonomy, social stigma) dimensions. This framework posits that technical dimensions will affect user competence and that human dimensions largely influence user acceptance. The user-friendliness of a technology therefore results from a smooth fit between technical and human features, with the fit varying between and within settings and individuals.

Such a framework may help to increase our understanding of how a given technology's design affects both treatment compliance and treatment effectiveness (Vicente 2003). As I have made clear earlier in this chapter, we of course must remember that this framework reveals only part of what happens with the use of health technology because, in practice, a variety of experts and lay individuals contribute to enacting both its desirability and meaningfulness.

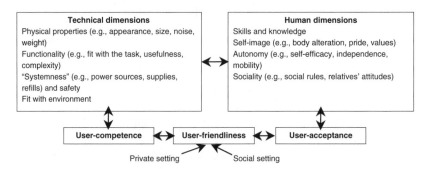

Fig. 3.2 Technical and human dimensions that shape the user-friendliness of health technology
Source: Lehoux 2004, drawing on Lun 1995 and Pippin and Fernie 1997.

Wanting Something for Others Out of Health Technology

In this chapter I have tried to clarify what humans want from health technology. For the sake of achieving a fuller understanding of the issue, I have dealt with this multifaceted question by parsing it into separate concerns: *whose* intentions and values shape the desirability of health technology, *how* the design process gives prominence to certain values and goals, and *for whom* those features are thought to be desirable. It is clear that although socially responsible design attempts to increase technology's appropriateness by emphasizing users' needs, local contexts, and power relations, at least when it comes to health technology it is often difficult to identify needs and expectations (Rip, Misa and Schot 1995). In some cases, physicians and nurses are clearly the main end-users at whom a given technology is targeted, whereas in other cases defining exactly who the users are (e.g., patients, family members, professional caregivers) is difficult. Health technology designers face acute challenges, and user-centered design might represent only a fraction of what socially responsible health technologies could be. It is therefore not surprising that health technology designers do not eagerly embrace en masse the currently emerging design approaches aimed at increasing user participation. Such approaches reduce neither the uncertainty nor the number of options and features that need to be considered—in fact, they do the opposite (Siu 2003). Even more striking is the fact that all the people engaged in the development and use of an innovation want things not only for themselves, but also for others.

These observations can help in the assessment of the desirability of health technology, as they foreground not only the normative dimensions of health technology but also, more significantly, the *relational* character of this normativity. Through design, users of health technology become objects to which culturally imbricated norms adhere. And, depending on the extent to which their views, assumptions, practices, preferences and values are taken into account, challenged or opposed by those who design and implement innovations, health technology users also become participants in that normativity. In the case of substantial innovations, the technological components are very often not the most crucial aspects to which project leaders will pay attention. "Resistance to change," "cultural shifts," or "clinical worldviews" preoccupy project leaders the most. Why? —because through such technology-based projects, managers, and reformers attempt to change *current* practices. They act normatively and, generally, in response to a current normativity that is deemed questionable (e.g., from a clinical, managerial or financial perspective). Hence, when I stress the relational character of technologically mediated normativity, it is in order to make more explicit the links among the actors who are judging what others ought to do and desire and who steer design processes accordingly.

As noted earlier, bioethicists have recently shown interest in exploring further the contribution of empirical research to moral theory. They suggest that empirical research may possess clues about values, the extent to which individuals and groups follow them, and the need to revisit some of the assumptions underlying ethical guidelines and principles (Molewijk et al. 2004). Taking a similar perspective, I argue that the empirical world is made up of technologically mediated ethical prescriptions, some of which may fall comfortably under one's own belief system and some of which may directly clash with one's sense of justice, fairness, or autonomy. When applied to health technology, this argument carries three implications.

First, there is a need to conduct in-depth research on the values, both implicit and explicit, that guide the development and use of technological interventions in health care. As Giacomini et al. (2004, 22) observe, "declared values can be powerful imperatives or toothless platitudes, honestly guiding or strategically misleading. Undeclared values can be either crucial or irrelevant, and in either case, it matters to know." Undeclared values operate profoundly, albeit subtly, on health care practices; we must therefore recognize that health technologies are crucial vehicles for encapsulating and reinforcing normative behaviors on the part of clinicians and patients. These authors (2004, 20) also showed that playing two substantial values against each other "echoes academic views (e.g., from economics, ethics) that consider values as goods that must be weighted against each other in a material world where we 'can't have it all.'" This point needs to be emphasized, as it is the basis for symbolically powerful discourses about health technologies, discourses that regularly pit desires against money.

Second, the scope of the "voices" that are given space in any design project as well as in any health care innovation must be scrutinized. Most obviously, pluralistic societies must be accommodated. More importantly, the range of choices and interventions now offered in modern medicine challenges the assumption that the physician acts as a trustee (a role physicians themselves may be increasingly reluctant to play). As Sang (2004, 187) emphasizes, "there is a growing desire to question whether long established health-care systems are ready and willing to break deep-rooted dependency cultures and open up public and private dialogues about the inherent risks and uncertainties of health-care transactions and interventions." Box 3.2 describes his idea of a modern participatory structure in which five groups each have particular roles to play in setting the health care agenda.

Box 3.2 Groups Likely to Influence Deliberations About Health Care

- *Civic entrepreneurs:* public servants who work as internal change agents and as valued partners with local people and their organizations, fostering an open participatory culture within the system.
- *Social entrepreneurs:* local people who facilitate capacity-building, active citizenship, and engagement in social-democratic, and service innovation.
- *Expert patients:* people with long-term conditions (disabilities and chronic disease, mental and physical) who learn to manage their own health journeys and, in so doing, work in partnership with service teams and services management on services development and improvement.
- *Independent lay advocates:* local citizens and independent practitioners who support marginalized and excluded people in participating in decisions that affect their lives.
- *Community engagement and governance:* independent means of ensuring effective, inclusive local democratic participation in decision-making, a necessary complement to corporate citizenship.

Source: Sang 2004, 188.

According to Sang (2004, 187), the purposes of these five groups vary and include "challenging health inequalities," implementing "continuous services improvement," and supporting "robust, transparent decision-making." It is immediately obvious that the private sector is absent from this scheme (I address this angle in chapter 4). However, what I wish to stress at this stage is the complexity of the institutional arrangements in which various voices relevant to health technology can be articulated. By underscoring the relational nature of technologically mediated normativity, my objective is also to highlight the impossibility of shifting the responsibility of technological interventions to a single group. As the example of the dialysis project showed, several individuals and groups—physicians, patients, relatives, and managers—may conclude that a given intervention is questionable without ever acting upon this shared belief.

The desirability of technology is therefore not only co-constructed by a range of actors; it may also be left intact through a tacit acceptance that it might represent the only available option (Sinding 2003). Understanding this irony is not easy, but we cannot conclude that if a technology were undesirable it would not be used. In other words, tacit acceptance should not be seen as deliberate approval, or, as bioethicists have stressed, we cannot derive an "ought" from an "is." STS and the other streams of social science research that I have summarized offer a theoretical means to challenge the perceived order of things. This type of research "can destabilize the dominant stories and ideologies. By unpacking that which has been simplified or buried, a rich complex empirical understanding of a case develops that enables sustained social and ethical critique" (Williams-Jones and Graham 2003, 290). Overall, increasing opportunities for different groups to deliberate over the value of various health technologies should enhance the clarity of the principles and preferences of those involved in shaping current health care practices, and may identify potential gaps between those practices and normative ideals (Molewijk et al. 2004).

Finally, by addressing the relational character of technologically mediated normativity, it becomes possible to envision new, stimulating approaches. We may, for instance, want to reflect upon the idea of transforming the ways in which health technologies are being designed by modifying, among other things, the perspectives that are brought to the process and by intervening in their articulation with one another (Garrety and Badham 2004). User-centered design does not really change what design entails—arbitrating between various constraints and interests—but it does influence the design process by making those arbitrations more visible and potentially inclusive.

Because the intentions of those who pursue such arbitrations may clash (Garrety and Badham 2004), it begs the question of whether researchers themselves play a role in such micropolitics? Timmermans and Berg (2003) suggest that sociologists need to break through disciplinary boundaries and become involved in the design, production, and implementation of technology, while maintaining a sociological perspective and identity. This multifaceted role would require, among other things, stepping away from the comfortable position of the external (descriptive) observer and critic. In order to avoid "us" telling "them," sociologists would need to cross bridges in language, culture, methods, and notions of evidence (Timmermans and Berg 2003). By and large, clarifying the micropolitics of the groups involved in, or implicated by, an innovation's design, may make it possible to alter its initial normative script: to render it more compatible with the values and intentions associated with meaningful health care practices, ones that operate according to the sense of appropriateness of clinicians and patients and that resonate with the societal principles of prevailing health care systems (an issue to which I return in chapter 5).

In this chapter I have tried to bring clarity to the idea that health technologies can be seen as embodying values and intentions as well as providing impetus for the integration of new ideals. Oscillating between what *is* and what *could be*, as well as between what *is* and what *ought to be*, remain pivotal to any design process, which is as much a creative as a normative undertaking (Bucciarelli 1994). Perhaps along the road to evidence-based medicine and cost-control initiatives we have lost a bit of the creativity required to deal with such challenges and to venture into uncharted ethical and political territories. If that is the case, I believe it is all the more crucial to position health technology as being necessarily embedded in broad socio-political practices that can be examined, called into question, and modified through appropriate policy initiatives and organizational incentives.

CHAPTER 4

Reconciling Competing Objectives

The Regulation of Health Technology

So far, we have seen that clinical, social, political, and ethical considerations shape health technology's development and use. This process is the result of a complex interplay among a number of different actors (e.g., designers, clinicians, patients, patient's family members, managers). We have also seen that values, preferences, and intentions are social constructs that pervade clinical interactions, influence the allocation of health care resources, and are themselves transformed by health technologies. I have argued that clinical practices are embedded in our normative understanding (tacit and explicit) of good health and illness and in the ideals we fashion around them. I have also contended that technology is a vehicle that is used to change or shift current health care practices toward different types of ideals. Finally, I have stressed that norms are relational, which means they are defined, enacted, ignored, criticized, and/or challenged in the course of social interactions. Thus, what we consider to be an *appropriate* use of health technology is, by definition, socially constructed, multidimensional, and subject to constant change.

These observations can be the seeds for productive change in health care. Up until now, however, this potential has received very little attention in the literature on health technology. In chapter 5 I offer an alternative framework for thinking about the problem of health technology and potential transformations. However, before turning to that analysis, we need to examine the current institutional arrangements in which key decisions about the regulation of health technology are made. This chapter therefore focuses on the perspectives of the four most influential organized groups involved in health technology regulation: industry, physician associations, patient associations, and decision-makers. My intention is to illuminate how different types of stakeholders—who often have conflicting stakes in health technology and varying levels of resources—define their interests and perceive the value and usefulness of health technology assessment (HTA) and other types of knowledge about health technology.

The Role of Organized Groups in the Health Policy Arena

Broadly speaking, the regulation of health technology involves deciding whether an innovation should be introduced into the health care system, which categories of providers should be allowed to use it as well as be reimbursed for its use, and which groups of patients could benefit from it and obtain insurance coverage (Battista et al. 1994; Giacomini et al. 2003). This regulatory process directly affects a variety of stakeholders (e.g., patients, industry, providers, taxpayers), all of who may lose or gain clinical, economic, and symbolic resources (Lehoux and Blume 2000; Giacomini 1999). Understanding the potential role of knowledge in reconciling stakeholders' competing objectives requires adopting a broad sociopolitical perspective that can articulate the interplay between these groups in the health policy arena. A closer look at what happens when scientific evidence is debated reveals more explicitly the norms and intentions of those who are supposed to act upon the evidence as well as of those individuals and groups that participated in the construction of the contested evidence (Abraham 2002; Knorr Cetina 1999; Williams et al. 2003).

In this chapter I expand upon some of the observations made in chapter 1 by delving more deeply into the policy arena in which technology-related decisions are made. I again draw on the research that explored six Canadian HTA agencies and their relationships with four categories of stakeholders (see Appendix B). These groups were selected from formal organizations representing health care providers, health care decision-makers, patients, and the biomedical equipment and pharmaceutical industries. As I explained in chapter 1, the first two groups are "usual" target audiences for HTA agencies. Patient associations and industry are more generally considered lobbyists, albeit some are more powerful than others. The missions of all these groups are to represent a more or less sizable constituency (i.e., their members), to defend certain interests, and explicitly to contribute to the formation of health policy (Light et al. 2003).

Table 4.1 reveals the importance attributed by the four groups to nine general issues related to health services and health technology. For the majority, access to health services was the primary focus (mean scores over 4.13). Not far down the ladder were the evaluation of health services and technology, the control of costs of both services and technology, and the development of new services. Somewhat contrary to observations made in the early 1990s, industry respondents highly valued the evaluation of health services and technology (4.13). Not surprisingly, patients and industry (3.71 and 3.40, respectively) were somewhat less concerned about costs than were decision-makers and providers (4.42 and 3.90, respectively). The data also show that providers, decision-makers, and patients were somewhat less interested than industry in the introduction of new technology and technology acquisition by hospitals (4.75 and 4.06, respectively). The renewal of current technologies did not rank high for any of the four groups (from 3.26 to 3.59), which is perplexing, given the rapid pace at which innovations are produced. The fact that the provider and decision-maker groups (2.83 and 2.73, respectively) did not consider R&D

Table 4.1 Importance of Issues Related to Health Technology and Services

Issues	Provider Assn.		Decision-makers		Patient Assn.		Industry	
	N	Mean	N	Mean	N	Mean	N	Mean
Access to health services	218	4.53	105	4.52	58	4.71	16	4.13
Evaluation of health services and technology	217	4.00	104	4.09	57	4.09	16	4.13
Control of the cost of health services	221	3.90	105	4.42	58	3.71	15	3.40
Development of new health services	219	3.84	105	3.72	59	4.03	16	3.50
Control of the cost of health technology	219	3.79	105	4.20	58	3.33	16	3.63
Introducing new health technology into the health care system	220	3.63	105	3.69	57	3.70	16	4.75
Renewal of existing technology	218	3.59	105	3.59	58	3.26	16	3.38
Purchase of new technology by hospitals	222	3.35	105	3.42	57	3.18	16	4.06
Support of research and development (R&D) activities in the biomedical equipment and pharmaceutical industry	218	2.83	103	2.73	58	3.40	16	4.69

Note: Mean scores were calculated using a five-point Likert scale: (1) not important; (2) somewhat important; (3) important; (4) very important; (5) extremely important.

to be critical was also somewhat surprising, given the efforts invested in "early warning" and "horizon scanning" initiatives by HTA producers.

In the following sections I will explore in greater depth the rationales behind the expectations and actions of each of these stakeholder groups, as described in the literature and as revealed by group representatives during semistructured interviews my colleagues and I conducted across Canada. By contrasting the perspectives of the different groups and by highlighting variations *within* each group, these findings clarify the broader institutional tensions between stakeholders who pursue competing objectives but are obliged to negotiate their interdependencies and the reflexive nuances that characterize the position each group occupies in the policy arena.

Taming the "Big Bad Wolf"

As I mentioned in the introduction, the role of the biomedical industry in technology use and policy-making is rather taboo in HTA. Of course, the broader issue of university–industry relationships has always stirred up controversy, especially in health research, where profit generation is often seen as being in direct conflict with the production of unbiased, critical knowledge (Blumenthal et al. 1996). The ability to produce this type of knowledge is perceived as the "university's most precious commodity"—its intellectual integrity (Lewis et al. 2001). Not surprisingly, industry is often portrayed, at least in academic circles, as the "big bad wolf." Because dubious intentions are ascribed to industry, it must be kept at a distance and firmly regulated. I believe we need to abandon this stereotype; it is shallow, and may even obscure or prematurely block valuable paths of action. However, this *does not* mean blindly embracing industry as a "partner." It requires, rather, serious examination of how relationships between health care (delivery, research, and policy-making) and industry are structured, in what ways they are problematic, which objectives are reached and which forsaken in the interactions, and the specific as well as overall affects on the health care arena.

To better appraise the issues at stake in such public–private relationships, we need to define who is involved and what kinds of relationships are actually being forged. The biomedical equipment and pharmaceutical sectors comprise a heterogeneous set of players, among which resourceful drug manufacturing and retailing companies are particularly feared by the academic community because they are seen as "invading" the research-funding scene as well as medical practice through their sponsorship of continuing medical education (CME) events. According to Mather (2004), making the drug pipeline more predictable requires that pharmaceutical companies control settings and activities outside the domain of industry by funding research programs, supporting scientific conferences, sponsoring roundtables and journal clubs, hosting CME events, and giving gifts. These firms are also very active in the policy-making arena, where they seek to influence regulatory decisions that affect market access (e.g., Food and Drug Administration [FDA] approval in the United States, listing of specific drugs on provincial formularies in Canada, reimbursement rules) and even subsidy and tax policies that may affect their competitiveness in certain geographical areas (Laupacis et al. 2002). Because pharmaceutical companies' interests (when compared with those of biomedical equipment firms) can be more easily pinned down (i.e., selling drugs) and their level of resources is generally very high, scholarly work has focused on examining their influence on medical training/practice and health research. In contrast, the biomedical equipment industry is, in terms of its interests and resources, a more heterogeneous subgroup within the broad "industry" category. It is also less well studied and understood by academic researchers.

As Blumenthal et al. (1996, 368) assert, while the biomedical academic community now feels slightly more comfortable about its relationship with industry than it did in the early 1980s, there are still "very scant empirical data about the prevalence of relationships with industrial concerns, their characteristics, or the risks and benefits for the parties involved." In their 1994 telephone survey with senior executives of 210 small and large life sciences firms based in the United States (69% response rate), Blumenthal et al. (1996, 369) observed that 90% of respondents had some relationship with academia, 88% had consulting contracts with university faculty members, 59% supported university research, and 38% supported the training of students and fellows. Further, they concluded, "the generally short duration of the relationships and the small amounts of funding involved suggest that the research they support tends to be targeted—that is, applied rather than fundamental." Relationships typically lasted two years or less, 71% of the firms gave less than $100,000 a year, and only 6% provided annual funding of $500,000 or more. According to these findings, it would appear that it is important for industry to establish relationships with academics, but that it seeks mainly short-term returns on its financial investments.

Interestingly, Blumenthal et al. (1996, 370) found that industry respondents "perceived themselves as depending on the academic sector more for access to ideas, knowledge, and talented potential researchers than for specific marketable products or services." The authors interpret this finding as reassuring for universities: "If these advantages explain the strong and continued interest of life-sciences industries in academic institutions, then the future of relationships between industry and academia generally, and those centered on research in particular, may depend in a major way on the intellectual vitality of the academic health sciences" (372). In other words, if industry is looking for intellectual vitality, universities can still hope to gain from such relationships because these companies' goals are compatible with universities' overall mission—producing original research.[1]

Blumenthal et al.'s (1996) survey also explored a number of obstacles and problems in university–industry relationships. The most common obstacles for concluding agreements were university bureaucracies (cited by 54% of the firms surveyed) and university regulations that interfered with contractual negotiations (cited by 49%). Also, 34% of the companies surveyed reported problems with intellectual property and 58% indicated that they required information to be kept confidential for more than six months in order to file a patent application. The authors interpreted such secrecy policies as problematic, particularly for students and research fellows, who need publications in order to secure their first academic positions.

The extent to which competing public and private objectives can be reconciled, and the degree to which university–industry collaborative projects should become more prevalent clearly warrant further scrutiny by researchers. Whereas some observers argue too quickly that "win–win relationships" (Sanders 1995, 1538) can be established, I believe that to pursue their mission properly and fully, universities should continue to support a large number of research projects that *do not* involve industrial interests. We must forcefully recognize that a single model of knowledge production (Gibbons et al. 1994) is not ideal, given that diversity in knowledge creation and application is one of the academic sphere's most precious resources. Furthermore, trying to persuade trainees, researchers, and funding agencies that collaborative, applied research projects with industrial participants are always harmonious and mutually beneficial is misleading. While such relationships can be very productive, they are often tense and conflict-ridden, and require significant compromises (Cooke and Khotari 2001).

In their aptly titled paper "Dancing with the Porcupine," Lewis et al. (2001, 783) conclude, "in its best form, academic participation in drug-related science both spurs innovation and, through the disinterest and skepticism that are hallmarks of the academic mission, provides a check on the premature enthusiasms of industry." Nevertheless, the authors insist on the need to carefully manage industry–university relationships: "The warrant for prudence is not that something *will* go wrong; it is simply that something *may* go wrong, and *has* gone wrong in several cases. The intimidations and lawsuits are only the tip of the iceberg" (784).

In an editorial in the *New England Journal of Medicine*, Angell (2000, 1903) reminded readers that drug companies, no matter how hard they advocate for a reduction of regulatory "barriers" (e.g., market approval requirements, cost and pricing control policies, length of patent rules), make enormous profits, greater than in any other private sector area:

> The top 10 drug companies are reported to have profits averaging 30 percent of revenues—a stunning margin.... According to a recent issue of *Fortune*, in 1999 the pharmaceutical industry realized on average 18.6 percent return on revenues. Commercial banking was second, at 15.8 percent, and other industries ranged from 0.5 to 12.1 percent. An industry whose profits outstrip not only those of other industry in the United States, but often its own research and development costs, simply cannot be considered very risky.

Angell therefore argues that an industry that enjoys extraordinary government protections and subsidies, and that is only partly innovative (e.g., the production of many "me-too" drugs), cannot hope to be taken seriously by the public and the medical community[2]. As a result of such open criticisms, the pharmaceutical industry has had to adapt to public, economic, and regulatory pressures over the past decades. By reducing the cost of some of their products, for instance, drug companies have reacted to critical analyses that emphasize the increased proportion of hospital expenditures devoted to pharmaceuticals (Laupacis et al. 2002). From the pharmaceutical industry's point of view, the economics of producing and marketing drugs is increasingly scrutinized; or, as Sanders puts it, the "name of the game is to become the low-cost producer" (Sanders 1995, 1538).

A physician by training and now working for a pharmaceutical company, Sanders also believes that the medical community and industry "share a great deal in common." His plea is rather typical of the current discourse surrounding the need to increase collaboration between various constituencies, wherein the patient is transformed into the perfect neutral third party around which such collaboration gains meaning and becomes less threatening:

> Although I happen to work in the pharmaceutical industry, we are concerned with patients. All of your work ultimately is focused on the patient. We are bonded together ineluctably in the service of the patient. If we work together, if we pull together in ways that

show we add value, that we are committed to innovation that meets unmet medical needs, then we can make a difference (Sanders 1995, 1540).

It is important to recognize that finding a pure, axiologically unquestionable aim such as serving the patient is a discursive strategy that physicians, nurses, and health care managers also use. Along the same lines, another reason some physicians may feel collaboration with industry is beneficial lies in the knowledge that pharmaceutical companies possess. Writing in the venerable *Journal of the American Medical Association*, another physician observed, "Representatives from the health care industry can be a valuable information resource for physicians. The potential for this information to help patients creates a responsibility on the part of the industry to share pertinent knowledge with physicians so that it can be used to raise the level of health care delivery" (Tenery 2000, 391). This physician also emphasized that the physicians' need for CME has substantially increased with the complexity and pace of technology renewal, and that "with no other apparent alternative, funding from industry has almost become essential" (Tenery 2000, 392). In other words, technological and scientific advances make ongoing learning for physicians a lifelong responsibility *and* make them dependent on industry for acquiring requisite up-to-date knowledge. Indeed, drug companies' sponsoring of CME events has so far represented the most prevalent point of entry for interacting with medical practitioners. In recent years, the "fancy meals" and "attractive packages" offered by industry (Tenery 2000) have transformed the medical culture around knowledge and training. It is noteworthy that, in reaction to perceptions of undue influence resulting from CME initiatives, many jurisdictions have begun to implement stricter policies (see, for instance, the policy of the Royal College of Physicians and Surgeons of Canada: www.rcpsc.medical.org/publications/index.php).

The physician–industry relationship is, of course, not unidirectional. Adopting an anthropological perspective, Mather (2004, 1324) argues that "the physician–industry relationship is a special type of gift-giving relationship known as a total prestation." This type of relationship reconverts economic capital into cultural capital and back again. Physicians are "obligated to reciprocate the gifts they receive from industry" by providing cultural capital that is controlled and produced only by medical practice, and to which drug companies would otherwise be denied access (Mather 2004, 1324). To explore this line of inquiry, Mather carried out fieldwork and interviews (n=54) as part of an ethnographic study in the Department of Clinical Neurosciences at a Canadian university teaching hospital. In this department, physicians could not avoid contact with industry because they were obligated to attend industry-sponsored CME and scientific activities (Mather 2004, 1331). Commenting on such environments in which relationships with industry are institutionalized, Mather observes that ethics is seen as a matter of personal judgment. For instance, physicians stressed that they did not "check their scientific judgment at the door" before entering industry-sponsored events, thereby emphasizing their intellectual independence (Mather 2004, 1328). Also noteworthy was physicians' lack of trust in the very institutions—universities—that were, not so long ago, seen as symbols of medical ideals and moral integrity. As one physician suggested, authorities in universities could also be seen as ethically compromised:

> Who supports the department? Who provides financial support for our conference? I disagree … that the university should control these sorts of events. In the past the university could be a centre of truth but not anymore. Where does the money go and come from? The university profits from the relationship between drug companies and physicians (quoted in Mather 2004, 1329).

This physician's comments resonate with two ubiquitous claims found in the literature: universities no longer sufficiently support training and research activities, and universities have sold their souls by consenting to large increases in the private funding of their activities. This quotation also suggests an ambiguous position: because everyone else is engaged in ethically equivocal relationships with industry, neither academic institutions nor individual clinicians should refrain from participating as well. This position is a result of the complexity of current institutional arrangements in which health care research and practice unfold, and of the increased interdependence among various parties (Berg et al. 2004).

Interviews my colleagues and I conducted with representatives of the Canadian biomedical equipment and pharmaceutical industries support these contentions. They indicate that public–private relationships are more complex than they have usually been portrayed in the literature; that is to say, it is far from clear that these arrangements are simply a question of "good guys" versus "bad guys." Furthermore, the practices and decisions of industry, physicians, and health care authorities are deeply intertwined. Consequently, any policy intervention aimed at increasing rationality in health technology acquisition and use is doomed to fail unless it fully addresses the interdependencies among these various constituencies (Light et al. 2003).

These points can be illuminated by considering the point of view of the industry, particularly as it pertains to the dynamics underlying the introduction of innovations into health care systems, the macroeconomics and regulatory mechanisms that affect industry, and the potential for collaboration with knowledge (including HTA) producers. The interviewees we recruited for our research included representatives of a range of associations active in both the drug and medical devices areas. As is so often the case, these people wore several hats—most spoke from the standpoint of the individual firm at which they were employed as well as that of the associations they represented. Within the pharmaceutical sector, we also encountered a significant range of perspectives. For instance, supporters of generic drugs tended to highlight themes such as social inequality and system efficiency, topics not mentioned by those representing mainly branded products, who emphasized issues such as the cost of research and development (R&D). As one decision-maker said of industry, "They're a whole country unto themselves" (Decision-maker 1). Indeed, the heterogeneity of the issues that interviewees addressed illustrates the diversity of the dynamics structuring relationships among industry, physicians, and decision-makers.

One interviewee who worked for a multinational medical device manufacturer emphasized, at the outset, the large amount of money his firm devoted to R&D:

> If you're talking strictly about products, [our company] invests about 8% of our total worldwide medical revenues on R&D. And last year, we generated about US$6 billion in sales, so we spend about $500–600 million a year in R&D. So from a product development perspective, keeping abreast of the needs of physicians, particularly specialists like radiologists, cardiologists and oncologists, is obviously very important to us, as is keeping our products current (Industry Representative 1).

This interviewee also insisted on the need to keep up to date with technological advancements that medical specialists would likely demand. He explained, further, the two processes (health care pull and industry push) that shape product innovation and marketing:

> Interviewee: [We] introduce products either because the marketplace is demanding them and we've been working on them, or we bring a product to market that we think our customers need to know about and we make a conscious business decision based on a lot of parameters to do that. So the decision to introduce a

product is first and foremost market driven, then secondly, once you determine that there might be a market for it, you go through … obviously the product development kind of issues. But it really all goes back to an initial marketing decision as opposed to developing a technology for the sake of a new technology (Industry Representative 1).

Interviewer: Right, but the demand … I mean, does it come from the professionals?

Interviewee: That's what I mean when I say "the marketplace." The marketplace is the professionals. Or these days, it can be administrative people as well, but primarily our market is driven by the physicians that ultimately use our product, and that's why we have—in our company at least—customer advisory groups that spend a lot of time with us in Germany or in our other factories helping us understand what they require as physicians, what our equipment has to be able to do, and that helps drive our product development cycles (Industry Representative 1).

Despite emphasizing that technology is not produced simply "for the sake of a new technology," this industry representative did not refer to an appraisal of potential health needs that could be met by a technological innovation. While it should be acknowledged that his company manufactures medical imaging devices (defining the need for diagnostic tests is more elusive than the need for therapeutic devices; Laupacis 2005), in his view, medical specialists were the end users and, therefore, products were shaped according to their needs and the market was constructed through their use of the devices. But this brings us back to the problem of how physicians can know what they need from a new technology. And why do physicians feel they must keep abreast of clinical advances brought about by new technologies? In other words, who, exactly, is driving the innovation process?

Later in the interview the industry representative quoted above explained some of the intricacies of introducing a new imaging device into the health care marketplace when physician reimbursement has not yet been established:

So the market for PET scanners in Canada has been very low, because a PET scan is not … a reimbursable expense to a doctor or a hospital at this point. So certainly these kinds of decisions affect sales opportunities, that's for sure. The larger question, with respect to PET, however, is that it is a very expensive product to buy—about twice the cost of an MRI—but you have to look at the health economics. If a hospital, for example, uses a PET scanner, they can often avoid using a CT or MRI or some other modality, because it's much more accurate in finding certain kinds of diseases. However, when you look at the benefits of the downstream cost, the government is very reluctant to look at these because of the initial high up-front cost, and so looking at the overall impact on health care is something that's very difficult to get governments to do (Industry Representative 1).

These comments point to several financial factors. The first is the absence of physician reimbursement, which blocks market access. Second, the high initial acquisition cost for hospitals also acts as a barrier. Third is the "broader" economics argument that over the long run, PET scanners would incur fewer costs for governments because they would reduce the use of other diagnostic devices.

However, these financial considerations that seem to govern the ability of a manufacturer to introduce its innovation into the health care system—despite its best efforts to appraise the marketing issues in the first place—are not the only factors at play. Indeed, the same interviewee was keen to stress other, more subjective financial issues:

On the other hand, there's also a cynical view. When you look at radiologists, for example, they currently make a lot of money reading MRI and CT scans. There's also the view that if you went to a technology like PET, you would be reducing the number of scans required and therefore reducing physicians' incomes, and so you've got those politics as well. But from a government point of view … they tend to take a view of technology related only to the initial cost and not necessarily to the downstream impact cost on health care. So on one hand there's an impact on industry because we can't sell these products, while on the other hand, there's an impact on Canadians who may not necessarily have access to the most advanced technology available (Industry Representative 1).

The fact that physicians might not accept lower revenues so the government could reduce its spending on imaging tests appears to be an important issue. Furthermore, the interviewee believed that, ultimately, the losers were industry and the public. So what would a "win–win relationship" look like in this context? Should physicians be reimbursed for PET scans and all other tests they feel are clinically useful so that technology manufacturers can sell their products and patients can access the latest health care innovations? This scenario would require that government and hospital administrations allocate more resources to imaging devices. Is this what is really needed? And what would be the financial impact on other areas of health care?

The case of PET scans is a good illustration of the complexity of the macroeconomic forces that shape, and are shaped by, the evolution of health technology innovations. However, it only partially captures the interdependencies that sustain or impede the introduction of a new technology. The following comments were made by a representative of an association of pharmaceutical manufacturers. He provided a clear picture of the market dynamics driving drug manufacturing, and his remarks apply equally well to several other health care interventions:

> Certainly doctors do [have influence] because they are the actual prescribers. I mean, pharmaceuticals are a very different product than any consumer product, because for pharmaceuticals, for one you have a patient who's sick and therefore is in a heightened mind-set to want to take a drug. You're not necessarily always in a heightened mind-set to want to buy a television set. So, as soon as you're sick, your mind-set, your whole thought process, is: "If only I could take a drug ... ." No one wants to be sick. They want to feel better, so you have someone who wants the product, you have a doctor who is the decision-maker and the gatekeeper for the product, and that doctor is not affected by the cost of the product so he picks the product, not thinking about what the product is going to cost. Actually it's usually a pair—the government or an employer who also usually has no say in what is being prescribed. So you have a very interesting scenario that's different than for any other product in terms of decision-making (Industry Representative 2).

This industry representative stressed the pivotal role of physicians and suggested that the cost of a product does not affect (at least directly) their decisions. The patient is here cast as a passive recipient. As long as a drug coverage policy is consistent with a physician's choice of prescription, or as long as the cost of a drug is affordable, a patient is not seen, at this stage, as actively shaping the microlevel decision-making process.

Both pharmaceutical and medical device manufacturers emphasized the need to lobby governments:

> When the federal government ... forced Health Canada [Ministry of Health] to become budgetarily independent, it meant that some of the directorates of Health Canada started charging fees.

And they set up this process of getting license approval for products and as a result of that, we had to—as an industry—make sure that the new regulations and pricing structure were not overly onerous on the industry. So that was a battle that we fought, and I must admit Health Canada was very good—we didn't get everything we wanted, but they didn't get everything they wanted, and I think we came up with regulations that were mutually beneficial. Most recently, they have also started a process of regulating certain product lines more stringently, and the first one they started on was ultrasound. And I think what we're seeing is a tightening up of Health Canada's rules with respect to certain products. Again, they listen to us about ultrasound, and I think most people are quite happy with the rules and regulations that emerged. However, we have to be cognizant of the fact that other product lines are now going to be targeted by Health Canada for greater regulation and we have to make sure that we stay on top of those changes to make sure that they are good for the Canadian public obviously, but also that they are not overly onerous on industry (Industry Representative 1).

What seems most important here is the need for solidarity among manufacturers and retailers, for them to speak with a unified voice in order to fight government policy initiatives that might have cumulative, negative repercussions on the industry as a whole. The focus is on industry as a collective, rather than on a technology per se or its safety. The above comments also refer to a shift of (some) licensing costs from the public to the private purse and to *mutually* satisfying deals that can be struck through negotiation. The interviewee was careful not to bluntly attack the purposes and means of the regulatory mechanisms that were initially proposed, but he nonetheless anticipated that similar initiatives were likely to surface in the near future and he therefore stressed the need to remain vigilant. Finally, the interviewee alluded positively to the ability to strike a balance between regulations that are safe (for the public) but not too costly (for industry).

This interviewee did not, however, address the content of the negotiations that determine what is safe, fair, or good for the public. Nevertheless, one would certainly like to learn how the technical, scientific, clinical, social, and policy issues are commonly reconciled in such discussions and deal-making (cf. Giacomini 1999). Is the main emphasis on striking a deal that is satisfying for both parties? Or is it to establish effective regulations that are based on scientific evidence and that fulfill the public's expectations of public policies? According to Kent and Faulkner (2002, 205),

"How far promotion of trade jeopardizes the protection of public health is clearly a contentious issue requiring further investigation." Only cross-national comparative case studies could shed light on the degree of policy convergence and divergence in regulatory strategies (e.g., approval and postmarketing surveillance).

The final issues I would like to consider here are whether industry representatives believe they can collaborate with knowledge producers and whether they are receptive to the use of scientific evidence in policy-making and clinical practice. The opinions quoted below indicate that even though some groups may be keen to support research, securing collaboration with researchers is highly dependent upon political issues that reflect the internal diversity and economic complexity of the industry itself:

> As an association we have actually found it very difficult to have studies done because: 1) there's a lack of expertise available and 2) there may often be conflicts or just … a lack of willingness to do it because it's always seen as taking one side over another within the industry; for example, branded versus generic drugs. For example, some of the university organizations that we've tried to get contracts with have said, "Sorry, but if I do something for you, then I'll be shut out from doing research for the brands for the next five years." So we've actually had trouble getting universities, not because we're asking them to do anything disreputable, but because it's just hard for them to look at the available funding options and say, "Well, okay, I may jeopardize other funding" (Industry Representative 2).

Given the paucity of research on industry–academic collaboration, it is difficult to ascertain whether such hesitancy is widespread. These remarks nevertheless suggest that some groups may have more powerful arguments when it comes to convincing researchers to join their particular camps. More specifically, some representatives of the industry saw opportunities for collaboration with HTA producers, but wanted its focus to be shifted from the cost-effectiveness of a given technology to its policy implications: "So in fact maybe one way to help with decision-making is to focus more on the policy implications of making these decisions, rather than on trying to ascertain whether technologies are cost effective or not. Because I think other institutions are doing that at this point" (Industry Representative 3).[3] This quotation suggests that macroeconomic analyses would be more helpful than cost-effectiveness studies. According to this interviewee as well as several others, broader economic analyses would show that the government and the public can benefit from the introduction of a particular innovation, either in terms of industry health outcomes or cost savings. On this account, the public good is regarded as a *common* mission:

> [Our] companies do feel that we can collaborate with these technology assessment groups to make decisions and help inform policy ... because at the end of the day we have similar mandates, but if we work together in a more transparent and collaborative fashion, we will get a lot more done.... We're both in the business of trying to bring health care solutions to the Canadian public. And of course that means making the right decisions and informing policy in the best possible way. And so I think more collaboration with these agencies can only be a win–win scenario (Industry Representative 3).

As these comments suggest, the industry representatives with whom we spoke widely (though not universally) regarded collaboration as a mutual benefit. The industry representative quoted above expanded a little on why using scientific evidence in decision-making might prove to be a common objective worth pursuing:

> We know that our target audience may use some of the data provided or developed by these HTA groups and therefore it motivates us to do so. Because then it comes back to this whole approach—rather than working in parallel, let's try to see if there are some things we can combine and use to inform decisions, rather than always working separately. Because at the end of the day, it's only going to be able to help to inform the decision-making (Industry Representative 3).

Despite this optimistic outlook, however, it should be kept in mind that several industry groups frequently raised the issue of transparency because they felt excluded from HTA processes. These groups claimed they were informed of HTA results only when assessments had been made public.

While analyzing this set of interviews, I was repeatedly struck by the extensive range of negotiations that must take place for a given health technology to enter the health care marketplace, the centrality of the physician's role in that process, and the work required to articulate industry's concerns with regard to policy-making. More important, the interviews illustrated the complexity inherent in the institutional settings that are *collectively* responsible for making decisions about health technology, and suggested that HTA and scientific knowledge in general are welcome, although their use may take various forms (cf. Hivon et al. 2005).

Unpacking Physicians' Claims

As I alluded to earlier, when debating the value of an innovation, several claims can be made on behalf of the public good or patients' needs. This sort of reasoning can be used either to identify a valuable goal that is able to reconcile various groups' interests or as a means to reinforce expertise-based paternalistic control over decision-making. Moran and Alexander (1997, 578) point out that the professionalization of medicine and the concomitant increased use of science have created a comfortable niche for physicians:

> Modern health care systems are professionalized: the making and implementation of health care policy are deeply influenced by occupations that have succeeded in using the occupational strategy of professionalism for the defense of collective interests. Doctors have been the most important of these professions. They owe much of that importance to an alliance forged early in the present century with an emergent research elite in universities and with business interests.

According to these authors, over the past few decades, physicians' intimate connection with science has given them a persuasive claim to authority. But ties to professional knowledge can be manifold, and physicians often emphasize the value of clinical knowledge, as opposed to scientific knowledge, which mainly emerges from the literature and clinical trials. For instance, the following quotation suggests that physicians would pay more attention to HTA if it were both produced by clinicians and grounded in clinical contexts:

> [I'd rather have something] based in actual practice needs versus based on some researcher's view of the literature, which is very sterile. . . . You can't make decisions about new technologies simply from a non-clinical perspective, just on the basis of what the evidence in the literature says because there's too much clinical context. You need that input. [If HTA] was coming from representatives of the discipline, then we'd use it. Then I have more of a sense of how it fits in with other available technologies. . . . A clinician working in the area will know if there's actually not more

evidence for any of the other current technologies in use (Physician Association 1).

This interviewee was uncomfortable with scientific evidence that appeared out of context, preferring a medical specialist's opinion that had been forged through clinical practice. Without rejecting HTA input, he nonetheless stressed that meaningful knowledge must come from someone *within* the discipline of medicine. As these remarks illustrate, physicians' claims to authority are typically grounded in a kind of expertise that is first and foremost medical and intimately linked to the use and mastery of technological interventions.[4] The same interviewee also pointed to the difficulty of keeping clinicians' knowledge up to date: "Part of the problem is that we don't fund continuing medical education in this country. The public pays for undergraduate medical school; they pay for post-graduate training. They do not pay for the continuing professional development side. And yet it's a public health issue" (Physician Association 1). This comment touches on the paradox of physicians' reliance on the mastery of technological advances in order to maintain their privileged status and control over medical practice issues while at the same time needing to access, absorb, and apply new knowledge.

One interviewee working in the area of genetics observed that the exponential increase in technologies not only puts pressure on the research agendas of HTA agencies, but also calls for a different approach to assessment: "because [the HTA agency's researchers] were going disease by disease at some point and we said, 'Look, you have to prepare a monograph that looks at the whole general area because there are 3,000 diseases.' So we sat down with them to help decide what genetic diseases to study" (Physician Association 3). This person was particularly concerned about the introduction of genetic technologies into medical practice, and believed that part of the role of HTA agencies was to convince government of the proven efficacy of such innovations. That supposed mission explained why this association and its members had collaborated with a particular agency:

> [HTA agency] has produced a number of monographs in different areas of genetics and there have been different members of the genetics community invited to sit at the table and contribute to the monographs.... Since the mandate of the Office of Technology Assessment was to prove to the government that these were useful, there would be a way to get the government moving on implementation. I think most people would at least know ... about their monographs, and we're very hopeful that this will be used as objective support for implementation (Physician Association 3).

As became clear in chapter 1, the role of HTA is, for some individuals and stakeholder groups, mainly to validate technologies, to serve as a stamp of approval for their implementation. As might be expected, based on his earlier comments, the interviewee quoted just above provided confirmation of this view vis-à-vis the field of genetics:

> There's been a great deal of new information in the area of genetics, and in a way the government has been very slow in adapting this information to health care. It's new, they don't know when to adapt it, how much of it is going to be generally accepted. And part of our frustration is that, I think, the area of genetics has been held to a different standard than have other areas of medicine because it's become so politicized, with the discussion of DNA and what is life. I think a lot of things that we as physicians would consider almost routine—that have been shown to be of benefit elsewhere—should have been implemented already. Because there's this cautious approach. We just hope they move on with the studies more quickly, so that the government can say "Yes, this has been validated, and now implement it," especially for things that have already been introduced in other provinces or have become mainstream in other places (Physician Association 3).

This person clearly believed that politics plays a major, even detrimental, role in technology diffusion, leading to an overly "cautious approach" to the adoption of new technologies, a process in which scientific evidence becomes a form of argumentation (cf. Greenhalgh et al. 2004).

Another respondent provided a more detailed picture of the political and administrative channels that ultimately determine the diffusion of health technology. When asked which players he believed were influencing health policy in his jurisdiction, he replied:

> Well, the regional health authorities are number one, of course. They control the purse strings when it comes to what technology is going to be purchased for their facilities. Individual physicians who provide high-tech services in their offices make independent decisions about what they're going to use. Certain specialties, like radiology, have consensus groups within the province, so their society would no doubt be an important decider of what, for example, mammography technology would look like.... [The Ministry of Health] makes some decisions; they can't avoid questions about what new expenses in pharmacology to fund, and that's a really important one. When it comes to expensive drugs,

they're an important player, as is Blue Cross, the big public payer of drugs. [Our] college writes standards so it is a very important player when it comes to standards of practice. The nursing profession is very much part of any new technology that affects its members, like if somebody's bringing in ultrasound machines to look at the residual volume of urine in the bladder at a nursing home. There are user groups, like professional groups for laser technology, that would use the technology in their practice (Physician Association 1).

I choose to include such a lengthy quotation because it gives a clear overview of the diversity, complexity, and heterogeneity of the groups that influence policy-making. Those who have stakes in health technology policy possess varying levels of resources, authority, and expertise. And they are likely to belong to, or promote, organizational cultures that may structure how they perceive the role of knowledge in health policy-making.

Another respondent held a broader view of what informed health policy should look like. He insisted on the need to use scientific data but, more important, to develop a critical attitude toward information and its meaning: "I have to myself critically analyze a problem and ask others to do the same. Discussion groups are key. We call it 'communities of practice'—they have become increasingly important" (Physician Association 2). His emphasis on collectively sharing, discussing, and debating ideas and analyses was consistent with his stance on the training of physicians:

Our college emphasizes education, but so far I am not comfortable with the prevailing concept that focuses on knowledge, skills, and attitudes. One key element is missing—judgment. From my perspective, the problem-solving approach is very good for knowledge and skills development, but it's not the way to make good judgments. There's an emerging literature that stresses that judgment develops out of diversity, openness and, in fact, one has to think in new ways.... This is a value I would like to see our organizations adopt (Physician Association 2).

This interviewee not only addressed, from a broader perspective than did other representatives of physician associations, the role of evidence and HTA in bringing changes into health care systems, but also was critical of the fact that a small group of experts can, illegitimately, end up making decisions that affect wide ranges of stakeholders:

One striking observation about professional organizations, and not only with respect to physicians but also engineers, accountants and so on, is that they don't have a clue about what the people they represent really think. One major challenge for professional organizations is to better understand what their members think. So when a "select club" that happens to chair a given association decides to define and foster certain priorities, this isn't honest (Physician Association 2).

What Do Patient Associations Know and Expect, and for Whom Do They Advocate?

The emphasis on the role of expertise in policy-making is not unique to medicine. In many sectors (e.g., energy, environment, agriculture) policy-making increasingly depends upon expertise. Simultaneously, many policy-makers condescendingly regard lay members of society as ignorant or insufficiently knowledgeable (Beck 1992). The result is paradoxical: on one hand, policies are justified by referring to the public good or to patient well-being; on the other, the public is excluded from policy-making. In the case of health technology, the public is also frequently accused of being gullible in its demand for ineffective interventions. Cohen and Hanft (2004, 95), for instance, argue that "because most consumers are unqualified to judge the scientific validity of the information at hand, they often will uncritically accept reported 'findings.' ... In addition, the impact of patient advocacy groups on consumer demand for specific technologies should not be underestimated." But are such views not simply another way of buttressing experts' paternalism?

Right from the start it should be stressed that the terminology used to designate nonexperts is problematic. While "the public" is supposed to represent a wide (more or less neutral) civil constituency, the terms "patients," "patient advocacy groups," "clients," "consumers," and "users" often highlight the stake these groups or individuals hold vis-à-vis health care as well as their dependence upon medical experts. Such semantic designations can, however, blur identity nuances, since lay individuals can learn and master complex knowledge and professionals are also, of course, part of the public (as citizens or taxpayers) (Dyer 2004).

Notwithstanding these definitional difficulties, researchers have, of late, been paying increasing attention to the impact of such groups on medical practice and policy-making, and to patients who become experts with respect to certain health issues (Barbot 1998; Sullivan 2003). From a sociological perspective, "the growth both of discourses on the expert patient and the technology to facilitate a consumerist approach to health, illness and its treatment, suggests an agenda for research into how these innovations construct patient-hood and notions of normality and pathology" (Fox et al. 2005, 1300). Along similar lines, Kent, who has examined the controversy around breast implants and silicone-related disease in the United States and Europe, underscores the "marginalization and pathologization of breast implant recipients" that prevailed in the 1990s (2003, 416). She argues, however, that certain groups of women

> have been engaged in a form of identity politics, and the emergence of a single issue "social movement" has sought to challenge the view that they are obsessed with body image and are mindless and neurotic. Through the telling of breast implant experiences, a "lay epidemiology" and stock of knowledge has been produced, and many women have become "lay experts" (Kent 2003, 416).

Researchers also point out the need to examine the public's ease of access to, and understanding of, medical and scientific knowledge. As Calnan, Montaner, and Horne note, the lay public use some form of criteria for "evaluating health-care technology, such as its 'life-saving nature,' its 'quality of life' enhancing capacities, its 'iatrogenic' consequences and the degree to which it is viewed as 'immoral' or 'unnatural'" (2005, 1938). For some scholars, the ethical and social issues surrounding genetic testing highlight the need to improve the public's "genetic literacy" (Robins and Metcalfe 2004). Indeed, most patients' understanding of the results of genetic tests appears incomplete (Marteau and Lerman 2001), the availability of genetic counselors in many regions is limited, and general practitioners face multiple obstacles in their efforts to inform patients about the meaning and limitations of genetic technologies (Friedman et al. 2003). More globally, as Zimmern and Cook (2000) conclude, because genetic testing affects individuals' reproductive choices and can drastically alter, at the societal level, how insurance companies and employers define and avoid risks, the public needs to be involved in debates about the regulation of genetic technologies.

As a result of this belief in the importance of lay involvement, various initiatives to include public representatives in evaluation or policy-making have been implemented. For example, in 2002 the United Kingdom-based HTA agency, the National Institute for Clinical Excellence (NICE), set up the Citizen's Council. Thirty members were recruited (from over 4,327 applications), reflecting the diverse populations of England and Wales, according to criteria such as age, education, gender, ethnicity, employment status, and location of residence. The council held a number of three-day meetings during which experts were invited to speak and deliberative sessions were convened to identify and discuss key issues. The primary goal of the council was to provide information about the general public's views and the "motivations and values that underlie these opinions," as well as to help NICE make decisions about how the National Health Service (NHS) should administer treatments and therapies (NICE Citizens Council Report on Age, undated; www.nice.org.uk). And in Switzerland, a technology assessment agency has also been organizing citizens' panels, called Publiforums, to explore and debate broader ethical and social issues arising from new technologies (www.ta-swiss.ch). These panels promote a participatory method inspired by consensus conferences wherein public representatives can both obtain information and experts' views, and call scientific evidence into question.

The existence of such initiatives confirms the perceived need to engage the public in health technology decision-making, but also highlights the complexity of achieving this goal. After examining the role of lay members on Local Research Ethics Committees (LRECs) in the United Kingdom (survey: n=218 LRECs; interviews; n=45), Dyer (2004, 346) concluded that lay members may have a certain experience of being patients, but they do not have a monopoly on understanding the patient experience. She added, "Expert members, many of whom have day-to-day dealings with patients, can and do claim more expertise in public understandings of medicine and illness." Indeed, when the goal is to protect the rights and autonomy of patients (as opposed to understanding their preferences or rationales), the question of who can represent and defend the patient's view remains open.

In one study in which I took part (Hivon et al. 2005), we sought to understand what patient groups were promoting, what kinds of expertise and information they were using, and how they were defining their role in the policy arena. We observed striking differences among the various groups we contacted across Canada, both in terms of mission (e.g., raising funds for research, lobbying, offering information and/or services to patients and their relatives) and of views about the role of knowledge in influencing patients' behavior and policy-making (Barbot 1998). The following exchange, for instance, took place with a representative of a formally structured association whose principal mission was raising funds for research on lung disease:

Interviewer: Do you play any role in informing patients?

Interviewee: No. That's the doctor's role. Because we don't understand the patient. The doctor might know that the patient can't do this, or whatever.... So it's useful for the patient to be educated, but it's difficult to educate the patient. I guess the position we take is: If the device is, as I said earlier, mainstream, established, we tell people about it. And then, if they want to go to their doctor and ask for a specific thing, then the doctor will have to make a judgment about whether or not that would work for them (Patient Association 1).

This person's view was thus very compatible with physicians' expertise-based claim to authority, which is not entirely surprising, because his association mainly funded medical research. In sharp contrast, a representative of a large and formally structured association whose mandate is to support cancer patients (and their family and friends) provided a fuller explanation of her association's responsibility toward patients and the public:

Interviewer: So do you think that an organization such as yours is a good mediator for transferring research results to the public?

Interviewee: Yes, I think it is. For example, we took some research about men's experiences with prostate cancer and, with the help of others, turned it into a dramatic production. So we use novel ways of getting evidence-based information out to the public. We've also done that with information about hereditary breast cancer, based on our knowledge about how women want to have this information presented to them (Patient Association 2).

Here might be an instance of the best patient association partner HTA producers could hope to find. Its members not only are keen to use scientific evidence, but also integrate that knowledge into an accessible format that responds to patients' concerns. As another member of this association clarified, part of the group's mandate is scanning cancer-related issues addressed in the media and participating in public debates on these issues: "On a day-to-day basis, we are also engaged in active communication around public issues—things that are in the media … which sometimes means we have to understand the context and get additional information in order to respond adequately" (Patient Association 3). This interviewee's colleague added that patients want to be "involved in decision-making around what gets researched and what gets selected. They want equity. And sometimes they probably want things that aren't appropriate, like the PSA test available for everybody" (Patient Association 2). Again, this view resonates with the cautious stance of HTA producers toward innovations.

This interviewee also had a fairly precise idea of what matters to cancer patients:

Interviewer: Are there any particular issues that are important for people dealing with cancer?

Interviewee: I think they'd like less invasive tests. Or if you're talking about something like mammograms, they would like to have more specific tests. People don't understand when they know there's a better test out there, such as digital mammography, which can be used by the general population. I think there's a sense that people would like to think they're always getting the best of what's available, perhaps know that they're not because of the cost. And cost is always an issue for governments (Patient Association 2).

Clearly, these insights were grounded in firsthand knowledge of actual technologies and of the policy-making context as it relates to diagnostic testing.

Lobbying was, as might be expected, an important theme that surfaced throughout the interviews with patient association representatives. Some respondents were more careful than others when trying to articulate what they were lobbying for and on behalf of whom. When asked whether her organization was using research findings, one interviewee was a bit hesitant: "If I think about drug therapies, for instance, we advocated on behalf [pause] now how do I say this properly [pause]? We advocated to have all drug therapies as they became available added to our provincial formulary [the list of drugs reimbursed by the health care system]. And we could do that only because we had the information that there is a benefit to the people we're trying to serve, and that they're safe and approved" (Patient Association 4). This respondent refrained from saying that her association was advocating on behalf of a particular drug, preferring instead to employ more general phrasing. But she acknowledged that scientific evidence was useful in her association's plea for adding safe and effective drugs to the formulary, thereby facilitating patient access to beneficial therapies. Should this example be read as a sign that the evidence-based culture of decision-making has spread to lay groups? Or should one be concerned about the potential for increasing the symbolic use of evidence (e.g., selective or post hoc)?

Similarly, the representative of the association involved in fund-raising for lung disease research was rather equivocal when explaining what his group was promoting and how much of its work involved advocating *for* science or *through* science:

Well, we advocate on behalf of science as well as on behalf of people. It's mostly drug companies that want us to promote their products. We don't really promote certain products; we might advocate a class of medications. So as new technology in these areas becomes available, and again it's drug companies that are doing all the research—well, most of the research, or pretty much all the research. For instance, we would advocate that the government give everybody a spacer. This is the kind of thing we might advocate because that would be backed by science. For this particular device, the patent is held by 3M. There are several other devices that use a different technology, different shapes—these are all the result of scientific research and most … much of that science has been done by drug companies. So we're in a bit of a dilemma—should we be helping drug companies sell their product? Yes. Well, probably. If it's a good product. Yes, we probably should (Patient Association 1).

This person's struggle to define whether or not his association should promote a particular product is intriguing. First, he refused to advocate on behalf of a particular company and referred to promoting a class of medications or type of device, which is a strategy for deflecting any potential attack along conflict-of-interest lines. Second, he conflated research with investigations done by pharmaceutical companies. Third, he revealed detailed knowledge about a certain innovation, including the name of the company holding the patent, and stressed that the device was the result of science. Fourth, he thought out loud about whether or not it is ethically correct to advocate for a particular product, and concluded that it would be, if a device were beneficial.

Such statements—and their underlying reasoning and understanding of science—are a bit perplexing (at least for university-based researchers). But *why*? The principle that those who conduct research should be independent from those who fund research and from those whose products are being developed is a long-standing tenet in university-based science. Most university-based investigators therefore believe that research conducted by private companies is of inferior quality.[5] The conclusion arrived at by the interviewee quoted above, however, is not so different from that reached by proponents of evidence-based medicine. Both agree that if an intervention is beneficial, it is worth advocating. They simply disagree over which type of science should determine its value and, consequently, inform policy-making.

When asked about the ways in which his association was keeping abreast in the area of lung disease research, the same interviewee offered a vivid simile to explain why certain types of products were successful while others were not:

It's like rock stars. There are thousands and thousands of good musicians, but only one or two we know about. How did they get to be so famous? I don't know. The same is true for science. There are thousands and thousands of scientists all doing important work. How do one or two rise to the top to win the Nobel Prize? I don't know. But those are the ones we hear about. So how did they get there? I don't know. But they did. We read it in the [newspaper]: "New medication discovered for asthma." There are probably hundreds of new medications, but the only one we hear about is this one. And then people start to pressure us: "How do I get that medication? I need that medication. I want it." Then we, along with our medical advisors say, "Yeah, it's good!" And then we start to pressure people and all of a sudden you have a rock star! How did it happen? I don't know. You know, it's just the way it works. I don't understand it (Patient Association 1).

Here again, the interviewee conflated drug-related innovation with science. Furthermore, he used the rock-star simile to clarify that if certain physicians end up prescribing a given drug it is partly because that therapy had been successfully marketed to them:

Why does the doctor prescribe it? I don't know. He likes the "brand," somebody marketed it to him, somebody told him about it.... Unless they watch American TV, patients are in no position, at least in this country, to make any decisions about their medication because drug companies are not allowed to advertise to the patient. They can only advertise to the physician, whereas in the United States—if you watch any American TV, you will know—they do what they call direct-to-consumer advertising (Patient Association 1).

This person also pointed out that only in jurisdictions where direct-to-consumer advertising is allowed can patients obtain useful information and make decisions. This view is rooted in a strong belief that industry-driven research and advertisement are trustworthy sources of information. For instance, he knew that physicians regularly attend trade shows and conferences at which the results of clinical trials and new devices are showcased. For him, such marketing does not have a negative connotation, and is merely part and parcel of how innovations are diffused: "The health community ... often learn[s] about devices through manufacturers ... whether at conferences where people are giving presentations on clinical trials, or through displays or exhibits at conferences—in whatever ways these companies market their products (Patient Association 1).

Finally, we asked this person how influential, in his opinion, his association was in policy-making processes in his province. His answer was somewhat oblique, emphasizing the potential political weight linked to the number of votes his association represented:

> We have more credibility than a single person. ... We actually don't get a big response. We have 100,000 members ... I would be paying attention if I was the minister of health. We're probably more important than 1,000 people, maybe more important than 10,000 people. I don't know. So when we go to the government and say we have 100,000 supporters, they should pay attention to us (Patient Association 1).[6]

In some provinces, consultative and collaborative processes between the government and lay groups have been implemented, and we interviewed groups who had been involved in such activities. The following quotation gives a concrete example of such consultation and an enthusiastic, positive appraisal of the process:

> Interviewer: Do you feel that organizations such as yours can play a role in influencing policies in [your jurisdiction]?
>
> Interviewee: Absolutely! Absolutely! We've just been involved with our government on developing a strategy for [name of the] disease. [Our association] was at the table with regional health authorities, colleges and universities, and physician associations. Yes, absolutely. And we're in touch with different government departments as well. They don't give us any money [laugh] but they sure like to listen to us (Patient Association 4).

As the range of views we gathered shows, although initiatives to include patient associations in HTA and policy-making may prove fruitful in the long run, those who spearhead them require a better understanding of the types of activities they support, the sources of knowledge they favor and trust, their needs and abilities in terms of accessing and using scientific evidence, and their relationships with industry. Some patient associations depend largely on the private sector for funding, a relationship that may clearly constrain the kinds of claims and attitudes they bring to technology-related policy-making. Furthermore, as Light et al. (2003) note, it is important to distinguish between initiatives that include members of the public at large (e.g., NICE's Citizens' Council) and those that rely on representatives of established, organized groups.

We should perhaps also be reflexive about *why* some regard industry's support of patient associations as problematic. Indeed, HTA producers and university-based researchers in general may assume (too quickly) that the knowledge they generate is the best type of evidence and the only kind that ought to inform policy-making. Nevertheless, they may increasingly be forced to acknowledge that within their institutions' walls, industry is almost certainly already active and that several groups outside the academy trust and rely on privately sponsored research (Blumenthal et al. 1996). The points I am urging here are that the pervasiveness of industry in health care cannot be ignored and that more attention should be paid to the high level of interdependence among physician and patient associations, industry, policy-making bodies, and researchers (Kent and Faulkner 2002). These groups may all be keen to use research results to inform public policies, but they may vary in their views on what type of knowledge should drive decision-making (Barbot 1998).

Are Decision-Makers Victims of Their Own Cost-Control Initiatives?

I want now to turn attention to the pressures that decision- and policy-makers feel, the options they believe should be presented, and their perceptions of the usefulness of HTA and scientific evidence. In recent years the need to increase collaborative research between decision-makers, providers, and/or university-based researchers has been emphasized by knowledge transfer advocates. Coupled with this development, "attention has shifted from what either the producers of research or the users of research can do on their own to what the two communities can do together through interactive processes" (Ross et al. 2003, 26).

According to Golden-Biddle et al. (2003), four key elements are at play in collaborative research: the relational stance that researchers and decision-makers assume toward each other, the immediate purpose that creates occasions for developing and using knowledge, the knowledge-sharing practices for translating knowledge, and the forums in which researchers and practitioners access knowledge. These authors recommend adopting "a communicative perspective on research collaborations that emphasizes the members and the communicative elements called upon in knowledge-making and -using efforts" (Golden-Biddle et al. 2003, 21). The frequent misunderstandings that arise between researchers, decision-makers, and/or practitioners as a result of cultural differences underscore the importance of comprehending the communication elements of these relationships and interchanges. According to Bartunek et al. (2003, 65), academics and practitioners "do not share the same norms regarding scholarship and practice, and they often do not know well enough how to work with each other in a way that takes these different norms into account." As a way to overcome these differences, they suggest that "being involved in interpretation processes that take each other's viewpoints into account should facilitate the ability of each party to translate between, and at least partially integrate, their own and the other's frameworks" (66).

On this score, it is often argued that involvement in collaborative research can reduce the cultural gap between the two communities. For instance, in a survey of 350 researchers and practitioners active in the area of social research in Quebec, Canada, and funded under a policy initiative explicitly supporting collaborative research (formerly the Conseil Québécois de la Recherche Sociale, CQRS), my colleagues and I observed that "the views of researchers and practitioners regarding the dimensions of collaborative research seemed to converge. They agreed on the skills deemed necessary for collaborative research to be successful. They valued the development of activities with partners from the community sector and from health care organizations" (Denis et al. 2003, 49). In addition, both groups had a fairly positive sense of the ability of collaborative research to affect knowledge production and practices. One unanswered question, however, was what level of involvement would be required for their views to converge.[7]

Notwithstanding the enthusiasm for collaborative research, the need to preserve the autonomy of scientific practices is often raised in the literature. As one group of authors remarks, "The spectre of too close a relationship between the researchers and the government funders can become an issue" (Goering et al. 2003, 17). To what extent should this specter be a concern? This question points to the need to be clear about who the partners in collaborative research projects are and what their stakes in specific research or policy processes might be. As a result of their investigation into collaborative research, Ross et al. (2003, 33) observe that "in some situations the decision-maker partner was perceived to have injected a new kind of rigor into the process, a sort of ongoing healthy self-consciousness about the contextual implications of the research." However, as became evident in chapter 1, an HTA agency's credibility is affected by the perceived distance between its scientific mission and the cost-control policies that government officials pursue. A tension, in other words, exists between the need to maintain a close connection to policy-makers and the need to preserve academic independence in order to avoid being perceived as agents of government (Coburn 1998). Although scholars of collaborative research stress "the need for researchers to be genuinely committed to the activity and to be selective about who they engage" (Ross et al. 2003, 31), HTA's public mission forbids ignoring other stakeholders. Furthermore, each stakeholder group seems keen to have HTA agencies adopt its particular goals, but not necessarily those of other parties. Thus, a relationship that one stakeholder sees as distant, another might regard as too close for comfort.

This perspectival complexity reinforces the need to examine more intensely what happens during collaboration, because scientific autonomy may not be limited primarily by the *presence* of partners but, rather, by their relative weight in terms of input into the research process. Among other things, several authors recommend anticipating and managing potential conflicts of interest and having "clear, mutual expectations" about each partner's roles (Goering et al. 2003, 18). In this regard, however, the potential that HTA may end up with unclear recommendations could be problematic. When analyzing various ways of dealing with the lack of compelling evidence concerning the value of adopting certain innovations, Giacomini et al. point out that "when assessment determines that the value of a service is 'gray,' decision-makers have the option of making a 'gray' coverage decision in response. Specific coverage conditions correspond to specific 'gray' qualities encountered in evaluation" (2003, 312). It would be possible, for instance, to limit the use of a new technology to university teaching hospitals operating under detailed research protocols. As a result, further research on its efficacy and safety could be conducted and its wider diffusion could be postponed until more solid evidence became available.

For policy-makers, managing the diffusion process (e.g., by setting criteria and providing conditional funding) is a well-established strategy (Battista et al. 1994). Among our interviewees, some nonetheless argued that HTA results should be made available quickly and stressed that policy-making is performed under important temporal and legal constraints:[8] "timeliness is a major problem... HTA—the way it's being done now—is working at a very leisurely academic pace. So the two just don't fit together. I mean, in eighteen months we could be in a lawsuit" (Decision-maker 2). Similarly, another respondent stressed that the policy-making domain is erratic and changeable, and thus completely different from the world of science (Decision-maker 3). Some interviewees alluded to the unpredictability of the health policy arena and the haste that sometimes surrounds government decisions or interventions. For example, the same respondent explained why several of her peers declined an invitation to sit on a panel during a one-day workshop on HTA:

Well, part of it is laziness, but it's not just that.... Doing a panel discussion on top of everything else is just ... you know, I don't need this pressure. I think part of it is political for some people. There is a reluctance to appear in a forum that could put you in a very vulnerable position as an employee of [the Ministry of Health]. Sometimes you feel like you're a sitting duck. There's a feeling that you could be the target for anybody who's got a particular axe to grind (Decision-maker 3).

Nonetheless, several interviewees felt that it would be desirable to increase collaboration between HTA agencies and policy-making bodies:

I've certainly talked to [the HTA unit] about this myself. I think there are ways of better linking research and policy agendas. There's never going to be a perfect fit because health care is political and someone could raise some issue in the legislature and the minister of the day would have to deal with it. So I'm not talking about day-to-day issues, but when the government looks over the coming year, the main things it's going to deal with, it would probably be useful to regularly sit down with [HTA unit] and ask what they're doing, or what they could be doing, to help us with some of our policy decisions (Decision-maker 1).

As I discussed earlier, the number of people who are, ultimately, at the heart of policy-making can appear limited, or at least concentrated in hermetically sealed spheres. When asked what groups were influential in policy-making in his jurisdiction, one respondent from a regional planning body replied:

I would say that senior civil servants in the government are the pivotal people in terms of: A) policy direction and B) funding decisions. We have a deputy minister and a number of assistant deputy ministers, and a number of managers under that—they're called the senior management team—so I'd say there's about a dozen of those individuals and by far and away, they're the most influential in terms of a whole series of health related decisions. Now, outside of that fairly small group of people, there's sort of two groups of influential people. One would be the main hospitals and the leaders of those organizations, because they get huge amounts of money each year from the government and have a fair amount of discretion about how they spend that money. So in terms of what piece of equipment goes where and who does what, they have a fair bit of influence. Then, the physicians who aren't employees of the hospital are the other sort of very influential group of individuals. So I'd say those three—the heads of hospitals, the physicians, and the senior bureaucrats at the ministry of health would be probably the key people (Decision-maker 1).

Using very similar terms, a civil servant with the Ministry of Health in another jurisdiction emphasized that a limited number of individuals were in fact shaping health policies, but that these individuals were under pressure from other, larger groups:

Well, the caucus, the MLAs [members of the legislative assembly] and cabinet would be the primary ones, the minister in particular. Strictly speaking, in the [Ministry of Health] we don't make policy; we provide direction. We give advice, but we don't make policy; the MLAs and the minister do. There's a variety of people who influence them—professional associations, regional health authorities, etc., and that influence is proportional to their size (Decision-maker 3).

This last response introduces the notion that the *number* and *weight* of people included in a constituency, as an organized group, can influence from outside the governmental activities that produce policies.

Comparing and contrasting interviewees' perspectives also paints a more elaborate picture of the internal circuitry of policy-making. In certain cases, interviewees admitted they did not control much of what was happening:

Unlike a lot of the regional health authorities, *we don't actually receive the funding, so we don't get to hand it out.* So we really only *advise* on what should happen in our particular regions and, like all advice, you can take it or leave it [laugh]. So sometimes the government will act on our advice and sometimes it won't.… So I think that at the end of the day, we have some influence but it's certainly not the only influence, and there are others, like the ones I described, who have a fair amount of influence as well (Decision-maker 1; emphasis added).

For us, one of the paradoxes with HTA is that the [Ministry of Health] *does not provide health care services.* The [regional health authorities] do that. So with respect to the decisions we make—to some extent we can decide whatever we want, but they have to pay for it [laugh] or not, as the case may be. They're the ones who have to find the staff, find the resources, find the room for the machine, buy the doctor his equipment, buy the imaging equipment, get the nurses, get specially trained staff, look after the patients, open up another bed in ICU (Decision-maker 3; emphasis added).

The first respondent quoted above stressed that lack of budgetary control meant little or no influence over technology use, whereas the second decision-maker argued that resource allocation is not really what determines technology use. So to what extent should controlling the purse strings be seen as a pivotal issue? Across Canada's ten provinces there is significant variation in the level of decentralization and the type of power each administrative level holds. Perhaps, then, it should not be entirely surprising that, even for the civil servants working in those administrations, the degree to which resources for acquiring or using technology should be linked to knowledge about efficacy and safety is not always clear.

The following remarks suggest that when a technology is "established," the decision to fund it does not require thorough investigation:

A couple of years ago, one of our smaller hospitals wanted to introduce CT scanning and so they had to submit a proposal to us. But, again, because CT scans are a fairly well established diagnostic tool, neither us nor the hospital would have had to do a lot of health technology assessment to say that CT scanning is a good or bad thing—it's fairly well established. But for bigger equipment purchases or new services that a hospital hasn't had before, we do review their proposals. But if it's a large hospital and it's really a question of equipment replacement, then no, that's largely an internal process (Decision-maker 1).

On this understanding, it appears that the possibility for HTA producers to use scientific evidence to curb decision-making is stronger when the value of a new technology is controversial. If a given health technology is perceived as being part of standard practice, its adoption and use may be seen purely as an administrative matter, one that does not require scientific input.

For another respondent, who represented a health care employers association, technology was neither on the agenda nor seen as a salient issue in health care delivery:

We don't make any assessments of technological advancements, new procedures or specific interventions. Our organization doesn't look into that. We do not touch any patients, and we're not involved in analyzing whether or not the health delivery system is delivering quality care ... except with respect to the people side. Is it run efficiently? Are people being used properly? Do we have the proper scope of duties for people? Is there some way we can expand their scopes of practice for medicine or nursing in order to use them more effectively (Decision-maker, 4)?

These remarks are enlightening because they show that certain groups that play important roles in shaping health care human resources policies see their members' job functions as almost independent of technological developments. Given that technologies do, however, profoundly modify health care providers' clinical responsibilities, scope of action, and training needs, this lack of interest in technology may reflect a historical, institutionalized division of labor between various regulatory bodies (Faulkner et al. 2003; Foray 1997). Each group must adhere to a well-defined agenda, focus on its mission, and defend its interests. However, all these groups ultimately seek to influence the same thing: the health care system. As a result, health policy-making becomes a politically intense playing field in which everyone is trying to get the most out of the current situation and to steer the future in a desirable direction for the sake of their own group.

Here is a final dialogue in which a decision-maker described the relative power of industry and patient associations:

Interviewer: What about patient associations, do they have any influence at all?

Interviewee: Yes. I think there is a growing number of what I'll call consumer associations. I think in [name of province] the ones that will very soon have the most influence, if they don't already, on government will be the seniors associations. And that's just because seniors are growing in number because society is aging. So I think that politically, and in terms of votes, they are and will be the most influential (Decision-maker 1).

Interviewer: And what about the pharmaceutical industry?

Interviewee: Yes. I mean obviously—at least in [name of jurisdiction]. Drug costs are the single fastest growing cost in the Ministry of Health budget, and I don't think the government knows how to manage that because drugs are created and supplied through very large private companies, and while you can try to regulate that, and I think there are obviously some regulations, at the end of the day, people want to take drugs because they like a quick fix to whatever their problems are. So market demand isn't going to go away and will probably continue to grow. So they certainly have a huge influence on the health care consumer and so, indirectly, on the government (Decision-maker 1).

According to this individual, the demand for technology is fueled by patients, generates benefits for industry, and must be controlled by governments. Should we conclude, then, that the regulation and use of health technology is merely a question of politics? That the introduction of HTA or any other kind of scientific input into decision-making is doomed to fail? In accord with several other evidence-based policy-making proponents, I would answer "no" to these questions. However, it seems clear that decision-makers can easily become victims of their own cost-control initiatives when they attempt to curb what are seen as inappropriate uses of the collective health care resources. What remains obscure, however, is the ways decision-makers assess the need for high-tech medicine and appraise the validity of the demand for it.

The Gap Between the Evidence-Based Approach and the Empirical World

So far in this chapter I have explored the various rationales of four stakeholder groups—industry, physicians, patients, decision-makers—that are generally influential in health care policy-making in several industrialized countries. An examination of the Canadian situation has shown how these groups have pursued both common and conflicting interests. It has also made clear that each of these groups had a certain understanding of its ability, vis-à-vis the others, to influence and even shape policies. Indeed, they knew that the other groups could well be pushing in contrary directions, and this awareness may explain why some of the interviewees referred to their *weight* in terms of constituency size or number of votes. Less evident was their assessment of the relative cultural authority or economic power that certain groups possess, factors that are taken into account by the various parties when it comes time to strike satisfactory deals and to reach compromises (although the representatives of physician associations were more explicit about the types of knowledge, and therefore authority, they believed should influence health policies).

While each group referred to HTA as a useful input into decision-making, they seemed to hold different definitions of the dimensions (e.g., efficacy, safety, need, impact, cost) that should be assessed and inform technology-related policies. This divergence of opinion leads me to wonder whose perspective should be used when defining, once and for all, the appropriateness of a given health technology. While HTA producers may be able to provide some evidence regarding patient outcomes, risks, and cost-effectiveness, clinicians—who generally wish to optimize their work conditions and enlarge their repertoire of clinical tools (Blume 1992)—have no choice but to build convincing claims about their patients' needs. Industry, meanwhile, can forge alliances with physician and patient associations and emphasize how rapid access to innovations will benefit patients and the population in general (Gelijns and Rosenberg 1994). And added to all these claims is the fact that the value of health technology invariably remains an elastic notion, one that depends on the level of resources governments are willing to invest. Hence, desirability becomes, in large measure, a matter of affordability.

What role can (or should) HTA and scientific evidence play in such an intricate policy arena? HTA agencies are knowledge-producing organizations that often hold a societal perspective that is compatible with their public funding (Banta et al. 1995). As chapter 1 clarified, what differentiates HTA agencies from other knowledge producers (e.g., university-based research teams, private research laboratories) is the pursuit of a particular public mission (e.g., supporting the rational use and regulation of health technology) that requires an effective interface with the policy-making environment (Jasanoff 1990). Nevertheless, as I noted at the beginning of this chapter, while *access* to health technology is the prime issue for most stakeholders, various groups are tempted to reinforce their demands through both discursive (i.e., arguing on behalf of the patient's good) and factual means (i.e., arguing on behalf of evidence). Each of the four organized groups is aware of the malleability of scientific facts, but strongly supports and values independent science because it forms a basis for their advocacy, lobbying, and other policy-shaping endeavors. On this score, Kent (2003, 411) suggests that the controversy in the United States and Europe surrounding breast implants illustrates "the politicization of science, and demonstrates the limitations of science as an objective, quantifiable system of risk assessment, in formulating regulatory policy. In the context of scientific uncertainty, communicating risk and formulating policy became a highly contested *political* decision."

When it is part of a quest to persuade others of the legitimacy of certain claims, the use of HTA may prove mainly selective and symbolic (e.g., using only those study results that support one's claims or stressing the inconsistent outcomes of various studies to increase one's margin of maneuver) (Berg et al. 2004). Accordingly, HTA, and scientific evidence in general, may ultimately contribute to a shrewd increase in the discretionary power of those who make health care decisions. As more (potentially contradictory) knowledge is developed and circulated, groups find it easier to justify their positions through a selective use of that knowledge. The most pressing question, then, becomes whether or not the current regulatory processes pertaining to health technology can absolutely avoid misinformed and publicly illegitimate politics.

Figure 4.1 summarizes the ways different groups' claims can reinforce and contradict one another by stressing the desirability of health technology on the one hand and its affordability on the other. The interviews discussed earlier reveal strongly entrenched *institutional dynamics* that shape the health policy arena (e.g., defending an organization's interests, persuading others, sticking to an organization's mission, dealing with the interdependencies among all stakeholders). The interviews equally suggest that *reflexive nuances* about the complexity of the policy arena may be easily downplayed and even relegated to the background. First, from industry's perspective, R&D processes and all the actions required for accessing the health care marketplace strongly depend upon several groups, especially the physicians, who are the end users or prescribers of innovations. Second, physicians are both empowered by having access to the most advanced technologies and dependent upon industry's financial support for acquiring and updating the skills and knowledge required to use those innovations. Third, some patient associations can play a pivotal role in the translation of scientific knowledge into services and tools that can support and inform patients and the broader society; others can be more easily co-opted by physician or industry groups.

If we are to comprehend fully the nature of HTA in relation to health care decision-making, it is vital that these nuances be explored in greater depth. In chapter 5 I argue that the dynamics and views shaping the desirability of health technology must be challenged and renewed. If it were not so, pressure on governments and third-party payers would continue to escalate, and the likelihood that health technology would be used appropriately, fairly, and consistently among society's members would invariably decrease.

There is a great need in scholarship as well as in the world outside the academy to foreground other ways in which health technology can prove desirable (Webster 2004b). Accessing the latest and most sophisticated technological tool does not always correspond to the most pressing health needs. Preserving the sustainability and public nature of health care systems and fostering solidarity among citizens and belief in the legitimacy of public policies might also be important goals (Deber 2003). Pursuing

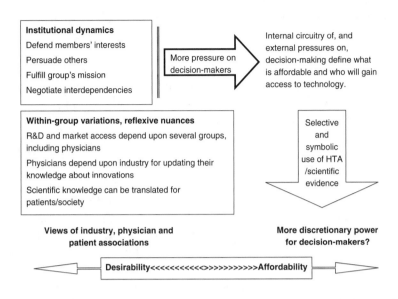

Fig. 4.1 Dynamics and views shaping the desirability of health technology.

such goals does not automatically imply using obsolete technologies, lengthening waiting lists, or practicing a form of medicine that lags behind that in other parts of the world. It does entail, however, giving more thought to the types of technologies introduced into health care systems and to their integration within *meaningful* health care services and practices. Because they are pivotal in professionals' "understanding of their responsibilities to the public affected by their work," Martin (2002, 548) argues that personal convictions and commitments "should not be dismissed as mere subjective matters lacking relevance."

In the following chapter I argue that institutional arrangements that support the regulation of health technology and health care practices must be revisited so they can allow for more ethical deliberation and practice as well as for socially responsible policies. That would be one way of creating more space in which to discuss the reflexive nuances mentioned above. Industry, physicians, patients, and government are just too interdependent for us to continue to ignore the problems associated with the inappropriate use and funding of health technologies. The pervasiveness of the private sector in university-based health care research, and in medical training and practice, must be recognized. It is too late to simply criticize or reject this participation altogether. As Lewis et al. vividly put it, "Some bargains are Faustian, and some horses are Trojan. Dance carefully with the porcupine, and know in advance the price of intimacy" (2001, 785).

I believe that everyone at the ball must learn to dance. I also believe that we are already paying the price of intimacy, although it remains largely unacknowledged because this form of intimacy is globally diffused, pervasive, and often institutionalized without being called into question. I therefore strongly emphasize the need to more fully explore the nature and characteristics of the relationships among industry, physician and patient associations, and decision-makers.

Throughout this chapter I have attempted to show that the goal and means of increasing the use of science in technology-related policy-making are often incompatible with the actual dynamics that shape the empirical world. In chapter 5 I address the fact that clinicians, decision-makers, and the public may all have particular, contingent reasons for adhering to various views about the value of health technology. That their views may not always fit neatly with what HTA producers see as appropriate does not necessarily reflect ignorance or intellectual laziness on their part. Their reasons may partly be rooted in concrete experiences (e.g., clinical practice, relatives' experiences, regulations in other jurisdictions) (Greer et al. 2002), epistemological frameworks (e.g., knowledge about a disease, a patient's ability to benefit), or political and organizational constraints and opportunities (Mol and Law 1994). Clearly, to my mind at least, the challenge is not to find the most effective way to get clinicians, decision-makers, and patients to comply with scientific evidence, but to understand how contrasting, challenging, and articulating multiple rationalities can help to move clinical practices toward more effective, fair, meaningful, and sustainable health care.

Health researchers cannot, in turn, continue despairing that clinical practice and policy-making are not based on hard evidence without recognizing that their own frameworks rely on a certain form of rationality. Strong emotional responses are likely to be encountered when restricting access to innovations equates with denying benefits to individuals (Johri and Lehoux 2003). Therefore, without proper mechanisms to secure the input of all stakeholders and the introduction of accountability in public and clinical policies, debates about the appropriate use of health technology will remain superficial, useless, or even, at times, deceitful (Giacomini 1999). And finally, to be politically legitimate, the regulation of technology must not only take values and preferences into account but also, and more importantly, identify robust, collectively endorsed practices. The regulation of technology needs, therefore, to be informed by social science research that examines why and how local practice deviates from evidence, and that illuminates the ways technology transforms clinicians and social expectations. This does not mean that scientific rationality is to be abandoned. But it should be rooted in, and articulated with, social, cultural and political ways of thinking and behaving. We have an urgent need to understand how multiple rationalities can contribute to and shape a more appropriate use of health technology. Only when such comprehension arises will HTA and science be able to foster genuinely fruitful debate around the value of medical innovations.

CHAPTER 5

An Alternative Framework

Rethinking the Problem of Health Technology

In the preceding chapter I drew on the Canadian health care policy arena in order to illustrate the typically complex and opaque institutional arrangements for regulating health technology found in advanced industrialized countries. I compared four main perspectives, emphasizing the multiple goals and interests pursued by industry, physician and patient associations, and policy-makers. Although far from homogeneous, these groups tend to defend their constituencies' interests at the *institutional level* and generally maintain that policy-making should foster access to new technologies. Providers, patients, and industry potentially benefit from evoking the familiar "for-the-patient's-good" argument. Meanwhile, often pitted against this notion of the common good, policy-makers are frequently seen as needing to be convinced to open the purse strings. At the same time, policy-makers recognize the pressures exerted on them and the limits placed on the means of controlling health technology use. Finally, within all these groups one can observe nuanced reflections about the less obvious interdependencies between the introduction of new technology and the acquisition and circulation of expert and lay knowledge among providers, patients, and the broader society in which they function.

Accordingly, the regulation of health technology—the norms, frameworks, guidelines, incentives, disincentives, and policies created and relied upon to control or shape its diffusion and use—should be seen as a *distributed* collective process of which interdependencies and the need to make persuasive claims are key features. Indeed, representatives from all four groups stress that scientific knowledge and health technology assessment (HTA) have the potential to inform health policy decision-making. Nevertheless, they tend to conceive of knowledge and evaluation as arguments (Weiss 1991) that can be mobilized in order to steer policy-making in particular directions. Upon entry into the policy arena, science is therefore transformed into a political entity (Jasanoff 1990). When it shifts from the context of its production to the context of its use, science is set loose from some of the critical principles and intellectual safeguards that typically govern its meaning and implications in the academic sphere. In this shift to another interpretive framework, using HTA to pin down the value of health technology is an equivocal enterprise. Moreover, although the "public good" argument is invoked to justify increasing access to certain technologies, in reality "the public" barely participates in deliberations involving health technology's regulation. In chapter 4 I therefore brought to light the main political processes and institutional structures that determine the introduction and funding of innovations, as well as showed how they contribute to framing access to health technology as an issue of affordability.

When combined with the social science insights addressed in chapters 2 and 3, these observations of the political and economic factors involved in health technology diffusion and use hold the potential of informing positive structural and procedural changes in health technology regulation. To date, however, such considerations have received little attention in the health technology literature. In this chapter, therefore, I begin by making the purposes, methods, and assumptions of the evidence-based approach to health technology more explicit. I then suggest five principles that could help refocus health technology research and policy on technology's desirability: explicit normativity, theoretically informed empirical insights, reflexivity, public input, and transparency. Finally, I clarify how these principles should be integrated within a deliberative democracy framework in order to overcome the challenges associated with the regulation of health technology in pluralistic societies.

Revisiting the Assumptions Underlying the Evidence-Based Approach to Health Technology

This book opened by characterizing health technology as a policy "problem" in modern health care systems and by suggesting that HTA, clinical practice guidelines (CPGs), and other evidence-based medicine initiatives are among the most salient scientific responses that have emerged in industrialized countries to address this problem (Faulkner 1997; May et al.

2003). Several chapters have also examined the social, ethical, and political dynamics that contribute to making the design and use of health technology problematic. Perhaps it is worth backtracking along this line of argumentation to ask whether health technology is inherently, and therefore unavoidably, problematic. Or, to put it in positive terms: What characteristics would make an innovation unequivocally better and *un*problematic?

Box 5.1 lists a number of attributes that, taken together, characterize medical innovations for which assessment and deliberative policy-making would appear to be superfluous. While these attributes constitute a utopian scenario, the process of making explicit an ideal situation helps to illuminate my rationale (and that of several scholars on whose work I draw) for considering health technology to be a "problem" in the first place. These criteria suggest that if health technology were affordable (and became comparatively more affordable over time), effective, safe, and ethically and socially neutral, it would not be problematic. The list suggests that cost, efficacy, safety, and ethical and social implications are relevant criteria according to which health technology's desirability must be defined. Taken as a whole, these concerns therefore reveal as much about the technological features that are valued as they do about the values against which desirability should be gauged. In a similar fashion, in what follows, I unpack some of the assumptions that currently underlie HTA production and use in order to elucidate how proponents of HTA, and of evidence-based medicine in general, frame the desirability of health technology and how I appraise the merits and limitations of their endeavor.

Box 5.1 What Constitutes A Better, Unproblematic Innovation in a Utopian World?

- A technology that is equally or more effective and costs less than its current alternative
- A technology that can be used safely and effectively by less skilled and less costly personnel
- A technology that can be used safely and effectively in any kind of setting and in all geographical areas
- A technology that solves a health problem permanently or that produces diagnostic certainty
- A technology that does not trigger side effects or reduce a patient's mobility or autonomy
- A technology that does not pose ethical dilemmas or give rise to equivocal social transformations

---

Chapter 1 offered a reading of HTA's recent history and development in industrialized jurisdictions. I also stressed there a number of challenges it now must address if it is to fulfill its mandate. Some of these challenges could be overcome by introducing incremental changes to the way HTA is produced, institutionalized, and used by decision-makers.[1] However, when one reflects on the issues addressed in this book, which can be genuinely examined as legitimate concerns only by adopting a broad perspective of what technology is and does, it becomes clear that the scope and relevance of those sorts of changes are insufficient.[2]

In the introduction and chapter 4, I emphasized the tension that frequently exists between health technology's desirability and its affordability. One might wonder why technological ingenuity seems unable to reduce this tension: "The fact that the prevailing political settlement in health care allows technology to produce inflationary effects creates a powerful tension: the dominant policy problem in health care is how to contain costs; medical technology has not been able to help solve that problem" (Moran and Alexander 1997, 574). Why, it must be asked, has technology failed to help contain costs?

Moran and Alexander (1997) argue for the need to complement microeconomic analyses of the incentives created by third-party payment that drive supply and demand with an examination of the political history of health technology. My approach acknowledges the importance of looking at the historical institutional arrangements that have shaped the desirability of health technology; however, it adds another empirical layer to the analysis: the institutional environment in which the desirability of health technology is perceived, constructed, and valued (both economically and ethically) by various groups who have a stake in its development and use. Examining the history of technology development and the social practices and structures that sustain, impede, or foster various uses of health technology have not typically been part of the HTA research agenda. That is why I have devoted so much space in this book to focusing on the insights and analytical tools that social science research has brought to the understanding of health technology and the critique of HTA.

There are a variety of reasons for carrying out such critiques. Some argue that there is sufficient evidence of HTA's failure to foster rational decision-making to justify abandoning it altogether (Berg et al. 2004). Others want to increase HTA's capacity to influence decisions and policies (e.g., implement tighter regulatory mechanisms between HTA and coverage policies) (McGregor 1992) or to create more informed consumers (Bero and Jadad 1997; Domenighetti et al. 1998). Indeed, for those who call for incremental changes, the pivotal issue becomes how the rational, evidence-based approach to health technology can be fully implemented in order to bridge the gap between current practices and more desirable ones. The principle at the root of this approach is that rationality and science can determine the "right" decisions and actions (i.e., fulfill a set of criteria pertaining to efficacy, safety, cost, and ethics).

While I do not advocate the complete abandonment of HTA, I do envision much more than incremental changes. I am especially concerned by the assumption, held by proponents of a "regulatorily stronger" HTA and by supporters of the "informed consumers" approach, that scientific rationality can and should help overcome current problems. Instead, if we return to the questions (introduced in chapter 1) that Cohen and Hanft (2004) regard as critical to health technology assessment, we can come to grips with the assumptions underlying HTA production and use today. My goal in reviewing each of these assumptions is to launch a better appraisal of HTA's epistemological and methodological underpinnings (see table 5.1). My aim is not to argue that these assumptions are erroneous, but rather to encourage a deeper awareness of the logic and framework within which HTA operates and to which any incremental changes designed to improve its relevance must of necessity be bound. As Bohman (1996, 219) astutely remarks, "Our values, modes of questioning, and ways of seeing things can become rigid and fixed, so that new aspects, new experiences, novel variations, and minority viewpoints are not even considered to be possibly relevant to deliberation." He emphasizes further that *disclosure* can help bring relevance to broader issues because it is "an act of expression that opens up new possibilities of dialogue and restores the openness and plasticity necessary for learning and change" (229). Paving the way for such "new possibilities" is, ultimately, what I hope to achieve with this chapter.

Three main points can be made about the assumptions outlined in table 5.1. First, HTA strongly relies on a postpositivist view of science in which the role of cost-effectiveness analyses is seen as both logical and authoritative (Giacomini 1999; May et al. 2003). Nevertheless, decision-making can be seen as unquestionably rational for a large group of people only for those innovations either that are less expensive and produce major health benefits or that cost a lot and generate fewer health benefits (when compared with established technologies (Wiktorowicz and Deber 1997; Laupacis et al. 1993). In addition, the time horizon according to which costs are considered adds another layer of complexity. According to Foote, there are powerful incentives for manufacturers to produce cost-reducing innovations:

Table 5.1 Key Assumptions Underlying the Evidence-Based Approach to Health Technology

Foundational HTA questions*	Related assumptions that underlie HTA production and use	Paradigmatic foundations
Economic impact: How are medical technologies changing the practice of medicine and affecting health care spending, and are they cost-effective?	There is a cost-effectiveness threshold that can distinguish "good" from "bad" innovations primarily on the basis of their health outcomes and costs.	Epistemic hierarchy: Quantification, clinical outcomes, and costs have truth-value.
Evaluation: Are technologies being evaluated appropriately?	Scientific information that can "freeze" the value of health technology is available or can be gathered, and the randomized controlled trial (RCT) is the scientific gold standard.	Science is rational and is the most desirable form of rationality for solving the "problem" of health technology.
Diffusion: Are technologies diffusing too rapidly (or too slowly) into medical practice?	There is an appropriate pace at which technology should diffuse and technology diffusion can be steered or controlled through science.	Deterministic conceptualization of what technology is and does: Health technology diffuses and improves according to a linear model.
Access: Is access to certain technologies impeded for some population groups by financial, geographic, cultural, or other barriers?	Health technology can be beneficial, but its benefits may not be distributed evenly across population groups because of "barriers" located in the individual.	Technology is in itself neutral, while society is a passive receptacle of technology.
Ethical choice: What ethical choices should guide the evaluation, adoption, and use of technologies whose long-term and short-term effects may be unknown or not clearly understood?	Ethical issues arise and must be dealt with after technologies come into existence. Ethical issues are linked to the effects of health technology over time.	

*(Cohen and Hanft 2004, 16)

(*continued*)

Table 5.1 *(continued)*

Foundational HTA questions*	Related assumptions that underlie HTA production and use	Paradigmatic foundations
Societal impact: How are technologies affecting societal behavior and organization, including society's basic demographic and institutional structures?	Health technology is an external entity that "impacts" society.	
Organizational impact: In what ways are medical technologies influencing (and being influenced by) organizational changes in the health care marketplace?	Health care systems are markets that are influenced by supply-and-demand dynamics generated by health technology.	Policy/regulatory stance: Health technology is an expertise-dependent commodity that circulates in more or less regulated markets.
Government role: What role (or roles) should governments play in attempting to deal with these issues?	Governments should not always interfere with market dynamics and clinical autonomy.	

*(Cohen and Hanft 2004, 16)

Because the DRG [diagnosis-related groups] system encourages hospital admissions but discourages long hospital stays, technologies that increase admissions for low-cost procedures may thrive; quality-enhancing innovations, which may have long-run benefits but increase present costs, may not. Even a technology that has long-run cost-saving potential may be discouraged in its early stages because costs and benefits may be uncertain (Foote 1986, 507).

HTA has prominently supported a scientific tradition that "freezes" the value of a given intervention by capturing, under controlled conditions, outcomes that are seen as amenable to quantification (e.g., mortality, morbidity, quality-adjusted life years, utilization of services) (Faulkner 1997). Recently, however, a number of observers have questioned whether patients' views should be included in order to recognize not only clinical outcomes but also the extent to which various outcomes (e.g., side effects, complications, physical losses) matter to care recipients (Coulter 2004). This suggestion is particularly warranted in the case of chronic care interventions, in the context of which mortality rates are not highly informative and coping with the consequences of various interventions depends on patients' individual preferences and lifestyles. In addition, initiatives to review and synthesize results from qualitative research, which some believe would better reflect the contexts in and processes by which health technologies are actually used, have also emerged (Dixon-Woods et al. 2004; E. Murphy et al. 1998; Leys 2003). Despite these fairly substantial theoretical advances, the postpositivist paradigm remains the basis for HTA reviews of economic analyses and clinical trials, and it operates according to a clear epistemic hierarchy comprising quantification, clinical outcomes, and costs.

A second point concerning table 5.1 concerns the way health technology diffusion is conceptualized. Asking whether a given technology diffuses too rapidly or too slowly assumes that there is an ideal pace at which it should spread. It also suggests that scientific results can specify that Platonic pace and be used to steer the process in a more rational manner, no matter what the context in which a technology is used (Mykhalovskiy and Weir 2004). This view is highly compatible with the false premise that society is a mostly passive receptacle of technology. Moreover, the debate over access to technology generally assumes that barriers to accessing a given health technology—be they financial, geographic, or cultural—are located in the individual, or at least are under her control, and are amenable to interventions targeted at the individual (e.g., patient training, financial aid). On such an understanding, it is not surprising that ethical issues are seen as generated by technology's *effects* and, consequently, as having to be dealt with after an innovation has come into existence. All these assumptions derive from a deterministic view wherein technology is seen as an entity separate from the social world (i.e., apolitical and axiologically neutral) that inherently improves over time.

A final point worth noting is that HTA producers have tended to adopt a conservative stance toward the health care marketplace. The guiding precept here is that technology regulation should be aligned with the dynamics that cause innovations to evolve in a market driven by the interplay among supply, demand, and capacity to pay (Coddington et al. 2000). Nonetheless, the demand for innovations is deeply enmeshed with claims to autonomy and expertise by medical specialists who work in large hospitals (Rocher 1990). As we saw in chapter 4, unless they are able to take control of the process, physicians typically resist most attempts to regulate technology acquisition and use. Health care managers can, of course, set financial limits as to what is affordable, but for strategic purposes they tend to generate delays and negotiate deals with those individuals and groups perceived as pivotal to upholding or expanding key clinical niches (Greer 1987). HTA can certainly play a role in such negotiations, but it is often used as a basis upon which to determine the value of a given technology as a commodity. While giving government a stronger role in the regulation of health technology is seen as legitimate in some jurisdictions (Battista et al. 1994), clinicians and industry in general still largely shape policy outcomes. However, each group depends upon the other; physicians need financial resources to update their skills and knowledge, while industry needs physicians to adopt its innovations. The evidence-based approach rarely recognizes that the alleged market in which innovations are supposed to circulate is in fact concentrated in urban centers and depends upon medical specialists. Hence, by ignoring the commercial and professional drivers of innovation, HTA remains toothless (Koch 1995).

Reviewing the questions posed by HTA and their related assumptions makes clearer the characteristics (and shortcomings) of HTA's scientific thrust and paradigmatic foundations. Completing this analysis requires examining the issue of its proper dissemination and uptake by decision-makers (Lavis et al. 2002). According to Lomas (2004, 287), although evidence-based proponents have revisited some of their initial assumptions and now promote a less credulous approach toward the role of science in decision-making, understanding of the ways in which research and decision-making processes can be articulated is still limited:

> We have moved away from the naïve individual rational actor view of evidence-based decision-making. The academic community is embracing the idea that individuals operate within a social milieu, that the characteristics of these milieus vary and must be better understood if we are to see how and when research evidence has a role, and that both research and decision-making are processes. Our missing information entails how and when to best intertwine these processes for evidence-based decision-making (Lomas 2004, 287).

As was proposed in chapter 4, the fact that several groups highly value technology assessment suggests that initiatives aimed at promoting evidence-based decision-making have already influenced the policy arena. What remains obscure is whether HTA or scientific evidence in general can be used in an apolitical manner to solve problems that carry political implications. Along these lines, Champagne et al. outline four limits to the rational use of evidence in health care: "rationality cannot replace judgment and politics in managerial and policy-making decision-making"; "technical rationality should not be pursued at the expense of social values"; "even at the clinical level, rationality may be inferior to some alternative decision-making processes" (e.g., intuitive synthesis skills); and "higher utilization may be gained at the cost of methodological rigor" (2004, 12). Each of these limitations stresses a specific lesson that students of research-based policy-making have learned. First, there is a need to acknowledge the political dimensions involved in decision-making. Second, an overly strong emphasis on quantification often leads to so-called technical rationality, which tends to obfuscate issues that are not factored into resultant measurements. Third, individuals often develop, in the context of day-to-day work, rules of thumb or expert judgment that are more appropriate than elaborate scientific analyses. Fourth, by blindly seeking to increase the usability of their findings, researchers run the risk of deviating from established methodological rules, and thereby compromise the rigor of their work.

Although even evidence-based medicine proponents have learned some lessons and accordingly readjusted most of their initial claims (e.g., those strongly criticized by clinicians and social scientists alike [Mykhalovskiy and Weir 2004]), it is worth pushing the analysis a bit further. When taken as a whole, all of the above-mentioned limitations reflect broader ambiguities. For example, it remains unclear what types of knowledge or processes fall under the rubric of rationality. Is only scientific knowledge rational? Is politics necessarily irrational? Are political dimensions not also involved in the production of science? Why is scientific rationality placed in opposition to social values? Can science be value-free? And, finally, why should rigor be the prerogative of science, as if policy-making could not have its own form of rigor? These implicit distinctions between the characteristics of science and those of policy-making need to be examined more critically (Denis et al. 2004). Indeed, when one acknowledges that both endeavors are the result of social practices, these distinctions appear misguided (Berg, et al. 2004; Jasanoff 1990); in fact, politics, values, and rationality operate in both. Therefore, treating HTA science as a "species of politics" could help further understanding of how we can introduce more accountability and reflexivity into its production (Fuller 2000, 146).

By now it should be clear that I strongly believe the presumption that clinicians, patients, and policy-makers behave irrationally and that science is the most desirable incarnation of rationality is deeply flawed. Clinicians' and patients' views also convey a certain kind of rationality pertaining to the virtue of health technology. If new technologies are constantly introduced into the market, it *must* be because earlier ones were not as satisfactory as they should have been; otherwise, why would innovation be called technological *progress* and why would medical research findings be regularly portrayed in the media as *breakthroughs*? Policy-makers struggling to control costs also obey a form of rationality. Considered together, if clinicians and patient advocates want access to more high-tech medicine and policy-makers want to spend less, is it not the case that all three groups are behaving perfectly rationally? And is this not exactly what we—as either patients or tax-payers—expect from them? So the next question to be answered is *Who* is being irrational according *to whom*?

While HTA researchers are usually comfortable arguing in favor of a collective approach to public health spending, dictating that only those technologies that have been proven effective and safe be adopted and reimbursed, it is important to recognize that such reasoning makes sense only when all its dimensions are made explicit and endorsed by all stake-holders. Among other things, it should be stressed that no evidence of benefits, risks, or costs has been produced and/or analyzed for many tech-nologies currently in use. The fact that it would be impossible to assess all technologies must also be acknowledged. Given these limitations, should the affordability argument hold only for a select few pieces of expensive new equipment? What about the desirability of other technologies?

As I argued in chapter 3, a single species of rationality does not govern clinical and social behavior. Rather, various norms structure the ways in which technology is adopted and used (or not used). Clinical practices are shaped by hierarchical expertise-based relationships and by the way uncer-tainty is defined and dealt with in the context of clinical encounters (May et al. 2003; Timmermans and Berg 2003). Social science research has shown that physicians and nurses can adopt practices that deviate from guidelines when they regard those policies as incompatible with clinical purposes and constraints. Moreover, clinical practice is not only context dependent but also relational (i.e., something performed through social interactions [Brown and Webster 2004]). Furthermore, sociologists of technology believe that innovations and their users are coproduced over time (Oudshoorn and Pinch 2003). This means that with every new tech-nology, new types of uses and users are created. Medical innovations transform clinicians by altering their knowledge, skills, and possible paths of action; they also create novel interdependencies.

Given this mutual reshaping, when HTA producers stress clinicians' over-reliance on technology (Laupacis, 2005), they are failing to acknowledge that high-tech medicine modifies clinicians and what is expected from them. And between prescribing expensive but reassuring diagnostic tests and deploying time-consuming clinical skills, who can say which is the more rational behavior? Between 1993 and 1999, the number of radiologists actively practicing in Quebec, Canada, remained basically unchanged (473 and 476, respectively: an increase of only 0.6%), while the number of diagnostic procedures they performed increased substantially (1,350,000 to 1,744,000: an increase of 29.2%) (Auditor General of Quebec 2001). Can this counterintuitive relationship between practitioner and procedure numbers be attributed to financial incentives? To patients' demands? To physicians' loss of clinical skills? By modifying its users' skills, knowledge, and opportunities to intervene, technology clearly transforms clinical practice and boosts the public's expectations regarding medicine's ability to provide diagnostic certainty. In the context of intensive efforts to foster and publicize progress in medical research (by health research foundations, hospitals, and the media), this should come as no surprise.

Increasing the role of rationality in the use of health technology will always prove difficult because it involves recognizing that rationality is largely context dependent and *inherently* multidimensional (i.e., evaluated according to criteria such as feasibility, effectiveness, cultural appropriateness, preferences) (Berg et al. 2001). Furthermore, the extent to which scientific evidence can or should supersede other decision-making logics remains obscure. Although I concur with HTA producers' call for greater reasonableness in the use of health technology, I doubt that scientific rationality alone can solve the situation. I believe that scientific rationality can bring about significant changes in health care only if it integrates reflexive consideration of underlying normativities and decision-making processes, and relies on transparent and genuine debate. Such reflexivity and productive scrutiny require time and sustained social interaction as well as the development of more elaborate institutional and political processes. These interactions should focus on examining current views and practices regarding health technology's desirability and use.

Ensuring that such interactions are able to take place can, I will argue later in this chapter, provide significant clues about ways forward for enhancing technology-related policy-making. Instead of abstractly defining what should be the appropriate framework for assessing and regulating health technology, the process of effecting positive change involves starting from what currently constitutes the empirical world (e.g., normative frameworks, professional ethos, organizational constraints) to generate propositions that are likely to resonate with or challenge actors' norms and practices (Reiter-Theil 2004). It also entails broadening the conceptualization of health technology; that is to say, recognizing it as a sociopolitical project.

Five Principles for Conceptualizing Technology as a Sociopolitical Project

Throughout this book we have observed that numerous players are directly involved in technology design, use, and regulation. Some of them are also indirectly involved through others stakeholders' claims or through actions other individuals and groups take on their behalf. Figure 5.1 outlines the network encompassing the most prominent groups that directly participate in or influence policy-making processes, and suggests that health technology regulation is the (more or less conflict-ridden) result of an ongoing interplay among those groups.

For most lay members of society, the deliberations of policy-makers, physician associations/colleges, patient associations, and industry lobbyists that lead to agreements on regulatory issues are obscure, if not inaccessible. Despite a few initiatives in industrialized countries to include nonprofessionals in health care governance structures, in practice the lay perspective is infrequently present. In addition, accountability mechanisms are often either nonexistent or too general to produce any truly informative records about the decisions made or the evidence/arguments supporting them. The main information sources pertaining to health technology regulation are therefore the electronic and print media and the experts who are called upon to comment on emerging issues or recent changes in health policies (Savoie et al. 1999). As Bohman keenly observes, "There seems to be little interaction between the public and the media analogous to the constitutional mechanisms structuring public input into the state, with citizens having less control over the systems of meaning and the purposes the media embody" (Bohman 1996, 235). In many cases a very small group of experts, officials, and lobbyists ends up influencing or making key health care decisions for the rest of society.

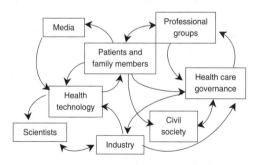

Fig. 5.1   The network of relationships that makes health technology contentious.

These current institutional arrangements need to be challenged, and new avenues for rethinking the purposes and processes of health technology regulation explored. In an effort to move these journeys forward, I have developed five principles that I believe could help to reframe the problem of health technology and to enrich the future of technology-dependent health care systems. Chapter 4 made abundantly clear the need to rely on more elaborate political processes to reconcile different, and at times conflicting, perspectives regarding the value of health technology. It illuminated the messiness inherent in policy-making processes, while highlighting that these processes are nevertheless not entirely devoid of rationality and reflexivity. Could these processes be improved? That is to say, could they be made more democratic and better fitted to pluralistic, complex, and ethnically diverse societies? I believe so. But that project requires carefully examining the structures and principles that enable civil groups to voice their concerns, to articulate their claims and reasons for wanting certain policies, and to reach compromises with respect to options that can foster the overall public good (Bohman 1996).

First Principle: Evaluation is a Process That Requires Making Values Explicit
Giacomini et al. (2003, 312) argue that HTA "has well developed methods for assessing means (effectiveness, efficiency) but less systematic approaches to assessing ends (purposes). New medical technologies' purposes and effects must be judged for their moral, social, or political value before technology assessment information can inform decisions in a meaningful way" (see also Heitman, 1998).[3] HTA producers' recent initiatives to better address the ethical dimensions of health technology (e.g., special issue of Poiesis & Praxis, 2004 [2]) point out the need to rethink their methods and theoretical underpinnings. As Grin suggests:

> Ethicists may contribute to reflexive HTA, if they combine a hermeneutic—and often also participative—methodology with a solid understanding of the relation between the health problem under scrutiny and more general critique of the health care system. Insights from the areas of science and technology studies, as well as from social philosophy, may be critical items in their tool kit (2004, 157).

These comments underscore why in chapter 2 I highlighted the various ways in which health technology embodies and reinforces values that contribute to the shaping of clinical practices. Technology is the result of creative, intentional processes that seek to "improve" the current state of affairs and change human behavior *through* technological means. Designers create technology in order to solve a problem, correct a situation, or prevent certain types of use or accident; their values are thus translated into their innovations. Because the end users of health technology are various categories of professionals and lay individuals, their values—either anticipated by designers or elicited through participatory design—are also incorporated into technology. Research on health technology should therefore seek to make explicit the ethical, social, and political values embedded in a given innovation and reinforced through its use. For instance, it could examine the extent to which an innovation exacerbates dependence on medical expertise, supports patient autonomy, or fosters social inequalities. It could also explore how the use of certain technologies reinforces or weakens institutional values (e.g., efficiency, accountability, responsiveness).

The principle of making values explicit should be understood as seeking first and foremost to foster open deliberations about the desirability of current practices. This undertaking requires creating opportunities for and vehicles by which stakeholders can explore and express the normative problems they encounter in daily practice. Chapter 3 emphasized the potential role of empirical ethics because of its primary interest in understanding real-world practices. Empirical ethics is "akin to what in ancient Greece was called *phronèsis* (practical wisdom): the insight or understanding born from and guiding experience and the capacity of, respectively, acting, judging and living accordingly" (van der Scheer and Widdershoven 2004b, 77). Because it acknowledges that moral judgments originate from and are to be found in actual experience, empirical ethics recognizes norms as dependent upon historical circumstances and cultural contexts. As a result, "new ways of dealing with normative problems can be developed by making explicit and by reflecting on what is experienced and by exchanging experiences in dialogue" (van der Scheer and Widdershoven 2004b, 78).

After agreeing on the need to discuss the embeddedness of values in health technology-related experiences, the next obvious question is Whose values should be elicited? This question touches on two issues that are crucial to any attempt to strengthen research on health technology. The first relates to political theory, because a robust framework that can accurately render the complexity of defining "representation" and eliciting values in pluralistic societies is needed. Researching the values embedded in health technology should not entail defining and choosing a single moral perspective capable of answering all the ethical dilemmas likely to arise in heterogeneous societies. I instead concur with Martin's (2002, 551) plea in favor of an ethical pluralism that could be deployed within the democratic settings in which any given technology is developed and used, an argument I develop further under my fourth principle.

The second issue relates to the ability of individuals and groups to be reflexive about their own normative frameworks. Values linked to health technology's use are far from discrete entities that can be analytically divorced from human desires, preferences, needs, and aims. Because some "practitioners may very well fail to see the problematic character of their own practices" (van der Scheer and Widdershoven 2004a, 89), it is vital to ensure that an extensive range of views is openly articulated. Furthermore, according to Melzer, a philosopher of technology whose views I introduced at the outset of this book:

> We lose our freedom to control a given means not only because it integrates itself into the world but also into ourselves. Objects we first choose as luxuries soon become necessities…. Our judgment is transformed by the very thing we are trying to judge. Thus, toward so pervasive and transforming a force as technology, we are unable to maintain a truly external and free relationship (1993, 319).

This keen observation can be reformulated and expanded using concepts drawn from science and technology studies (STS), which recognizes that social practices and technology are mutually constitutive. While it might prove impossible to maintain a free relationship with health technology (or an indisputable, neutral standpoint from which to assess its value), the fact that it shapes our judgment and that our critical faculties are likely to evolve over time and with experience in using it must be integrated into the processes and structures through which health technology is evaluated and regulated. This new approach requires reconceptualizing technology as something that exemplifies multiple normativities (see my second principle) and, more globally, encourages all participants to become more reflexive about their engagement with health technology issues (see my third principle).

Second Principle: Sociotechnical Networks Embody Multiple Norms
HTA's piecemeal approach presumes that technologies can be analyzed as discrete entities on the merits of their intrinsic qualities and properties. However, STS work has proceeded on a different basis, defining technology as part of sociotechnical networks wherein both human and technical components interact to perform various actions within specific contexts. This conceptualization holds three important implications for research

on health technology. First, health technologies are increasingly part of broader technical systems and the inherent interdependencies they necessarily create (Brown and Webster 2004). The efficacy and safety of a particular device depend upon the efficacy and safety of other technologies. Second, the knowledge and skills (usually possessed by humans) required to use health technology effectively and safely are key components that assessment cannot ignore (Lehoux et al. 1999). As patients are further transformed into users of health technology (e.g., chronic care) and as technologies migrate from institutional settings to community and private settings, the knowledge and skills that must be mastered by patients and/or their families and friends need to be taken into account. Third, there are an increasing number of "borderline" technologies (human–technology hybrids) that create regulatory hurdles because they cannot be conveniently classified as devices, implants, or technical aids. Regenerative medicine, for instance, relies on human tissue engineering and requires more complex forms of assessment (Faulkner et al. 2003, 1159). A similar argument can be raised about the fuzzy status of technologies whose main objective is not to treat a disease per se (e.g., "comfort" drugs) and technologies meant to reduce the effects of aging (Brown and Webster 2004).

By acknowledging these three implications, a sociotechnical approach is likely to offer more solid empirical ground from which to assess medical innovations. STS theorists have shown "the unstable identity and multidimensional status" of particular technologies that are not "singular objects that all stakeholders regard in the same way, as having a stable identity and purpose; rather, they are *multiply* defined innovations" (Webster 2004a, 63). This multiplicity in meaning and value has led some observers to stress that a rationalist approach to HTA "will always remain an illusion" (Berg et al. 2004, 36). Although I concur with the assertion that it is impossible to establish a single standpoint from which to assess all health technology, I believe the various meanings and normative frameworks that shape the desirability of sociotechnical networks could form the basis of vibrant deliberations if they were properly researched. In chapter 2 I highlighted the need to better understand what technologies do, and I recommended adopting, among other things, an ethnographic perspective that could highlight the fact that technology is always dualistic in nature, simultaneously enabling and constraining. Studies that take such an approach reveal the ways technologies empirically shape clinical practices as well as patients' expectations and very lives. As a result, a better understanding of how norms and ethical reasoning operate in the empirical world is extremely important

(Molewijk et al. 2004). We should first try to understand providers' and other relevant actors' (e.g., patients, families, ethicists, lawyers, managers) rationales and then redesign the sociotechnical networks in which they are embedded so as to reduce the gap between what *is* and what *ought* to be (Reiter-Theil 2004). These steps would require appropriate deliberative processes and a fine-grained analysis of the issues at stake. The effort would be worthwhile, however, because these steps have the potential of more clearly defining what is most desirable about sociotechnical networks, and to whom.

Accordingly, chapter 2 summarized three types of analysis that could facilitate opening the black box of health technology: epistemological, axiological, and sociotechnical. The first analytic type could help to define the relationship between knowledge/skills and health technology's appropriate use. It would also be able to clarify the assumptions built into the design of particular devices with respect to the cognitive abilities and responsibilities of their intended users (Prout 1996). Axiological analysis could help disclose the normative dimensions embedded in medical innovations (i.e., what types of information, interventions, and outcomes are implicitly valued and sought) and support comparative analyses of the ultimate purposes of various sociotechnical networks (Williams-Jones and Graham 2003). Finally, sociotechnical analysis could be used to examine how the power and performance of health technology rely on an effective delegation of knowledge, tasks, and skills among human and technical components. This approach would strengthen understanding of why and how local practices, organizational settings, and user education and support mechanisms influence the effectiveness, safety, and appropriateness of particular technologies (Lehoux et al. 1999). More broadly, it would also highlight the technical and sociopolitical ramifications that enable some innovations to work, spread, and become irreversible (May et al. 2003).

Conceptualizing medical innovations as sociotechnical networks would thus provide a framework capable of more accurately reflecting their normative characteristics and implications, one that recognizes that both humans and technologies are necessary for a technology to perform smoothly. This conceptualization stresses the ambiguity of proclaimed benefits by also emphasizing constraining features. Furthermore, within an evaluative approach, it enables the impact of values and norms in action to be examined (i.e., how they are socially and technically enforced through medical innovations, and how individuals and groups can contest, circumvent, or reject them [Molewijk et al. 2004]).

Third Principle: Reflexive Science is Produced Within Sociopolitical Projects

In the twenty-first century, knowledge is increasingly being called upon to provide guidance for a large range of policy issues. The importance of introducing reflexivity in scientific practices is thus crucial. On this account, Elzinga points out that closer collaboration with decision-makers and practitioners can transform researchers' views: "Working closely with 'practitioners' in the worlds of policy and politics involves not only a flow of concepts and ideas from the analyst to the decision-maker, but there is also the reverse process of getting influenced by the latter's interests and images in the policy arena" (2004, 955). It should also be noted that social scientists themselves are sometimes "consenting victims" or creators of trends and fashions that shape their research agenda. As Brown and Webster argue:

> Many historians of "assistive technologies" critically observe that disabled people's experience of machines has been neglected for years largely because it is seen as simply not up-to-the-minute enough to have attracted concerted scholarly attention. Indeed, the recent social science and humanities fascination with cyborgs is, they note, evidence of academic myopia that too often privileges accounts of the exotic over those of the mundane and the everyday (2004, 119).

Faulkner has similarly pointed out that the plasticity of HTA's mission, oscillating as it does between clinical and public health perspectives (but also emphasizing rational resources allocation), can lead to unforeseen results in decision-making and health care governance: "The workings of power are evident within and between the disciplinary discourses of HTA. The health technology metaphor serves the state by enabling the participation of the agencies of knowledge production required by the vision of a knowledge-based health service" (Faulkner 1997, 202). This explains why health technology researchers (from both the HTA and STS spheres) must be reflexive about the topics they choose to pursue, the methods they use, and their relationships with those who use their results. Elzinga goes even further and emphasizes that researchers become part of the processes that "orchestrate politics." He cautions that "it is easy to fall prey to the technological scenarios of power elites, especially if weaker actors lack the institutional clout to make a real difference in technological choices. It is not only a matter of intervention, but also a question: By whom and for what?" (Elzinga 2004, 955).

Furthermore, for HTA producers and social scientists to play a thorough role as scientific experts in policy-making, they need to make their assumptions more explicit and rethink the extent to which their own rationality should supersede the other decision-making factors that shape health care systems. Indeed, the ability to establish a dialogue between competing perspectives and to foster public deliberation is intimately linked to the ability of each actor to be reflexive about her/his own values and ends (Stengers 1993). Otherwise, these individuals and organizations might lack the capacity to understand, recognize as legitimate, and integrate into their own thinking the views expressed by others. Successful dialogue also requires being able to formulate one's own argument into what Bohman calls "public reasons" (i.e., "reasons that are generally convincing to everyone participating in the process of deliberation" [Bohman 1996, 5]). A public reason does not necessarily represent the good for everyone, but it is a reason that is answerable to one another:

> Citizens deliberate together before the audience of all other citizens, who must be addressed as political equals. This audience sets certain constraints on reasons that are public. They must be communicated in such a way that any other citizen might be able to understand them, accept them, and freely respond to them on his or her own terms (Bohman 1996, 26).

Moreover, if researchers want to play a greater role in steering public policy, they must be reflexive about the political and moral standpoints from which their claims are developed and acknowledge that they do not entirely control how their knowledge will be used and by whom. This explains why conceiving of science as a practice that operates *within sociopolitical projects* is important. If one takes this perspective, knowledge matters as much as social inequalities because dialogue is the preeminent means for building mutual trust and understanding, as well as for establishing accountability within and between various individuals and institutions that either produce or apply scientific knowledge (Fuller 2000).

Fourth Principle: Civil Society is Pivotal to Deliberations Concerning Health Technology

As the use of science in policy-making increases in step with the promotion and development of a knowledge-based economy, experts are increasingly seen as using their knowledge partly to pursue their own interests (Faulkner 1997). It is also becoming clear that "far from reducing uncertainty, more information also has the effect of making people aware of the complexities of science and that science does not speak with one uniform and necessarily coherent voice" (Brown and Webster 2004, 113). Although blind faith and trust in science have eroded across several sectors (Beck 2001), medicine triggers mixed reactions: "Western societies in the late twentieth century are characterized by people's increasing disillusionment with scientific medicine and yet, paradoxically, there is also an increasing dependence upon biomedicine to provide the answers to social as well as medical problems" (Calnan et al. 2005, 1938).[4]

For Bohman, who advocates a deliberative approach to policy-making, public trust is a moral resource that "*increases* through use" (1996, 169). This may explain why he suggests that "mechanisms needed to maintain trust may also preserve *equality,* since experts cannot be effective unless they convince non-experts of their claims" (Bohman 1996, 169). If scientists are asked to make their claims both public and more accountable, it should be easier to assess the value of various scientific claims. Similarly, Fuller[5] argues that "the fundamental problems facing the governance of science today rest on issues of representation: both how science represents its own interests and how it represents the public's epistemic interests. Answers to these questions can be given only once we specify who can participate in science, and how" (2000, 155).

Because many regard the current sociopolitical implications of scientific and technological advances as fraught with complexity and uncertainty, increasing interaction between scientists and the public and involving the public in health policy-making have been widely promoted (Abelson et al. 2003; Pivik et al. 2004). More precisely, there are at least two areas in which deliberations about health technology could solicit the involvement of civil society: HTA activities and policy-making. I briefly discussed a few examples pertaining to the first area in chapter 4. Preliminary assessments of these initiatives reveal useful information about their shortcomings and suggest areas for improvement. As an illustration, the United Kingdom-based Health Technology Assessment program includes consumers[6] on various panels and committees (e.g., research prioritization meetings, research proposals reviews, research reports reviews). In their report on this initiative, Royle and Oliver observe that while consumer involvement made a valuable contribution, it had to be supported by a mentor system, guidelines, and help sheets to orient panel members. This was despite the participants' previous experience in consumer organizations that regularly dealt with research and policy-making issues. Commenting on this difficulty, one participant said, "It is a bit like sending a message to Mars, not knowing whether the recipients want, need, or can relate to what one has written!" (quoted in Royle and Oliver 2004, 496). This remark highlights the role socialization plays in making what remains a *research-driven* endeavor function smoothly. Consumers usually have limited experience with discussing research methods, and even completing reviewing forms—a mundane task for researchers—can be a challenge:

> Consumers invited to comment on draft final reports ... found the reviewing forms inadequate and irrelevant to the main thrust of their contributions. Even so, consumers have been able to highlight issues about patients' views, social contexts, information and support needs, long-term outcomes, and dissemination of research findings to consumers (Royle and Oliver 2004, 495).

Royle and Oliver also reported having "faced difficulties in quickly identifying appropriate consumers" (2004, 497). They outlined a number of criteria, excluded individuals who were in conflict of interest (e.g., health practitioners, managers, or researchers), and recruited representatives of "volunteer-led organizations, major charities, campaigning groups and self-help groups" (495). As suggested in chapter 4, these are organized groups that pursue a particular mission and are therefore not, strictly speaking, "ordinary" citizens. Nevertheless, in their recent systematic review, Oliver et al. concluded that "more success might be expected if research programs embarking on collaborations approach well-networked consumers and provide them with information, resources, and support to empower them in key roles for consulting their peers and prioritizing topics" (Oliver et al. 2004, 103). This position more or less implies that for these particular sorts of lay individuals to become proficient and useful in a research-driven environment, they may have to be "reconfigured" (e.g., be better equipped or supported to carry out the research-oriented tasks delegated to them). It also begs the question of the extent to which such individuals and groups can really express their own concerns in their own ways. In other words, perhaps further experiences in public involvement in HTA should also examine ways to maximize learning from lay individuals instead of making them "fit" into inflexibly structured research-driven endeavors.

The second area in which the public could be involved is the broader policy-making process. Such a proposition almost always, however, raises the issue of the public's scientific literacy. In Canada, a national survey conducted in the early 1990s by the Medical Devices Review Committee (MDRC) found that "the public has a high level of confidence in the safety of medical devices and faith in the system to ensure the safety and effectiveness of medical devices" (Finlay et al. 1994, 189). The Canadian public reportedly believed that all medical devices were subject to evaluation before entering the market, whereas, according to the researchers, only about 5% of such innovations were subject to regulatory assessment. Since the early 1990s, several major incidents in Canada and Europe (e.g., HIV and the management of the blood supply, bovine spongiform encephalopathy [BSE], severe acute respiratory syndrome [SARS], hospital-acquired nosocomial infections) have attracted widespread media attention, which may have contributed to a weakening of public trust (Kent and Faulkner 2002; Kent 2003).

Although "it seems to be assumed that public trust will follow from having lay people involved" in advisory or policy committees, as Dyer notes (2004, 346), the concepts of expertise and laity must first be investigated and defined. Extending this point to determine the relevance and impact of public involvement in policy-making, we need to examine how representation is achieved, the type of procedures used, the information base supporting the process, and the outcomes in terms of policy (e.g., legitimacy, accountability), decisions, and impact on participants and decision-makers (Abelson et al. 2003). It is also important to reflect carefully about exactly what representatives of the public are being asked to comment on and to achieve when they participate. The assumption that their mere presence gives credibility to public decisions must be challenged. Can individuals really represent a *collective* opinion? Can a *consumer* group define the public good?

Issues such as these underscore why injecting political theory into the mix would be useful; that is to say, it could serve as a basis for designing thorough public involvement mechanisms. Otherwise, public involvement initiatives could be reduced to mere focus group marketing exercises[7] on the satisfaction with health care services and technologies or the readability of scientific reports. While such issues do matter, what I really envision when I imagine "civil society" as a pivotal participant in discussions on health technology are deliberative processes that can substantively address health technology as a social project and explore ways in which the public good can be achieved. Beyond punctual, highly visible public consultation exercises, formal mechanisms to support continuous and sustained discussion and interaction between lay groups and decision-making bodies are required. Such mechanisms would be aimed at overcoming the power, communicative, and political inequalities that create deliberative inequalities among citizens in the first place (Bohman 1996).

Another important dimension that requires further articulation through public consultation is the imperfect overlap between the common good and individual desires and aspirations. Although health care systems in several international jurisdictions now emphasize individuals' right to choose which medical interventions they do or do not want, the long-term outcomes of this trend could be disappointing (Fox et al. 2005). An overemphasis on individual rights cultivates the idea that health technology is first and foremost a private good that private persons should acquire (Coddington et al. 2000), and it discourages any attempt to publicly define what should be part of common (publicly funded) health care. Such a focus on individual rights and autonomy will inevitably lead to an emphasis on the ability to pay as the driving force behind technology use. And if I am doubtful about the capacity of scientific rationality to introduce appropriateness and consistency in health care practices and policies, I am equally concerned about the impact of a laissez-faire market approach that will principally benefit the more affluent members of society. Resourceful and wealthy people have a greater probability of achieving more, and are also more likely to thrive in favorable environments (Bohman 1996). I also reject the tyranny of the societal perspective if it cannot be responsive to individuals' preferences and values at the same time it is publicly accountable. Civil society must be called upon in order to increase rational deliberation on the use of health technology, but in a way that acknowledges social diversity and leaves room for individual autonomy.

Perhaps recognizing the interdependence among individual and social freedom and welfare is necessary for such an endeavor to succeed. As illustrated in chapter 4, every stakeholder group in Western health care systems (including the industry) attempts to influence other groups that, they believe, possess power over decisions related to health technology. Without a doubt, several observers would conclude that such power plays cannot be avoided. When Bohman reflects on the political pessimism surrounding contemporary democracy, he stresses that critics often overemphasize social complexity and its accompanying difficulties, and "ignore the *interdependencies* between social institutions and the publics that constitute them and constantly reinterpret their basis. The question for deliberative theorists is how to make these social interdependencies more democratic" (Bohman 1996, 152). The goal, accordingly, should be to rethink the institutional arrangements that presently impede the broad expression of public reasons and, consequently, tend to facilitate discretionary decisions and policies by a handful of experts, lobbyists, and policy-makers.

Fifth Principle: The Private Sector's Role in Publicly Funded Health Care Systems Must be Made Explicit

Despite the importance of the private sector in health technology issues, only a few scholars have systematically addressed the reasons why certain innovations emerge and others do not, as well as the implications of using public funds to assess or use technologies that generate profits for manufacturers and revenues for clinicians (McKinlay 1981; Moran and Alexander 1997). I believe that the ties binding industry and high-tech medicine are not only pervasive but also impossible to escape. Even university-based research increasingly depends on private funding:

> In 2000, "business enterprise," which was almost exclusively the pharmaceutical industry (although Statistics Canada does not break down the figures), accounted for about 43% of gross domestic expenditures on research and development in the health field. ... Universities and teaching hospitals received $161 million from industry, which was more than the amount from provincial governments combined and over half the amount received from federal sources (Lewis et al. 2001, 783).

This trend toward ever-increasing private sector involvement began a few decades ago. In the United States, for instance, $8 billion was spent on biomedical research in 1980, and "industry had about 30% of that eight billion, whereas the National Institutes of Health had 60%. In 1993 industry's component had risen to 48%, whereas the National Institutes of Health, although rising in absolute dollars, had fallen to 40%" (Sanders 1995, 1539).[8] Specific technological and market opportunities profoundly modify the ways health care companies invest in research, as indicated by the fact that in 2001 "the top five biotechnology companies spent an average of $89,400 per employee on R&D, compared with an average of $31,200 per employee for the top drug firms" (Cohen and Hanft 2004, 64). Private-sector investment in research and health care innovation is also partly due to changes in the sociopolitical and business environments. Some of the most significant innovations in diagnostic imaging are adaptations by military equipment firms that sought new business as traditional defense markets shrank. As Moran and Alexander (1997) note, all the major military contractors—IBM, General Electric, and McDonnell Douglas—are also leading health technology contractors.

Ignoring such ties is paradoxical on the part of HTA producers: they are content to argue that only cost-effective innovations should be adopted, yet refuse to recognize that the private sector largely (and increasingly) shapes both the ability to provide evidence and the innovations introduced into health care. And here I am not arguing that market-driven innovations are bad per se, or that the private sector's interests are necessarily in direct conflict with health care principles and needs. What I would like to see is a more sophisticated conceptualization of the private sector's role in publicly funded health care systems and research that could tackle the tensions and issues that contribute to narrowing the problem of health technology to mainly a question of affordability. As Moran and

Alexander stress, we need more subtle analyses of the interplay between health care providers and technology developers that generates certain types of innovations: "Technological innovation is not simply a matter of one group of petty capitalists—inventors—endangering the skill base of another group of petty capitalists, doctors: it involves competition and conflict between organized industrial and professional interests" (Moran and Alexander 1997, 582). They add that technological innovation can provoke struggles between medical specialists and the inventors, and between groups of specialists. As a result, technological projects that threaten a clinical practice can be sidelined.

Regulatory mechanisms also play a role in the emergence of innovations (Abraham 2002). For example, when the risk-based classification regulatory system in Canada was revised, one of the criteria taken into account was that the industrial competitiveness of the country's medical device industry must not be compromised (Finlay et al. 1994, 193). But exactly what would such compromise entail? What safety threshold would a national regulatory policy accept?

Examining the way commercial strategies can generate unexpected consequences, Kent and Faulkner (2002) found new governance regimes that affect prosthetic devices (e.g., the Trilucent breast implant and the 3M Capital hip prosthesis) and induce changes in regulatory structures. Brown and Webster comment on their findings:

> ... adaptations [to the existing devices] arose because the industry needed to maintain competitive distinctiveness within the market for implants and could only really achieve this by introducing relatively novel innovations into the otherwise routine technologies. And yet, even these minor changes were sufficient to destabilize their safety and efficacy. The artifacts showed some signs of premature failure, and doubts were raised about the design changes on which their commercial innovativeness had been built (2004, 122).

Kent and Faulkner argue that the proliferation of many different models of the same type of device is not dictated by clinical needs. Although such proliferation may be regarded as offering "more choice" to consumers, surgeons typically remain the key decision-makers (2002, 191). They further stress that medical devices must be understood in an international context:

> Like other industrial sectors in the global economy, medical device manufacture is big business and evidence from pharmaceuticals suggests that business interests have a powerful effect on

regulatory policies. The driving force for harmonization of standards in this area, as with pharmaceuticals, is the reduction of obstacles to trade and the creation of a strong European market (2002, 205).

A more elaborate conceptualization of the private sector's role within health care organizations should also go beyond the dichotomy that views public institutions as "essentially devoted to public goods" and corporations as mostly preoccupied with private goods (W. Martin 2002, 556). Both public and private organizations rely on the production and use of both types of goods (e.g., salary, prestige, power, solidarity, caring, equity). In addition, health technologies are not, strictly speaking, either public or private; they generally depend on the injection of both public and private resources (e.g., government subsidies, shareholders' support) and can produce both public and private benefits (e.g., health, profits and revenues) and costs (e.g., morbidity, litigation). Researchers should therefore examine the broader flows of public–private resources, benefits, and costs that arise in the context of concrete technological development projects. Such analyses would clarify whether the overall desirability of various health technologies is compatible with socially negotiated ideals, including the perceived need to foster industrial competitiveness. After all, as Webster suggests, it is possible to bring to the fore multiple dimensions that define the quality of health technology. Commenting on the discussions that arose during a workshop addressing innovative health technologies, Webster notes that the most important question that began to emerge was

> How can we best discern the direction of health innovation and how to determine the quality of the innovation itself? "Quality" was seen to relate both to *sustainable* health innovation but also [to] that which might be seen to be demonstrably a (therapeutic, curative, preventative) *public good*. Herein, as suggested by a number of participants, lies the possibility of a critical but constructive intervention by social scientists in the health policy arena. Claims made on behalf of novel innovation can be assessed against such criteria (Webster 2004b, 2; emphasis added).

Rethinking the criteria Webster identifies might indeed prove promising because it would thrust some key objectives of health care systems, such as sustainability and public orientation, into the analysis. Solely emphasizing such public dimensions may, however, prove counterproductive. Revisiting the criteria defining innovation could make it possible, for instance, to

Table 5.2 Strengthening HTA and Research on Health Technology

Proposed changes and their goals	How such changes could be implemented
Broadening perspectives Goal: Build a better understanding of the implications of health technology in society in order to tackle the issues that matter from a public policy point of view.	Developing joint studies with anthropologists, sociologists and political analysts of technology and health Integrating social science research findings by learning how to refer to the relevant literature and by hiring social scientists in HTA agencies (see "redesigning HTA structures" below) Making explicit the political, ethical, and social issues embedded in technology (e.g., actors, flow of resources, knowledge, and power) Identifying and contacting groups affected by a given technology who have not yet been heard
Expanding methods Goal: Produce assessments that are informed by the multiple "rationalities" and values that prevail in a given society.	Integrating qualitative research methods in assessments Documenting in more subtle ways patients' and communities' experiences of technology Developing health indicators and/or educational material with patients in order to better reflect what matters to them Articulating different views (e.g., patients', experts') in order to identify potential contradictions, interests, and conflicts
Redesigning HTA structures Goal: Create an organizational structure in which HTA can establish legitimate and productive relationships with social organizations and industry as well as potentially trigger concrete actions.	Establishing in-house multidisciplinary teams of evaluators Establishing advisory committees with social organizations and industry representatives in order to circulate information and debates about technology Enabling patients' involvement in HTA design or in technology implementation and follow-up Stimulating and informing public debate by organizing seminars and public forums (on methods and content of HTA)
Reconsidering the object of inquiry Goal: Comprehensively capture the socio-political issues relative to technology's stages of development, diffusion, and use.	Identifying technological and/or social alternatives Describing the socio-political configuration of given technologies Conducting broader economic analyses (e.g., market structure, profitability, flow of resources)

Source: Adapted from Lehoux and Blume (2000).

acknowledge more exhaustively the private, industrial dimensions (e.g., market [dis]incentives, innovativeness, exportability) that are currently structuring (albeit in a more or less obscure manner) many countries' regulatory environments (Australia, Productivity Commission 2005). In addition, the temptation to reduce the decision to use health technology to a private matter must be resisted. "Accountability increasingly, it seems, resides in the contractual relationship between the providers and users of technologies rather than via a wider social accountability" (Brown and Webster 2004, 84). The downside of this individualization of accountability is that it may serve to increase social inequalities and the instability of public policies (Cookson and Maynard 2000). There is, therefore, a need to acknowledge the plurality of beliefs, values and practices that animate and steer private and public institutions and interests in particular ways and that might (or might not) be aligned with one another. Articulating some of the objectives of industry with those of (public) health care systems and rethinking the commercial and regulatory constraints and incentives that shape certain types of innovations should help to clarify why certain technologies are worth developing more than others.

I firmly believe the five principles I have outlined could inspire concrete changes and, ultimately, strengthen research on health technology and HTA (see table 5.2). They aim at broadening the epistemological basis of assessments, at establishing fruitful dialogue among health technology researchers and groups that have a stake in health technology use and regulation (including industry), and at repositioning the analysis of health technology's value in the context of public policies. More particularly, fine-grained analyses that can illuminate the roles of the private and public sectors in health technology development and use should help policymakers to devise incentives and strategies that promote more meaningful innovations. Equally important is the capacity to produce reflexive science that can appraise and readjust its means and purposes within social and political projects. And it is this capacity that will largely determine the relevance and outcomes of an increased reliance on scientific knowledge in policy-making.

An Alternative Framework That Integrates Deliberative Processes

The five principles I outlined above seek to go beyond the current scientific and policy debates that, as I described in the introduction, contribute to a misleading framing of the problem of health technology. The principles are thus rooted in and further develop the issues I said were key to understanding health technology in modern health care systems (see table 0.2 in the introduction). Figure 5.2 summarizes the relationship between

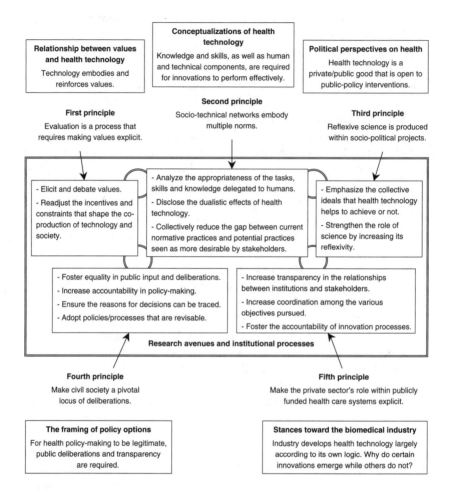

Fig. 5.2 An alternative framework for thinking about health technology.

these issues and the five principles for conceptualizing health technology as a sociopolitical project. This framework also incorporates a few research avenues (to be described in the conclusion) and the institutional processes that are necessary to enrich academic and policy-related thinking about health technology. One objective of the framework is, eventually, to ensure that efforts to increase rationality in health technology use and regulation are democratic and legitimate. The rest of this chapter will therefore focus on how deliberative processes can be made integral components of that alternative framework.

The framework should help to establish a dialogue among several groups that can regenerate the "epistemic community" that so far has framed the problem of health technology only in terms of affordability. As Campbell observes:

> "Epistemic communities" are responsible for generating new ideas and disseminating them among national policymakers as well as others in the international community. Epistemic communities are networks of professionals and experts with an authoritative claim to policy-relevant knowledge, who share a set of normative beliefs, causal models, notions of empirical validity, and a common policy enterprise (Campbell 2002, 30).

In particular, we need to revisit HTA proponents' claims that ignore the changing institutional environments in which health technologies are designed and marketed, on the one hand, and the role of science in social governance, on the other.[9] This is one of the reasons I emphasized the importance of integrating reflexivity into the production and use of research, including HTA and STS. If both fields are able to play pivotal roles in increasing knowledge about health technology, neither can be relieved of the responsibility of accounting for its objectives toward, and impact on, social policies and practices.

Another equally important reason for regenerating the health technology epistemic community is to reach, and to respond to the concerns of, a broader group of participants. Enriching the framing of health technology policy and ensuring it will remain at least somewhat grounded in the empirical world require new institutional processes more likely to speak to practitioners, patients, manufacturers, health care managers, and public interest groups as well as to facilitate their engagement in science-based policy-making.

The health technology policy arena is one of the most pressure-laden in industrialized countries. An increasing use of economists and lawyers in policy debates (Moran and Alexander 1997) adds to the complexity and diversity of the claims made in this policy arena. These claims involve overlapping and competing issues of safety, cost, clinical benefit, liability, the moral responsibility of facilitating access, and the reasonableness of delaying introduction. Given the interdependencies among stakeholders, the protection or expansion of one group's interests means that other groups must accept its claims as legitimate and/or its authority as significant (Light et al. 2003). Because of medical technology's clinical, technical, ethical, and political complexity, these claims, including those rooted in science, often introduce confusion over determining value.[10] The only way to reduce confusion and to learn about technology's desirability is to deliberate openly and frequently.

A deliberative approach to health technology would be capable of generating not only wider input into policy-making, but also accountability and transparency in the process. The objective here would be to render more explicit the rationale behind key decisions in health technology policy-making and the compromises that stakeholder groups make on behalf of broader social interests (Garcia-Altes, et al. 2004). Increasing public accountability for these decisions should make it possible to strengthen a collective and pluralistic rationality in the use and regulation of health technology. Such a change would also avoid the trap of resorting to science as the exclusive foundation of policy, which often amounts to doing politics *through* science with little respect for democratic principles.

Bohman suggests that four main difficulties confront deliberative democracy in contemporary societies: "cultural pluralism, which undermines the possibility of a general will, a unitary common good, and a singular public reason"; "social inequalities, which may produce a vicious circle of exclusion from effective participation in deliberation"; "social complexity, which makes it necessary for deliberation to take place in large and increasingly powerful institutions"; and "community-wide biases, which restrict public communication and which also narrow the scope of feasible solutions to social conflicts and problems" (1996, 238). These four problems are particularly acute in health technology policy-making. Devising one-size-fits-all policies is, in fact, an impossible task in culturally diverse societies (Reiter-Theil 2004). Social inequalities are also central concerns in modern health care systems that increasingly require resourceful patients and informal caregivers, and that often struggle with equitably distributing scarce resources across various groups (D. Martin et al. 2002). In addition, the number, size, and complexity of institutions (e.g., hospitals, professional colleges, regulatory bodies, insurance companies, community-based services) involved in health technology delivery, management, and use often lead to significant variations in access. Finally, misunderstandings and a lack of space in which to deliberate and voice concerns often reduce the collective capacity to find creative solutions to systemic, technology-related problems (Oliver et al. 2004).

The importance of these difficulties in the future of health care systems can easily be underestimated and tossed aside as pressing day-to-day issues absorb health care providers' and managers' efforts and energy. Nevertheless, they are not likely to lessen over time. This is why deliberative processes are both promising and necessary—they generate a collective dialogue on health technology and help to set in motion productive next steps.

Drawing on and expanding Habermas's theory of discursive action, Bohman develops a model for deliberative processes in which "it is crucial that citizens (and their representatives) test their interests and reasons in a public forum before they decide. The deliberative process forces citizens to justify their decisions and opinions by appealing to common interests or by arguing in terms of reasons that 'all could accept' in public debate" (Bohman 1996, 5). On Bohman's account, dialogical deliberation is needed to resolve atypical problematic situations and breakdowns of coordination. Lack of coordination in health technology policy and use can explain both maintenance of the status quo and unexpected moves forward. In such situations, dialogue has failed and decisions may not have passed the test of reasonableness with a large group of people.

For Bohman, dialogue is dynamic, pivotal, and transformative:

> In dialogue there is movement. Each speaker incorporates and reinterprets the other's contributions in his or her own. After a sufficient length of time, speakers begin to use expressions that they did not employ before; the process of trying to convince others may alter one's own mode of expression but also the reasons one finds convincing. One often hears oneself say things when made accountable to other specific actors that one might not have endorsed otherwise (1996, 58).

According to this understanding, dialogue can transform both the individuals who express their ideas and the people who receive them. It can create accountability for a speaker as much as it does for those who listen. It may also spark innovativeness and creativity. When new individuals contribute their views, they may reframe the issues or make relevant certain aspects that have hitherto been marginal.[11] The key principles underpinning deliberative democracy are increased accountability, broader input, sharing of views, and continuous processes that are both flexible and open to revision.[12] As Bohman goes on to say:

> Citizens will be more likely to overcome their myopia and ethnocentrism and to think of their democratic practices in an inclusive and future-oriented way, knowing that their decisions may have to be revised to maintain publicity and equality. They will also regard themselves as potentially occupying the minority position; even if they are in the majority for now, this alone does not lend their arguments epistemic force as necessarily the better ones (1996, 184).

A vibrant public sphere makes changing beliefs and attitudes possible through continuous dialogue, but it must also be able to alter the framework in which deliberation takes place. The emergence of what Bohman calls "new publics" (i.e., new coalitions or social groups) can alter citizens' established relationships to democratic institutions, thereby facilitating a renewal of deliberative processes and frameworks. Indeed, according to Light et al. (2003), the spread of political skills and new technologies to the wider population has helped mobilize such new interests.

The objectives and principles of Bohman's theory of deliberative democracy are similar to propositions put forward by several political scientists and philosophers of science (Rouse 1991). Fuller, for instance, suggests that the governance of science in modern societies should adopt principles drawn from political theory. He highlights three in particular. First, *coalitions* involved in the production of knowledge (e.g., universities, government, corporate interests) should clearly state their positions and should "treat research programs as party platforms" (Fuller 2000, 147). This approach would force scientists to reflect on the ways various constituencies might have a stake in the outcome of their research and increase their awareness of the consequences of knowledge production. Second, *contestation* should be made possible, and it should be facilitated by creating forums for managing conflict publicly and for evaluating and comparing various research programs openly. Third, a form of *election* should be devised that would create incentives for reporting and accounting for research programs on a regular basis (147).

The call Fuller and Bohman make for expanded public accountability and transparency in the institutions that govern the production and use of knowledge in policy-making is compatible with political analyses of how changes in the health care policy arena come about. Based on their examination of the links between the biotechnology and pharmaceutical industries, social movements, and grassroots organizations, Light et al. conclude that when "organized voices" are heard and groups exert social leadership, a series of mainstream policy changes can be initiated: "These movements articulate principles by which corporations can serve the best interests of consumers and society as a whole. They are changing the culture, the political economy, the terms of the debate, and even the regulations" (Light et al. 2003, 498). Such observations converge in a clear acknowledgment of the more open, unstable policy networks that characterize contemporary industrialized societies in which advocacy groups are becoming active at the same time as political entrepreneurship increases and government sponsors the creation of such groups.

Because increasing collective rationality in health technology use and regulation requires more than passively acknowledging the continuous emergence of social movements, a deliberative democracy framework offers a useful array of principles and processes that could be applied to health technology research programs and health technology-related institutions. The main goals would be to increase coordination and to manage interdependencies. In such an endeavor, however, consensus is not, and should not be seen as the overarching goal of deliberations. Participants are not obliged to convince and persuade others; rather, they must ensure that their claims can be understood and answered by a wide range of other individuals and groups.

Another important aspect of Bohman's deliberative democracy framework lies in its reflexivity about its very nature: "By irrationally believing in the powers of reason, including rational political deliberation, deliberators fail to acknowledge the limits of reason and thus to apply the self-critical capacities of reason to public reason itself" (Bohman 1996, 157). In other words, reason and deliberation cannot solve the whole problem of health technology.

What they can accomplish, however, is significant. In the context of pluralist societies, if the effects of inequalities are not dealt with, "those who are the most successful and competent in deliberation could well be those who are already the most well off" (Bohman 1996, 105). Correcting such inequalities in and through deliberation would enable more thorough reflection on the types of technologies that are introduced into health care systems and their integration within meaningful health care services and practices. Deliberative processes could form the basis of a renewed approach to the regulation of health technology. Introducing and acting upon the five principles I described earlier should help to reframe the problem of health technology and deepen academic and policy-oriented thinking about the relationships between health technology and providers' practices, patients' lives, and modern health care systems. As I mentioned in chapter 4, the main challenge for the future of health care systems is not to find the most effective way to get clinicians, decision-makers, and patients to comply with scientific guidelines. Rather, the principal hurdle to overcome is to fashion ways to contrast, challenge, and articulate the multiple normativities and rationalities that shape clinical practices and health care policies. Only when this obstacle has been overcome can we hope to move toward the delivery of effective, fair, meaningful, and sustainable health care.

Conclusion:
Toward Better Innovations

The Desirability of Health Technology

In chapter 5 I laid out an alternative framework for thinking about health technology in modern health care systems. In so doing, I set forth five principles intended to increase the relevance and integration of various streams of research on health technology. These principles were meant to address the five issues I identified in the introduction: the relationship between values and health technology, conceptualizations of health technology, political perspectives on health, the framing of policy options, and stances toward the biomedical industry. In chapter 5 I also underscored the importance of implementing deliberative processes capable of strengthening the nature and scope of the knowledge and normative assumptions involved in research, clinical, and policy debates on health technology.

Throughout my research on various health technologies, I was repeatedly confronted with the seminal question "How and when do we know that a given innovation is *better*?" In response to this foundational concern I argue that certain innovations in health care systems can be both different *and* better. They are merely "different" when the burdens and benefits of their use are shifted across time or groups. They are "better" when the rationale that has led to their creation as well as their coordinated application in real-world scenarios are explicitly consistent with stakeholders' normative expectations. Thus, determining the value of innovations requires reflexive, inclusive, and transparent research and deliberation.

This requirement explains why the framework I have developed seeks to enable thorough discussion of the desirability of medical innovations and the meaningfulness of current health care practices. Unlike current policy and research initiatives such as health technology assessment (HTA) or the evidence-based medicine movement in general, the main thrust of my proposed framework neither imposes nor forces upon the empirical world a predefined system of normative beliefs that I claim are more rational than all others. Rather, the framework should be seen as a tool whose purpose is to open intellectual and deliberative spaces in which various views can be expressed, contrasted, and negotiated. I developed it based on the key recognition that current practices are normative and that technology plays a pivotal role in defining, enticing, and prolonging the expression of certain values and preferences in clinical practices and, by extension, in society. By making these normative dimensions explicit and by discussing in a structured and accountable manner the ways things could be better—including for whom and with what implications—the framework's primary function is to support new conceptualizations of health technology's *desirability*.

It is now time to bring some closure to the intellectual journey on which this book has traveled. The initial objective was to examine and articulate two main bodies of literature—HTA and science and technology studies (STS)—in order to understand and then reframe the problem of health technology. In an effort to fashion a new intellectual space that creates dialogue between these two fields, I have also found it necessary, of course, to integrate concepts and insights from other streams of literature (e.g., political theory, governance of science, ethics). Such an interdisciplinary bricolage is, however, never straightforward. In this concluding section of my study I have thus chosen to synthesize the main arguments of the book and suggest new research avenues, to discuss the book's limitations, to offer a few key policy recommendations, and to explore what adding intelligence to innovations could mean for the future of modern health care systems.

Health Technology in Modern Health Care Systems

Tables 6.1 to 6.5 summarize the main arguments each chapter of this book has advanced with respect to the five ways that health technology "matters" (issues that were first raised in the introduction and then further discussed in subsequent chapters). In what follows, I highlight the key points for each of these issues and offer suggestions for further research.

Table 6.1 Summary of the Relationship Between Values and Health Technology

Chapter 1	Chapter 2	Chapter 3	Chapter 4
HTA has been defined as multidisciplinary research even though, in practice, the emphasis is on epidemiology and economic analysis	The social sciences offer additional points of entry and intellectual lenses that help to define the value of innovations	The design process articulates needs and expectations regarding appropriate and useful health interventions and seeks compromises that can rally those who have a stake in the marketing and use of health technology	Accessing the latest and most sophisticated technology does not necessarily correspond to the most pressing health needs, while preserving the sustainability, fairness, and legitimacy of health care systems can prove to be important goals
Less than 25 percent of the HTA reports available in Canada from 1995–2001 discussed ethical and social issues	Non-medical variables influence the effectiveness of health technology (e.g., emotions, knowledge, values, beliefs, cultural practices, social interactions, organizational structures and processes, financial incentives, and regulatory frameworks)	Current practices are largely shaped by needs, desires, values, and intentions that are co-constructed by clinicians and patients	
Two key tensions result: 1) The societal purpose of HTA's promotion of a rational use of scarce resources does not converge with the interests of *every* stakeholder. 2) When defining the value of health technology for society, HTA presumes that effectiveness and costs are authoritative criteria	Health technology mediates life, risks, identity and kinship, knowledge and uncertainty, power, mobility, autonomy, and death	Technology-mediated norms are relational	
		Health technology embodies current values and intentions and is the original impetus to new ideals	
		Oscillating between what is and what could be, as well as between what is and what ought to be, remains pivotal in any design process. Such balancing acts are as much creative as normative	

Chapter 5 – First principle: Evaluation requires making values explicit.

The Relationship Between Values and Health Technology

In chapter 1, I focused on the recent development of HTA, examined the content of assessments, and summarized the expectations of various stakeholders toward HTA (see table 6.1). I also showed that the literature on HTA does not offer a trenchant discussion of the values underpinning technological change in health care systems. In chapter 2 I explained how social science research can supplement HTA by providing insights into the ways in which values affect health technology's use. Next, in chapter 3, I extended this idea by examining the normative dimensions that designers import into health technology and by stressing the fact that clinical practices are co-constructed by providers' and patients' values, beliefs, and intentions. Furthermore, this chapter emphasized the *relational character* of the norms mediated through technology, which both embodies current values and triggers new sets of ideals with respect to what others ought to do and value. Then, in chapter 4, I argued that the discussion of health technology's value can hardly ignore or downplay the broader goals that (public) health care systems aim to achieve. The desirability of health technology should thus be appraised in terms of innovations' ability to help meet (or compromise) these other objectives.

By outlining a framework for thinking about health technology, in chapter 5 I suggested that *eliciting and debating values* should become integral to research on health technology (especially in HTA or other types of evaluation). This approach would involve clarifying how a wide range of individuals and groups (e.g., managers, providers, patients, the public) perceive the desirability of various technological ends and means in the realm of public health. According to Brown and Webster (2004, 168), "The *immediacy of the clinical encounter is the medium through which the technology is experienced,* whether as a one-off or a multiple series of interactive events." Thus, in order to better understand the nature and implications of a relational normativity, one ought to examine the ways various types of social interaction enable (or not) certain individuals and groups to express their normative preferences and/or to shape others' desires. This project would also require paying close attention to the ways in which the real-world use of health technology fosters or clashes with values. Instead of conducting debate strictly on economic grounds, such evaluative research would bring us closer to what actually matters to individuals and their societies. This is why I believe that the usefulness of such research does not lie merely in its publication through regular academic vehicles but, perhaps more important, in its being widely circulated and debated in various public forums. By being more broadly injected into public debates, such knowledge can help to create feedback loops between society, researchers, and those who make key technology-related decisions (Giddens 1984; Beck 2001).

Conceptualizations of Health Technology

In chapter 1, I observed that the field of HTA has, to date, been focused mainly on strengthening its methodological foundations while rendering its purpose and epistemological basis largely undertheorized (see table 6.2). The quest to quantify HTA has left a number of key issues only slightly addressed (e.g., ethical and social issues, the role of context in technology use). Chapter 2 explained how social science insights, especially those derived from ethnographic studies, can help to reframe our understanding of what technology is and does. In particular, the "technology-in-practice" perspective enables looking at the broader sociotechnical networks wherein important tasks and skills are delegated to human and technical components. I also stressed in this part of the book that technology is always concurrently enabling and constraining; it generates both gains and losses simultaneously. Such a conceptualization of health technology is significant because it brings both users and technical devices into the analysis, and examines how their relationships and outcomes are transformed, both positively and negatively, across settings and time. In chapter 3, I suggested that it is important to pay attention to medical innovations' user-friendliness in order to better understand the contextualized implications of their design. Up until now, the health research literature has not sufficiently called into question the form and characteristics of technology. The material examined in chapter 3, meanwhile, highlighted the fact that health technology becomes part of the fabric of social interactions in and around health care settings. In that chapter I also repositioned the patient's view within clinical and social interactions, a move that should further our understanding of how patients' appraisals of the benefits and drawbacks of health technology are shaped, in part, by clinicians' and lay individuals' perspectives. I expanded on this point in chapter 4, which emphasized the extent to which the appropriate use of health technology must be seen as context-dependent, multidimensional, and malleable. As a result, although knowledge about efficacy, safety, and cost is significant, it appears increasingly clear that such a scientific, rational approach to technology must be connected to the various forms of reasoning that currently shape health care practices.

Two research avenues regarding the conceptualization of health technology were proposed in chapter 5. First, there is a need *to better analyze the appropriateness of the tasks, skills, and knowledge delegated to individuals* through the design of health technology and new health care delivery

Table 6.2 Summary of Arguments About Conceptualizations of Health Technology

Chapter 1	Chapter 2	Chapter 3	Chapter 4
Phase I in HTA development focused on reinforcing the methods of the field; however, very few attempts at *theorizing* the goals and epistemological basis of HTA were made	A fundamental reason to turn to the social sciences lies in their ability to entirely reframe what technology is and does	Examining the user-friendliness of health technology may help to increase knowledge about how the design of a given device affects both treatment compliance and effectiveness	What constitutes an appropriate use of health technology is socially constructed, multi-dimensional, and subject to constant change
Phase II is concerned with HTA dissemination and increasing its impact on decision-making, goals that require a better understanding of the regulatory mechanisms that facilitate or impede the uptake of HTA's recommendations	The "technology-in-practice" perspective relies on ethnographic studies that examine what technologies do. This perspective recognizes that technology always emerges from, and operates within, heterogeneous networks comprised of various actors and technologies	Technology becomes active in, and part of, the social fabric that constitutes everyday life in health care settings, a facet that emphasizes the need to clarify whose values and intentions are reflected and encapsulated in a given technology	Scientific rationality should not be abandoned. It should be rooted in, and articulated with, the social, cultural, and political norms and reasoning frameworks that shape health care systems and clinical practices
	Three forms of unblack-boxing are helpful for 1) understanding how technology works, 2) disclosing technology's inherently political nature, and 3) examining how the power of technologies lies in their associations with humans	The patient's view is a relevant angle from which to appraise the value of innovations; however, clinical encounters should be seen as socially enacted practices because other social interactions contribute to patients' views	
	Trying to disentangle whether a technology generates either positive or negative effects is pointless because it is likely to do both depending on the knowledge mobilized and the context in which it is used (i.e., its dualistic performative dimension is crucial)		
	The deployment of socio-technical networks involves defining which tasks can be delegated to a device and/or to a human, and what knowledge and skills a user will or will not be obliged to master in order to operate the technology safely and effectively		

Chapter 5 - Second principle: Socio-technical networks embody multiple norms.

models. Technological complexity often increases the level of knowledge that users (e.g., providers, patients, family, and friends) require and the scope of their responsibilities (Vicente 2003). Sophisticated medical technologies may be symbolically and technically appealing, but they demand highly skilled staff and tend to concentrate resources in urban centers. Other forms of health technology have also emerged that tend to reduce geographical barriers by reaching settings and users across large distances (e.g., telemedicine, high-tech home care, personal monitoring systems). On this score, Brown and Webster remark that new technologies are *"mobilized through non-clinical networks* as sites through which health is produced and consumed" (2004, 171). As cost-control initiatives pursued by various governments increasingly push the frontiers of traditional health care settings toward ambulatory and home care (e.g., by shortening and/or avoiding costly hospital stays), and as private initiatives relying on direct-to-consumer marketing strategies bloom, fundamental questions arise: To what extent (and for how long) are patients (and their families and friends) appropriately supported in order to become active users of medical technology? And in what geographical contexts? The implications of and answers to these questions are far-ranging, from immediate safety issues to long-term social integration.

If one takes seriously the observation that health technology generates advantages and disadvantages simultaneously, *disclosing the dualistic effects of health technology* becomes a key avenue for further research. As I explained in chapter 2, when appraising the worth of various scenarios, most people tend to draft two separate lists of pros and cons, and then try to determine which list outstrips the other. This approach may prove satisfying because it helps one to reach and justify decisions. Nevertheless, even if one comes down on the side of the pros, the cons do not simply disappear. In the case of health technology, various drawbacks can easily be swept under the carpet or even tossed aside. They remain, however, profoundly influential. Side effects, for instance, must be dealt with; ethically equivocal situations must be managed; and patients whose quality of life is seriously compromised must endure tremendously difficult experiences. How, in light of even just this short list of serious considerations, can health care system managers and technology promoters continue to pretend to be concerned about patients' well-being? Faith in modern medicine relies largely on a demonstration of its wonders, whereas its failures are downplayed. Would it be possible to provide research that sheds light on the dualistic effects of health technology, thereby drawing a more realistic and exhaustive picture of technology-mediated medical practices? Such an endeavor would require going beyond a dichotomous pros-versus-cons analysis to engage more fully with the multifaceted dynamics underpinning technology use.

Political Perspectives on Health

In chapter 1, I argued that HTA agencies' societal mission remains problematic because the producers and the stakeholders of HTA hold competing political perspectives on what such a mission ought to entail (see table 6.3). Do the societal mission and its axiom of rational use of scarce collective resources conflate with governmental cost-control objectives? Some HTA agencies operate almost like autonomous university-based research groups, whereas others are geared toward delivering user-oriented knowledge products to their funders. As a result, although the science of HTA has gained acceptance, its political autonomy and impact on health care systems are frequently called into question.

As I suggested in chapter 1, in order to become a more mature and reflexive regulatory science, HTA should seek to articulate more clearly societal objectives that have clinical, context-dependent objectives. It should also develop a compelling conceptualization of the health policy arena. As a preliminary response to the first issue, chapter 2 showed that various types of health technology (e.g., prevention, treatment, rehabilitation, occupational health) possess different sets of health implications, some of which could be seen as more valuable than others when considered as part of a portfolio of public health interventions. As a preliminary response to the second issue, chapter 3 indicated that health technology's desirability must be unpacked by examining, among other things, the ways certain groups influence the medical innovations that others are supposed to desire and are permitted to access. On this subject, in chapter 4 I highlighted the interdependencies of the lobbying activities of various groups that tend to reinforce their claims for a broader access to medical innovations by using a selective mix of facts and arguments. Because of the malleability of scientific facts and their meaning, this chapter cautioned against HTA being used as a means to increase the discretionary power of elites that make decisions about health technology.

Two research avenues dealing with political perspectives on health can be derived from chapter 5. First, because it is commonplace to focus on the individual (clinical) benefits that health technology generates, *clarifying the collective ideals it helps achieve (or not)* should help to develop a more balanced understanding of their desirability. Certain types of health technology (e.g., food and drug regulatory policies, occupational health interventions, environmental health controls) may contribute to reducing health-related inequalities by intervening in the social determinants of

Table 6.3 Summary of Arguments About Political Perspectives on Health

Chapter 1	Chapter 2	Chapter 3	Chapter 4
HTA agencies can be situated on a spectrum ranging from "scientific autonomy" to "user-centered mission" For HTA stakeholders, the agencies' scientific rigor and credibility are positively perceived, but their political autonomy as well as their ability to bring about changes in health care systems remain debatable Two areas require development: 1) Articulating context-dependent and societal objectives needs a truly interdisciplinary understanding of the real-world use of technology; 2) A broader conceptualization of policy-making should strengthen HTA's ability to become a fully mature regulatory science that can engage more reflexively with stakeholders	Each category of health technology (from screening tests to occupational health interventions) carries different implications, which are of more or less value when compared with each other. Judging their relative value requires comparing alternatives and examining their desirability within a public health perspective	Examining the ways certain groups can exert influence on what others will or might want, and will or might have access to, makes more explicit why the issue of health technology's affordability remains deceiving unless one unpacks the ways its desirability is enacted	Understanding the role of knowledge in reconciling competing objectives requires adopting a socio-political perspective that articulates interplay among stakeholders in the health policy arena Because accessing health technology is the prime issue for most stakeholders, they may reinforce their demands through both discursive and factual means. The use of HTA in this quest to persuade others of the legitimacy of certain claim(s) can be selective and symbolic HTA may ultimately contribute to increasing decision-makers' discretionary power

Chapter 5 - Third principle: Reflexive science is produced within sociopolitical projects.

health across socioeconomic groups and/or in specific vulnerable groups. Developing a richer knowledge basis about the various effects of health technology (e.g., how it supports societywide solidarity and fairness) could help to counterbalance the highly emotional rhetoric supporting the individual's right to access high-tech medicine, a discourse that tends to legitimize ability and willingness to pay as natural drivers of technological change.

Further research should also explore how *adding reflexivity to science could help to strengthen its sociopolitical role*. If HTA and other types of scientific output are considered to be interpretively flexible, and therefore potentially conducive to symbolic and political manipulation, it is imperative to understand more precisely how science itself can account for and respond to such uses (Beck 2001). Furthermore, the recent call for increased knowledge transfer in health care research and the assumptions of the evidence-based medicine movement must be seriously examined. Such endeavors, if conducted naïvely and blindly in a context in which both industry and decision-making bodies become pivotal to funding research, could have profound, long-term effects on the nature of scientific production. Rather than bluntly refusing to engage in such a rapprochement (which nonetheless remains a legitimate option[1]), I recommend increasing scientists' reflexivity regarding science and its role in society. Such a move implies, first and foremost, consolidating knowledge about the effects of interactions between scientists and their "partners" on science itself. An open reflexivity, as outlined by Beck (2001), could introduce new dynamics in the processes underpinning science's use in policy-making and might push decision-makers and scientists toward greater accountability. In other words, if science were called upon to play a larger role in the political sphere, I would hope that scientists would become more politically astute and examine how their endeavors do or do not contribute to societal projects and problems.[2]

The Framing of Policy Options

When exploring various groups' use of HTA, chapter 1 stressed that HTA is but one source of information among others that contributes to the rationing (in contrast to the rationalization) of health technology (see table 6.4). This result typically involves negotiating the affordability of an innovation and who deserves access to it. I also underscored the fact that several barriers limit the overall impact of HTA on decision-making. Nevertheless, this limitation cannot be seen as a failure on the part of HTA because bridging the gap between science and policy obviously requires policy-makers to fulfill their part of the relationship. I also in chapter 1 stressed

Table 6.4 Summary of Arguments About the Framing of Policy Options

Chapter 1	Chapter 2	Chapter 3	Chapter 4
HTA is a source of information used in decision-making; however, several barriers and the potential lack of convergent regulatory mechanisms limit HTA's overall role	Medicine maintains its status by developing new knowledge and technologies that render physicians essential, while other health care providers are relegated to subordinate roles (reciprocal relationship between medical innovations and clinical expertise)	While some individuals and groups obviously want things for themselves, they also often want things for others	Health care stakeholder groups possess a diverse range of views and, therefore, hold multiple attitudes toward knowledge
A limited impact of HTA on decision-making cannot be considered a failure, however, because the use of HTA remains a shared responsibility of HTA users and producers		Technology frequently becomes a vehicle for shaping others' perceptions, needs, values, and practices	Although each group values and refers to HTA as a useful element of decision-making, they hold different definitions of the dimensions that should be assessed
HTA's challenge is formidable: the number of technologies to be assessed outstrips capacity; incentives must reinforce the use of HTA; most technology issues cannot be boiled down to black-and-white decisions; and limiting access to an innovation that provides benefits, even small and diffuse ones, is ethically and politically challenging			Health technology's desirability becomes a matter of affordability, and most attempts to rationalize access to technology are met with obvious discontent by a large group of institutions and individuals
			Only when HTA's scientific rationality is articulated with other reasoning that shapes practices will HTA be useful for fostering fruitful debates regarding the value of medical innovations

Chapter 5 - Fourth principle: Civil society is pivotal to deliberations concerning health technology.

HTA's ambitiousness. It is far from clear that all technology requiring assessment can be fully considered. In addition, the decisions that need to be made are multidimensional as well as ethically and politically challenging. Although HTA proponents have always recognized the importance of ethical and social issues, in chapter 2, I suggested that social science studies have addressed such issues in a more meaningful and instructive way. Among other things, medical innovations should be seen as pivotal to maintaining knowledge-based hierarchies in modern medicine, a role that partly explains why HTA remains poorly equipped to anticipate and provide guidance to the sociopolitical controversies surrounding technology's dissemination and use.

Chapter 3 expanded on this situation by emphasizing that innovations are vehicles for shaping perceptions, needs, and expectations. In other words, beyond its efficacy, safety, and cost, any given technology transforms the symbolic, ethical, and political environments in which it is used. Following this line of thought, in chapter 4 I explored the diversity of views about technology's desirability across stakeholder groups and, by extension, about the knowledge needed to make decisions concerning its regulation. Rationalizing access to health technology rarely gains the favor of all groups who put forward various reasons (e.g., clinical need, broader macroeconomics, entitlement to health care, need for hope) to justify initiating, maintaining, or increasing access to medical innovations. In order to enrich the repertoire of policy options pertaining to health technology, instead of trying to persuade all stakeholders of the superiority of HTA's scientific rationality, it is necessary to articulate these arguments and claims.

Stances Toward the Biomedical Industry

As chapter 1 made clear, by seeking to implement knowledge-based changes in health care systems, HTA directly and indirectly affects several groups, including the biomedical equipment and pharmaceutical industries (see table 6.5). In spite of this well-known fact, HTA agencies and health research scholars have not clearly explained why and how industry's concerns should be dealt with or ignored. The minimal response by HTA agencies has been to explicitly avoid conflict of interest by limiting interactions with industry and by asking their researchers to declare any potential sources of conflict (e.g., the International Network of Agencies in Health Technology Assessment's checklist; http://www.inahta.org). A tacit recognition that tension and misunderstanding are likely to be provoked by HTA's quest for evidence (which, according to some, may impede innovation) is prevalent among HTA critics.

Table 6.5 Summary of Arguments About Stances Toward the Industry

Chapter 1	Chapter 2	Chapter 3	Chapter 4
HTA seeks to implement knowledge-based change within health care systems. Such change affect: health care providers, governments, patients and the public, and the pharmaceutical and biomedical equipment industry	The competing and/or converging claims of medical experts, biomedical engineers, shareholders, policy-makers and patient representatives regarding the value of medical technology should be made more explicit	Several groups play an active role in the emergence of innovations The design of health technology is an intentional process that lies at the confluence of the public and private sectors' value-laden endeavors Needs are usually enmeshed with perceptions, desires, and values, and influenced by the existence of other technologies. An innovation cannot be seen as an unproblematic response to a specific demand, let alone a particular health need By designing technology in particular ways, designers impose/entice certain behaviors upon/from others. Technology acts normatively on health care systems, clinicians' practices, and patients' lives	The regulation of health technology affects several stakeholders who posses varying levels of resources and who may lose or gain clinical, economic, and symbolic resources through that process A large range of negotiations must take place for a given health technology to enter the health care system. The physician's role in these processes is central, and work on aligning and articulating the industry and policy-making sides is required Although including patient associations in policy-making might prove fruitful, it requires a better understanding of their activities, needs, and capacities in terms of using scientific evidence, as well as of their relationships with industry

Chapter 5 - Fifth principle: Make the private sector's role within publicly funded health care systems explicit.

In chapter 2, I recommended making more explicit the converging and/or competing claims, including those of industry, that contribute to defining the value of medical innovations. I then expanded on this proposition in chapter 3 by highlighting the intentionality that pervades design activities, which emerge from and are largely constrained by private sector interests, as well as the fact that a particular technology is rarely a straightforward response to a specific demand or health need. This chapter also underscored the fact that designers shape technology users' behavior and expectations by including certain features, characteristics, and functions in their innovations. These various elements have a direct impact on the organization and evolution of health care systems as well as on clinicians' practices and patients' lives.

Chapter 4 shifted attention to the broader processes through which industry influences health care systems by intervening more or less directly on the regulation of health technology. For a given innovation to enter the marketplace, several groups must promote it and gain access to physicians and policy-makers. Patient associations can play various roles in that process, ranging from being a silent group on behalf of whom claims are made to active lobbying entities whose purposes and methods may not always be transparent.

The Perils of Making Recommendations

The various chapters of this book have brought to the fore the sociopolitical complexity of technology-mediated changes in health care. Part of my aim has also been to stimulate scholarly work capable of enriching our understanding of the value of medical innovations. Along the way I have also made a few provocative statements and pinpointed a number of areas in which, I believe, both minor and major improvements should be sought. But, it remains to be asked, could formulating and following through on recommendations for change ever be that straightforward?

As I argued in chapters 1 and 4, improving HTA's epistemological, methodological, and institutional foundations is necessary because, in most jurisdictions and for the time being, HTA is the most readily available form of independent expertise capable of guiding policy-making. This book has, nonetheless, sought to push beyond an analysis of HTA's achievements and shortcomings in order to engage with issues that call for broader academic reflections and policy interventions. This is why a substantial portion of my comments has drawn on STS. By establishing a dialogue between these two fields, I called into question the impact of technology on patients' lives, health care providers' practices, and health care system governance.

Other approaches, of course, could have been adopted.[3] On one hand, it could have been possible to examine HTA's achievements around the world more systematically in order to identify the most successful organizational models and technology policy initiatives. Such a book would have brought a valuable contribution to HTA producers and policy-makers, but would have missed the opportunity to critically reconsider the object of evaluation—technology. On the other hand, if this book had relied exclusively on STS to examine health technology and had not brought in HTA's concerns and aims, the problem of health technology would have been analyzed without a consideration of the need for policy and regulatory changes. It would, thereby, have been addressed mainly as a sociological phenomenon that can be examined and criticized, but not necessarily with the aim of stimulating *improvements*.

My aim in bringing these two fields of inquiry together was somewhat more normative: I wish to see improvements in the ways medical innovations are designed, disseminated, assessed, and regulated in health care systems. For various reasons, this desire does not necessarily constitute an intellectual path or a political position that all STS scholars would endorse, let alone follow or adhere to. Their reasons for not doing so can be grouped under two broad categories.

The first set is epistemological, since it concerns the validity of the claims that scholars can make about desirable futures and ways to bring them about. My endeavor indeed runs the risk of falling into the trap of a form of positivist technological determinism (as introduced in chapter 2), which presumes that its own story about health technology (or construction of reality) possesses epistemological authority (Grint and Woolgar 1992). For several STS scholars, pretending to have a more valid or compelling story about the role of technology in society is not only naïve but indefensible. Any normative forecast in regard to technology is flawed because there is no "essential technical core" on which to firmly anchor such predictions (Grint and Woolgar 1992, 376). For Grint and Woolgar, technological capacity is indeterminate; therefore, influential narratives can be elaborated but they remain social constructs: "They do not derive their force from transparently (re)describing the technical capacity of technology but by providing a (more or less) persuasive and socially constructed narrative" (1992, 369).

By laying out policy recommendations that I believe could change the manner in which health technology is designed, disseminated, assessed, and regulated, my book could be understood to rely on the presumption that technology can be shaped by external incentives and is able, in return, to steer society in a predetermined direction. From an epistemological standpoint, however, there is a crucial shift between observing the dynamics that currently forge certain technological trajectories and assuming that if particular variables were modified, then other (more preferable) technological trajectories would arise. In other words, from a relativist perspective, empirical observations of current practices cannot straightforwardly inform policies that are aimed at transforming such practices. Either policies will be too narrow to capture a phenomenon's entire repertoire of contextual dimensions or the intrinsic properties of the phenomenon will be modified, thereby affecting its development. But then, is it not yet another form of determinism that takes precedence and assumes, in return, that attempting to shape the future will always be defeated by a logic that escapes all kinds of intellectual constructions?

As I emphasized in chapter 3, I prefer to see my scholarly role as an informed and engaged participant in the construction of society, even though such a role means that the desirable futures I envision might not materialize entirely or yield the exact outcomes I value. My position would at least, however, be coherent with the basic premise that researchers should engage in socially responsible research programs.[4]

Critics of research programs that lack political commitment are usually concerned by an "action imperative" that aims to influence policy and to interfere in technological projects. However, those in favor of relativist and deconstructionist stories avoid telling others what to do; they seek, rather, to debunk dominant discourses (Grint and Woolgar 1992, 368). This latter position—which indirectly influences public debates—can, of course, be seen as a subtle form of political activism.[5] For instance, by criticizing the policy processes that underpin health technology-related decisions, relativists can further observe (and deconstruct) the ways technology and society mutually evolve, and whether this co-production is affected by policy interventions.

Nevertheless, for relativism's critics, it is not enough to play the role of the court jester and merely destabilize the policy arena's foundation. According to Kling, eluding the powerful infrastructures that give rise to technological innovations and the historical hierarchical and discriminatory organizational practices from which they emerge is absurd (1992a, 361). Similarly, Stengers emphasizes the need to avoid surrendering one's social responsibility as an STS scholar too quickly: one should conceive of sociotechnical networks as "raising, in certain areas, the heroic necessity to be neither lazy, conformist, nor respectful, so as to avoid being gullible" (1993, 142; my translation).[6] Kling also strongly disapproves of Grint and Woolgar's (1992) refusal to venture into normative recommendations:

They cherish the "radicalism" of their thoroughgoing interpretativism. It is like the radicalism of an uninhibited comedian who freely debunks all social actors: rich and poor, powerful and weak, sacred and profane, even himself. Comedy gains force by restructuring social boundaries, reconfiguring conventional labels and narratives, transforming improbable situations into likelihoods, and accepting nothing as sacred. Comedy is an important genre of literature (and form of social action). But debunking and unraveling does not form a complete literature or a complete sociology (Kling 1992b, 383).

Such debates between relativists and anti-relativists are fascinating, and no doubt could go on forever because there is not a single valid view of what an academic discipline should be and aim at. As Fuller puts it, "All disciplines are normative, though rarely self-consciously so.... A self-consciously normative discipline is one that makes the ends of its inquiry an ongoing subject for negotiation" (1993, 211). To my mind, refraining from formulating recommendations strictly on the basis of an epistemological standpoint is intellectually valid but lacks political nerve. This lack of engagement creates a false dichotomy between two equally unsatisfying stances: telling stories devoid of authority and reverting to "truth" claims to give one's scientific work political weight. I do not believe the salient issue is whether or not researchers should decide to *either* debunk dominant discourses *or* to reveal historical structures. Both approaches appear compatible and complementary, although the false epistemological dichotomy between a descriptive and a normative stance may obscure the possibility of a third option (Hirsch 2005).

Is it not possible to acknowledge, on one hand, the potential fallibility of researchers' claims and, on the other, the need to move policy debates forward? Such a dual approach would mean taking seriously the role of knowledge—albeit always incomplete and uncertain—in social governance and creating opportunities for reflexive and constructive interactions among various perspectives. Furthermore, this approach would involve rethinking how a critical stance is to be both researched and framed. One thing the debate between the relativists and anti-relativists has taught me is to avoid jumping too quickly to conclusions regarding who is weak and in need of being defended and who is powerful and deserving of attack (Lehoux 2000). Such conclusions are rarely valid and accusatory positions often encourage defensive responses, with the net effect on research and attempted dialogue being nil (Stengers 1993). I have therefore sought throughout my research and this book to forge the basis of a serene engagement with technology-related issues instead of an "angry rebellion" that could fuel unqualified opposition (Melzer 1993, 320).[7]

I have also sought to do epistemic justice to the multiple dimensions and perspectives that contribute to the problem of health technology, thereby seeking to foster a "shared perplexity" (Stengers 1993).[8]

The second set of reasons that (STS) scholars might refrain from engaging in policy recommendations is bounded by the academy itself. In the introduction, I alluded to the audiences whom scholars address. Disciplines create for themselves particular audiences and sometimes underestimate the influence these publics exert over intellectual production. Building an argument *for* one's peers involves a certain set of communicative skills, norms, and habits; establishing oneself as a respectable scholar involves knowing what one's peers are likely to pay attention to and value. In some social science quarters, adopting a critical standpoint toward medical expertise and technology is necessary and often sufficient; the emphasis in this type of scholarly work is on theorizing. Being understood by those about whom one is constructing theories and providing useful guidance can easily be downplayed. In contrast, in the research that has gone into this book I have not only interacted with a range of audiences, from clinicians to biomedical engineers, but my work has also relied heavily on interviews and observation. I have spent time listening carefully to what actors say about what they do and about what they believe health technology should provide. My role as an analyst is to compare and contrast these views and to raise issues that are problematic as well as questions for further investigation.

I have attempted to provide what Fuller (1993) describes as a "non-opportunistic criticism," a type of scholarship that bears responsibilities toward the actors one observes and to whom ones listens. "The social epistemologist cannot get the normative side of her project off the ground unless she cultivates *ethos* and *kairos* with her audience. In other words, to get their attention, she must show that she understands their interests, and to get their action, she must show that they have a stake in the fate of her proposal" (Fuller 1993, 214).[9] In other words, I have sought to translate my observations into a language that will be understood by a range of scholars, students, health care practitioners, and policy-makers. As Lomas remarks, enhanced opportunities for "cross-learning" between researchers and various audiences could "significantly alter the future trajectory of evidence-based decision-making" (2004, 288). This observation explains, in part, why I wished this book to reach HTA producers and various health care practitioners on their own grounds, and why I pushed elaborate theorization to the sidelines. I concur with Berg et al., who stress that "formal policy fails to draw upon the repertoire of personal skills of those concerned in health care, and their experience, imagination and intuition" (2004, 36). One way to begin addressing this deficit is to publish articles and books that can speak to several audiences.

In my research I have also tried to maintain a broad perspective on the impact of technology in modern health care systems, an approach that may bother those who possess a profound knowledge of specific aspects that become somewhat lost or diluted in the "big picture." Although I hold a deep respect for scientific rigor, mastery of details, and disciplinary advancements, I am often perplexed by the tendency to circumscribe research areas into separate, disconnected epistemic islands, as if the world operated according to a set of entirely independent registers of action (Serres 1991). I therefore made a number of decisions that, I hope, have enabled this book to avoid the trap of technological determinism through an emphasis on deliberative processes and empirical research that ought to remain inclusive and reflexive and, thus, indeterminate. In favor of a thorough form of reflexivity, I have insisted on the need to disclose the embeddedness of normativity in current technology-mediated practices and to make one's own norms and values explicit. For some researchers, especially anthropologists, normative systems represent an important focus of observation and interpretation. However, in general their own systems of norms, against which they implicitly contrast their selective observations, are not systematically discussed; if they are, it is often in terms of Byzantine, ironic, or somewhat shamefaced reflexivity (Hammersley and Atkinson 1983; Pinch and Pinch 1988; Woolgar and Ashmore 1988; Woolgar 1988). In other disciplines, such as management, evaluation, or public health, actors' norms are often deemed irrelevant, nonexistent, or simply wrong: researchers are the experts who produce the relevant (science-based) norms. In both cases, researchers set aside the influence of their own normativity, as if the interpretation and production of norms could be a self-effacing exercise.

In this book, I opted instead to make as explicit as possible a personal form of intellectual engagement in a topic that I see as extremely important for the future of health care and societal well-being. The potential academic vulnerabilities inherent in such a position are numerous, but at least they are discernible and open to debate. As Fuller suggests, participants in a debate can learn to recast their interlocutors' positions in a "more comprehensive light, namely, by revealing the conditions that enable them to have a genuine *disagreement*" (Fuller 1993, 216). I certainly hope I have made my views—and my reasons for holding them—explicit throughout.

Policy Recommendations: Devising More Sophisticated Political Processes to Regulate Health Technology

In chapter 5, I presented and discussed governance-related principles that could be vital to renewing the way the problem of health technology is framed. The last two principles—to make civil society a pivotal locus of deliberations and to make the private sector's role within publicly funded health care systems explicit—are associated with a number of institutional processes capable of more directly enriching health technology policy. I want now to spend a little time clarifying their potential relevance for health care policy-makers.

To Readjust the Incentives and Constraints that Shape the Co-production of Technology and Society

Stressing the indeterminate nature of both technology and society, as well as their mutual shaping, makes it clear that there cannot be any truly informed *ex ante* evaluation and choice with respect to a nascent health technology. Rather, one should expect differentiated *learning processes* in which individual and collective interactions with an emerging medical innovation are likely to unfold. From a policy perspective, this observation suggests creating opportunities for examining, questioning, debating, and regularly reconsidering the rationale and embedded normativity of innovations while they are still in the process of being designed. Currently, regulatory mechanisms generally emphasize safety and effectiveness at the point of a technology's entry into the health care system (Kent and Faulkner 2002). In these pages I have argued that it may prove extremely counterproductive to expect social and ethical issues to surface only later, in the adoption and dissemination stage. These issues *are already partially present* in the design stage; they are embedded in clinical practices, health care systems, and social dynamics, and they are part of the research and development (R&D) ethos, market incentives, and technological opportunities.

If one takes the position that technology and society are co-constructed, intervening in the articulation of technology as well as in social desires and practices emerges as a significant practice (Rip et al. 1995). Doing so requires dealing with the underpinnings of how and where technology and society become intertwined. Brown and Webster (2004) observed both continuities and discontinuities in the emergence and social use of new medical innovations (e.g., technology-assisted human reproduction, implants, transplants, and technologies of dying). Continuities tend to reinforce the prevailing arrangements that clinical experts desire and uphold. Such arrangements revolve around a contractual relationship between a physician and a patient, and they are imbued with a strong symbolic power linked to the prolonging of life and the delaying of aging and death. Discontinuities are intimately linked to the broad spectrum of possibilities generated by various bodies of knowledge (e.g., genetics, neurosciences), new technologies, and the culture of experimentation that promotes and makes visible exotic practices (e.g., cloning, xenotransplantation, cryogenics).[10] Given the importance of such dynamics, deploying policy regulation that goes beyond issues of effectiveness and safety and deals with evolving social and individual ideals and responsibilities appears to be warranted.

To Collectively Reduce the Gap Between Current Normative Practices and Potential Practices Stakeholders Regard as More Desirable

In chapter 3, I introduced some of the principles of empirical ethics, a field concerned with the normative beliefs and behaviors that characterize the observed world. Proponents of empirical ethics argue that important first steps in sorting out the normative dimensions associated with (new) health technology are to elicit and debate current normativities and to identify how individual and collective actions could make future practices more meaningful and appropriate. Brown and Webster observe that recent experimental and applied research has led to "strange couplings" between technologies and humans, "a significant discontinuity related to the transgenic modification of species, or the prosthetic reworking of the self via body–machine hybridization" (Brown and Webster 2004, 170). New technologies are also mobilized in networks that tend to "*extend the spatiotemporal* boundaries of life and the entities that 'have' life, both organically and culturally, and carry thereby more or fewer rights and more or less status as moral entities" (Brown and Webster 2004, 170). Fetuses, stem cells, genetic information taken from a given individual, and tissues that are frozen for future use all possess such unstable status.

From a policy perspective, addressing ethical issues implies setting forth deliberative processes that would not merely focus on the features of an innovation that are seen as potentially problematic, but also would ground analysis in what humans actually do and believe. I also emphasized that an ethical pluralism capable of being deployed within democratic, diversified settings ought to be developed. Along with this, it is necessary to establish mechanisms to contrast, challenge, and articulate the multiple normative beliefs that are active in diverse societies and that shape clinical practices and health care policies. Moving toward the delivery of effective, fair, meaningful, and sustainable health care will not be possible without the integration of such mechanisms into policy development.

To Foster Equality in Public Input and Deliberations

In chapter 4, I stressed the need to avoid reinforcing social inequalities by setting up deliberative processes that would prove inaccessible to vulnerable or marginalized groups. This chapter also stressed that the organized groups that at present successfully attempt to influence the health policy arena might not represent all the relevant stakeholders whose practices and lives are affected by health technology.

From a policy perspective there is a need to rethink how a large range of groups can be consulted and involved in technology-related decision-making, instead of simply letting those more organized and vocal groups occupy the public sphere and monopolize public debates. It might also be necessary to abandon public consultation exercises that offer limited opportunities for voicing genuine disagreement (Fuller 1993) and that exert little weight in political decision-making, especially if one wishes to build trust (and avoid its fragmentation) across social groups.

To Increase Accountability in Policy-making

Medical innovations are often portrayed and can easily be seen as "*developments that will enhance individual choice over health care* and the management of illness and disease" (Brown and Webster 2004, 169). Because social and ethical issues are considered to be complex and less amenable to "hard" science, there has been a tendency among policy-makers and HTA producers to favor an individual informed-consent approach that returns the decision-making ball to patients' hands and avoids policy-makers taking a sociopolitical stand (e.g., prenatal testing for Down's syndrome). As shown in chapter 3, however, allegedly micro, individual decisions are always shaped by larger normative systems (e.g., medical expertise, legal frameworks) and economic and organizational constraints (e.g., coverage criteria, access to health care, counseling and social services, level of education).[11] As a result, the individual approach could do more harm than good.

The diversity and unpredictability of technological opportunities, coupled with related pressures from their promoters to reduce regulatory hurdles and to accelerate access to medical innovations, often create a sense of urgency in the policy arena. At the same time, given the importance of the short- and long-term implications of medical innovations and the visibility of recent public scandals and incidents (e.g., contaminated blood supplies, ruptured breast implants), health care policy-makers have come under strong pressure to increase their responsiveness and accountability. Doing so requires not only relying on a broader scope of disciplinary evidence (e.g., epidemiology, sociology, ethics, law) but also ensuring that policy-making processes remain socially legitimate and responsive to citizens. Similarly, third-party payers should seek to define and systematically apply coverage rules that take into account the boundaries of individual autonomy and the extent to which a sense of collective solidarity can be preserved.

To Ensure Traceability of the Reasons for Decisions

In chapter 5, I revisited the assumptions behind HTA and the evidence-based medicine movement, and I suggested that the promoters of these research initiatives tend to create false dichotomies between science and policy. These more or less implicit distinctions do not always hold, and might even conceal important similarities in terms of values, preferences, and ideologies (Denis et al. 2004). Among other things, politics, values, and the use of reason operate in both spheres. Thus, increasing accountability in health technology policy-making should not mean simply enforcing the use of HTA, which, as suggested in chapter 4, is at risk of symbolic manipulation. From a policy perspective, if the locus of controversy shifts from arguing over the value of health technology to the value of evidence, not much is gained.

Instead, it would be preferable to emphasize the complete rationale supporting a given decision (i.e., the full set of criteria and implications that were considered). If medical innovations "deepen the medicalization of the lifecourse and wider society" and tend "to confirm the power of the biomedical model" (Brown and Webster 2004, 168), one must strengthen the democratic basis upon which decisions are made. Cost-effectiveness alone is an unstable and unevenly applied criterion for backing up public policies (Faulkner 1997). In addition, it will be handily defeated by the complexity of the innovations that will emerge in the near future. Increasing the traceability of the clinical, economic, social, ethical, and commercial reasons behind decisions represents a vital component in enhancing democratic decision-making.

To Increase Transparency in the Relationships Between Institutions and Stakeholders

While writing this book I became ever more deeply aware that health technologies are not, strictly speaking, either private or public goods. They emerge from mixed alliances and they produce both private and public benefits and costs. In these pages I have also stressed that it is paradoxical for HTA producers to argue that only cost-effective innovations should be adopted but to refuse to recognize that the private sector largely (and increasingly) shapes both the ability to provide evidence and the innovations that are introduced into health care that require assessment.

It is therefore urgent that we develop policy initiatives that can bring together private and public interactions in technology-related endeavors and that we introduce transparent mechanisms for monitoring and readjusting those objectives. Furthermore, within government itself, civil servants responsible for trade and industrial policies, which often promote medical innovations, may rarely (if ever) interact with those who design health policies (which often restrict medical innovations). To revisit the specific contradictions and overall incoherence underlying such a "schizophrenic" policy nexus would prove to be a major policy initiative (Lehoux 2002).

To Increase Coordination Among the Various Objectives Pursued

In chapter 4, I compared the regulation of health technology in modern health care systems to a *distributed* collective process within which interdependencies and the need to make persuasive claims are salient. If all the objectives various stakeholders pursue cannot be reconciled, there is a need to make those goals more explicit and to begin addressing interdependencies between those in favor and against specific innovations. It will also be necessary to find ways to better coordinate use (selective use or nonuse) of those innovations. By recommending an increase in deliberations around the value of medical innovations, I realize that I am not offering a completely satisfying solution to the problem of coordination. However, one important aspect of deliberative processes, as set out in chapter 4, is that consensus is not the overarching goal of deliberations. Debaters are not obliged to convince and persuade others; rather, they are called upon to be cooperative and to make their claims answerable.

Ensuring cooperation between researchers, decision-makers, industry, medical practitioners, patient advocates, and civil society should be seen as the first step toward producing more meaningful and sustainable technology-mediated health care. This rapprochement should emphasize the broad spectrum of goals that public health care systems pursue, and ought to rely on clear negotiating criteria and transparent processes for appraising how medical innovations help them to meet those objectives.

Adding Intelligence to Health Innovations

From the outset, I have stressed the need to reconsider the meaning of technological progress and its tendency to subordinate ends to means. That is why chapter 3 focused on the exploration of what individuals and groups want from technology, and for whom. In the introduction, I raised another consideration that might, at first glance, seem to contradict this emphasis on the ends of technological changes. By quoting a fiction writer about the experience of a youngster learning to pour milk from a cardboard container, I alluded to the ingenuity and beauty of means. These technological aspects—which are at the core of biomedical engineering and design—have not, I admit, been fully addressed in this book. Nevertheless, the potential to increase the *intelligence* of medical innovations lies in closely examining the ways biomedical engineering's technological features and organizational dimensions affect the nature and characteristics of health technologies that are ultimately introduced to the market. Several of the issues that the HTA field struggles to appraise and that matter to policy-makers (e.g., cost-shifting, safety, impact on hospitals, level of skills required to use technology, types of settings in which a technology can/should be used) are largely determined upstream (e.g., during the R&D process). Would it be possible to establish more systematically the features that make a medical innovation better in the context of public health care systems? I believe so. Here again, however, bringing together different streams of empirical inquiry is required.

First of all, most of the literature concerned with innovation processes and the management of technology-intensive firms adheres to a business research tradition, wherein design is posited as a means of providing competitive advantages. Petre (2004), for instance, has examined various innovative teams, taken stock of innovation paths, and listed a number of success factors.[12] What remains unclear, however, is the way success should be measured in the case of medical innovations. Some observers have broadened the business-oriented perspective a little; for example, they note there is social and economic relevance in exploiting and developing expertise in design, "given the importance of design as an added-value economic factor and as a key factor in quality of life" (Cross 2004, 425). Christensen et al. (2000) go further by arguing that "disruptive technologies" could "cure" health care systems by bringing about sweeping changes. Their main argument is that technologies that are less expensive and simpler to use can be designed and marketed by emerging firms that are entering relatively established markets. These technologies are labeled "disruptive" because they disturb private preserves in the medical technology market by simplifying both the organizational contexts in which technologies are deployed and the level of skills required to use them. The development of low-intensity mobile radiology units is a prime example of such disruptive effects. These units are inexpensive (10% of the cost of conventional radiology equipment) and can be used by nonspecialized care providers. According to Christensen et al. (2000), the introduction of this technology met with resistance from the big players in the medical imaging market and clashed with mainstream corporate mentalities.

Another example—one that deserves more detailed examination than I can accord it here—is the technological evolution of diabetes management. A series of innovations (e.g., injection devices, blood glucose monitors, automated monitoring of physiological parameters) has made it possible to expand the role of patients while simplifying and reducing the procedures and materials required. While not being free of difficulties for patients and caregivers, such innovations do modify the policy landscape as it pertains to health technology.

Among other things, examining R&D processes can lead to a reconsideration of the market logics that preside over technological development. Market logics impose constraints that may be detrimental to the spread of certain types of technology. Why would firms commit to producing technologies likely to reduce the market share of other products they manufacture? Or why would small- and medium-size businesses risk developing a technology that generates little profit and whose sales are expected to be low? Nevertheless, given the fact that most Western industrialized societies, on one hand, expect a great deal from technologies and, on the other, are reluctant to spend more money, is it not necessary to call into question some of the sociopolitical forces that drive innovation? By examining more closely the flow of private and public R&D funding, one might well conclude that the development of technologies that more clearly contribute to public health might have to be supported by regulatory incentives other than simply market incentives such as sales volume and profitability. Guaranteed markets, tax credits, and special subsidies could, for example, be granted in order to reduce commercial constraints that now stand in the way of these initiatives.

The second stream of inquiry that would help to define the intelligence of innovations is found in ethnographies of design and engineering practices. Bucciarelli (1994) offers a fascinating analysis of the design process as requiring the combination of multiple microtechnological worldviews. Objects and their technical properties and behaviors contain several "object worlds"; for example, "the domain of thought, action and artifact within which participants in engineering design ... move and live when working on any specific aspect, instrumental part, subsystem, or subfunction of the whole" (Bucciarelli 1994, 62). Designers and technicians differently explore and exploit these object worlds, which they see as possessing heterogeneous properties. Bucciarelli offers the example of a book page to illustrate this point:

> Or consider this page in front of you. It is an object. A naïve empiricist would sense its weight and estimate its size; another

reader might note its color or texture; a chemist on the design team would describe its resistance to discoloration, its acidity, and its photosensitivity. A mechanical engineer would be concerned with its tear or its tensile strength, its stiffness, and its thermal conductivity. An electrical engineer would speak of its ability to conduct or to hold a static change. All of these attributes of the object, the same artifact, are understood within different frames of reference, and they all might contend in a design process (1994, 71).

Design also involves teamwork, hypothesis-testing, integration of more or less complex and diversified human and technical components, a strong trial-and-error culture, and working within financial and temporal constraints. Throughout team-oriented processes, a wide spectrum of issues will be discussed, debated, and negotiated before a final product can be brought to market. Bucciarelli emphasizes that "ambiguity is essential to design process, allowing participants the freedom to maneuver independently within object worlds and providing room for the recasting of meaning in the negotiations with others" (1994, 178). In other words, when observed more closely through an ethnographic approach, practices that could be seen as "merely technical" reveal a pivotal social core and the intentionality, uncertainty, and creativity that pervade most R&D processes. For Bucciarelli, designers seek to bring harmony to an artifact. They do this through repeated negotiations, the mobilization of various resources found in the broader environment, and successful maneuvering within a field of constraints: "The quality of the final design and artifacts … will then depend upon the social process engaged by participants, the competence of participants working within object worlds, and also the infrastructure and its vital, sustaining ecology" (Bucciarelli 1994, 187).

Thus, if the intelligence and quality of a medical innovation are reframed as residing in its desirability for society at large and in its capacity to increase the fairness and sustainability of a health care system, the social processes underpinning design practices and their broader regulatory, technical, financial, and political environments become important topics for further research. Might it be possible to introduce into design processes (and their regulatory environments) arguments (and market and policy incentives) that would lead to the design of more intelligent innovations? Bucciarelli does not make this claim directly, but his observations bring to the fore the concerns, aims, skills, and social organization of engineering teams. He underscores the significance of values as they are expressed through technical tropes such as "force," "energy," or "efficiency," considerations that emphasize certain technological features over others. From this angle, the metaphors, viewpoints, and organizational incentives that shape what engineering teams do, how they think about technological improvements, and how they test their hypotheses could (and perhaps ought to) be reconsidered.

Asking design teams to rely on a clearer "theory of use" (i.e., a substantial rationale about why and how a device should/can be integrated into users' daily routines) (see Lehoux, Sicotte, 2002) and to keep in mind a population health perspective, could bring about innovations that would be different and, eventually, better. Of course, they may prove merely different if they just shift the benefits and burdens toward different groups and/or if they displace these in time. Invasive interventions and devices that enable avoiding the death of extremely low-birth-weight babies, for example, tend to offload part of the burden onto parents and social services. Only over time and across contacts with other care providers (e.g., rehabilitation and specialized education) can the value of such interventions be fully understood.

An innovation could be different *and* better if it helped to solve a health problem and maintain a healthy population with fewer or lighter interventions. Indeed, innovations that combine technical, social and organizational creativity could prove superior. Very often, what designers and promoters of health technology are trying to achieve—and sometimes do achieve—with technology could be accomplished by reconfiguring tasks and increasing communication and coordination among providers and/or patients. For example, in remote areas nonspecialized staff can take pictures of the retinas of diabetic patients by using a digital camera, which does not require pupil dilatation and thereby reduces both risk and the need for authorized health care providers (Baker et al. 2004). These images can be transferred electronically and help clinicians to identify cases of retinopathy. Patients can then be transferred to a medical eye specialist who performs eyesight-saving laser surgery. This type of innovation requires fine-tuned coordination between human and technical components, and it relies on a clear clinical and population health rationale. Of course, like any other sociotechnical network, such screening practice is neither flawless nor devoid of (im)practicalities (Neyland 2005). Nevertheless, its shortcomings might be preferable to certain side effects and technological hurdles, and it could inspire new ways of thinking about what constitutes a desirable health care delivery model.

An example of innovative technology such as this leads me to believe that the design of high-tech medicine can take a different turn, one that would be both more creative and more socially responsive than is the norm today. If critical observers of technology design have questioned the masculinist ethos that pervades certain engineering practices and that gives shape to invasive and powerful technologies, the issue of whether this culture has evolved (or is currently evolving) because of worldwide concerns about renewal of energy forms, overconsumption, and environmental damage remains open. Pacey (1999) contrasted two main forms of technology design: people-centered and object-centered. The former involves an explicit attention to users, society, and the environment (i.e., caring for, as opposed to controlling), whereas the latter focuses on technological performance and issue compartmentalization (i.e., adopting an analytical, detached stance). As Martin astutely notes, Pacey's dichotomy fails to capture subtle nuances, and ignoring the strength of compulsive drives that come with puzzle-solving and creative challenges might be misleading (M. Martin 2002, 553). Nevertheless, a framework that integrates people-centered and object-centered features could pave the way for new design practices.

Thus, here again, the main concern likely is not whether designers of health technology should concern themselves *either* with people *or* with objects. Rather, striving to connect various technological features with meaningful human practices may represent a more inspiring and productive challenge for the future. As I have shown throughout this book, blunt ideologies and claims to universal principles may offer reassuring messages, but they rarely (if ever) solve the problem of health technology. If "creativity springs from around the edges of words" (Bucciarelli 1994, 173), perhaps what we need is many more words, ones that are fully grounded in a multitude of reflexive thoughts and actions.

Appendix A: Methodology of the Research Projects on which this Book Draws

Canadian Health Technology Assessment (HTA) Agencies Study

The overall goal of this study was to analyze the production and dissemination strategies of six Canadian HTA agencies and the relationships they established with four organized groups of stakeholders in their respective jurisdictions: provider associations, governments and administrative bodies, patient associations, and the pharmaceutical and biomedical equipment industry. A multiple case study combining qualitative and quantitative data from four sources of information was undertaken.

Agencies Included in the Study

In 1999, chief executive officers (CEOs) from eight important groups that produce HTA across Canada were invited to participate in our research. Six agencies (of the eight operating at that time) formally agreed to participate. An advisory committee that included all the CEOs from the participating agencies was appointed. The committee's role was to comment on research methodology, facilitate access to informants and useful documents, comment on preliminary findings, and provide feedback on the results of the study to their staff. The study began in January 2001 and ended in 2004.

Table A.1 provides general information about the structure and resources of the six HTA agencies. These agencies were located in five Canadian provinces: British Columbia, Alberta, Saskatchewan, Ontario (one provincial and one federal agency), and Quebec.

Table A.1 Structure and Resources of the Six Agencies (2001–2002)

Jurisdiction	Federal	Provincial	Provincial	Provincial	Provincial	Provincial
Date of inception	1989	1992	1993	1992	1990	1988
Type of structure	Private, nonprofit, government-funded	Arm's-length government agency	Arm's-length government agency	Freestanding, nonprofit, government funded	University-based	Arm's-length government agency
Scope of mandate	Technologies Drugs Systems Procedures	Technologies Drugs Services	Technologies Services	Technologies Drugs Services	Technologies Drugs Services	Technologies Drugs Services (incl. mental health)
Budget	$4.3 million/year	$1.1 million/year	$650,000/year	$4.5 million/year	$600,000/year	$1.5 million/year
Staff	27 FTE	13 FTE	10.65 FTE	35 (incl. scientists holding university appointments)	7.5 FTE	10 FTE
Staff devoted to dissemination	Yes	Yes	No	Yes	Yes	Yes

Note: FTE = full-time equivalent.
Source: Lehoux et al. 2005.

Interviews with HTA Producers

A total of 40 individuals distributed across the six agencies were interviewed (executives: 9; researchers: 21; communications staff: 7; information specialists: 3). All executives and communications staff were interviewed, and evaluators who had a minimum of three years' research experience were recruited. The interviews were designed to elicit detailed information on the following five issues: agency organization, report production, relationships with stakeholders, dissemination strategies, and institutional operating environment.

All semidirected interviews, which lasted between 35 and 90 minutes, were recorded and transcribed in electronic format. The software NUD*IST was used to code and selectively retrieve verbatim extracts. Some verbatim extracts were translated from French to English and slightly edited for clarity and to preserve anonymity.

Content Analysis of HTA Documents

The document analyses presented in chapter 1 draw on the official HTA documents published by the agencies between 1995 and 2001. All six agencies provided us with a list of their outputs, including HTA reports, rapid technology assessments, scientific papers, and, when available, copies of oral communications. For further analysis, only peer-reviewed documents (in English or French) were included. A total of 187 HTA documents was obtained directly from the agencies or from their Web sites.

These documents were coded using a predefined scheme inspired by the one proposed by Menon and Topfer (2000). It comprised (1) document type; (2) type of technology assessed; and (3) issues addressed. The first item included three mutually exclusive subcategories: full HTA reports, reports jointly published with another organization, and short documents (e.g., technical briefs, rapid assessments, updates). The second item included six mutually exclusive subcategories: diagnostic and/or screening technology, devices, procedures, drugs, health services, and general essays and/or research tools (e.g., reliability of a given database, guidelines for economic assessment). The third item, the assessment scope, was defined through subcategories that were not mutually exclusive: costs, effectiveness (including efficacy), cost-effectiveness, quality of life, safety/ethical/social/cultural issues, legal issues, state of current practices, and "other outcomes" (e.g., management of a given health problem, impact of a given health reform).

Definition and Selection of Stakeholder Groups

Respondents were selected from *formal* organizations representing four points of view: health care administrators, provider associations, patient associations, and the biomedical and pharmaceutical industry. The first two groups are HTA agencies' usual target audiences, whereas agencies do not view the other two as direct *users* of their reports. Patient associations and industry are more generally considered lobbyists (some much more powerful than others).

For both the interviews and the survey, we selected stakeholder organizations according to two steps. This was achieved for each jurisdiction in which the HTA agencies operated. Because one agency operated at the national level, its stakeholders were selected from national-level associations and the federal government. First, we created an inventory of stakeholders from each jurisdiction, using inclusion and exclusion criteria (see box A.1). Then, using the agencies' mailing lists, we added each organization that met our criteria but that had not been identified through our inventory. For each organization, we targeted individuals at the highest administrative level and whose responsibilities were directly relevant to HTA (e.g., technology-related policy, quality of clinical practice). This sampling strategy enabled us to obtain a range of viewpoints that reflected the various information-use practices of key organizations across the country.

BOX A.1 SAMPLING CRITERIA FOR STAKEHOLDER GROUPS

- **Health care provider associations:** Formal organizations of physicians or nurses mandated to safeguard the quality of clinical practice and protect the public. Excluded were bodies whose function was strictly to defend members' interests (e.g., unions).
- **Governments and administrative bodies:** Formal associations of government health care administrators and decision-makers located at ministries of health, regional health authorities, and university-based teaching hospitals. Excluded were regional associations and associations representing members from a subset of a larger organization.
- **Patient associations:** Formal associations of patients with a specifically health-related mandate that was sufficiently broad in scope and that represented a large number of individuals (e.g., heart disease, cancer, mental health). Excluded were regional associations and associations representing small groups (e.g., people afflicted by a rare disease).
- **Pharmaceutical and biomedical equipment industry:** Included not-for-profit associations representing the interests of pharmaceutical and biomedical equipment firms appearing on the mailing lists of HTA agencies.

Interviews with HTA Stakeholders   In total we contacted 86 organizations and conducted 46 interviews with a range of HTA stakeholders (providers: 11; decision-makers: 17; patients: 14; industry: 4). Face-to-face or telephone interviews, which lasted between 45 and 90 minutes, were conducted between May 2001 and October 2002. All interviews were audiotaped with the consent of the interviewees and transcribed in electronic format. We used the NUD*IST software application to categorize verbatim excerpts and created comparative tables to contrast the opinions expressed by the various groups.

Survey of HTA Stakeholders   A survey was developed in order to document the views of a broader group of HTA stakeholders. We included a large number of organizations belonging to the four groups across the country. However, each agency had its own particular research portfolio resulting in the production of reports that likely would be of interest only to very specific groups (e.g., planners of genetic services, midwives). The implication for the survey development was the creation of various sets of items that fit respondents' level of knowledge about the HTA agencies and their reports. The self-administered survey was developed in the light of eight exploratory interviews with stakeholders, the literature on knowledge utilization, and a survey developed in another study on collaborative research (Denis et al. 2003).

The survey (available upon request from the author) comprised six sections: the perception of health technology and services, the sources of information used, the relationship with HTA agencies, the experience regarding the use of knowledge, the institutional environment affecting policy and practice, and the mandate of the organizations, and the respondent's duties. Most questions were closed and used a five-point Likert scale. For provider associations, patient associations, and industry, the final survey was mailed to each organization's CEO. For health care administrators, the survey was sent to the heads of departments in hospitals. For departments/ministries of health and regional health authorities, it was sent to the chiefs of the relevant divisions. Survey data were collected from January 2002 to June 2002. Two reminders followed the first mailing. Table A.2 indicates an overall response rate of 27% (n=405).

Examining the profile of our survey respondents, we found that about half were top-level managers. Their organizations relied on a wide range of human resources. Whereas half of the provider and administrator groups employed more than 500 full-time equivalent (FTE) staff members, close to half the patient associations employed 10 FTE or fewer. Finally, except for the administrators' organizations, up to two thirds of the organizations had existed for more than ten years.

Table A.2 Survey Response Rates for Each Group and Jurisdiction

	Provider Assn.		Decision-makers		Patient Assn.		Industry		Total	
	N	%	N	%	N	%	N	%	N	%
National	48/95	51	28/111	25	19/35	54	7/10	70	102/251	41
British Columbia	24/107	22	11/76	14	9/42	21	2/8	25	46/233	20
Alberta	14/52	27	8/40	20	3/23	13	1/1	100	26/116	22
Saskatchewan	8/32	25	14/42	33	4/16	25	0	0	26/90	29
Ontario	77/304	25	21/120	18	6/54	11	1/32	3	105/509	21
Quebec	52/196	27	23/47	49	19/57	33	6/18	33	100/318	31
Total	223/786	28	105/436	24	60/227	26	17/68	26	405/1517	27

Source of Funding Medical Research Council of Canada (now Canadian Institutes of Health Research) (grant number 42499; January 2001–January 2003). Study title: Institutionalization of Knowledge-Based Change: A Case Study on Six Canadian HTA/HSR agencies. Investigators: P. Lehoux, J.-L. Denis, A.-P. Contandriopoulos, and M. Hodge.

Publications Derived from this Study

Lehoux, P., Denis, J.-L., Tailliez, S., and Hivon, M. 2005. Disseminating Health Technology Assessment: Identifying the visions guiding an evolving policy intervention in Canada. Journal of Health Politics, Policy and Law, 30(4): 603–641.

Hivon, M., P. Lehoux, J.-L. Denis, and S. Tailliez. 2005. The use of Health Technology Assessment (HTA) in decision-making: The co-responsibility of users and producers? *International Journal of Technology Assessment in Health Care* 21(2): 268–275.

Lehoux, P., S. Tailliez, J.-L. Denis, and M. Hivon. 2004. Redefining HTA in Canada: Diversification of products and contextualization of findings. *International Journal of Technology Assessment in Health Care* 20(3): 325–336.

Lehoux, P., J.-L. Denis, M. Hivon, and S. Tailliez. 2003. Dissemination and use of health technology assessment in Canada: The perception of providers, health care administrators, patients and industry. Report no. R03–01, GRIS, Université de Montréal. www.gris.umontreal.ca/publication2.asp?fromwho=gris&no=8975

High-tech Home Care Study

This study examined the extent to which primary-care organizations (called centres locaux de services communautaires [CLSCs]) in Quebec, Canada, had been involved in the provision of high-tech home care, and the technical, human, and organizational challenges faced by managers, providers, and patients. This study combined qualitative and quantitative data sources: interviews with CLSC home care program managers and staff (n=41); a survey of all CLSCs in the province (n=140); interviews with patients (n=16) and caregivers (n=6); observation of home visits by nurses (n=16); and content analysis of patient manuals issued by manufacturers and hospitals (n=26). We selected four technologies that were used frequently and that showed a wide range of technical and clinical characteristics: antibiotic intravenous (IV) therapy, oxygen therapy, peritoneal dialysis, and parenteral nutrition.

Interviews with Patients For interviews with patients (n=16), our sampling strategy was intended to diversify the viewpoints. We sought to survey patients from both high and low socioeconomic brackets, and from both urban and rural settings. All IV therapy and oxygen therapy patients were recruited through CLSCs. Due to the relatively small numbers of patients using peritoneal dialysis and parenteral nutrition, these participants were recruited through specialized home care programs managed by hospitals located in Quebec's largest urban center (Montreal), but which also provided services to patients in rural areas.

The interviews explored eight features that could both enable and constrain the use of technology: ability to learn how to use the technology, patients' skills and knowledge, safety measures, perceived autonomy, nature of the patients' responsibilities, fit with the home environment, and maintenance of patients' professional and social lives. Interviews lasted between 60 and 120 minutes, and were audiotaped with the interviewees' written consent. The interviews were then transcribed in electronic format. The NUD*IST software was used to code and selectively retrieve verbatim extracts, thereby facilitating constant comparative analyses.

Source of Funding   Medical Research Council of Canada (now Canadian Institutes of Health Research) (grant number 15472; April 1999–April 2001). Title: User-friendliness and Organizational Framework of High-Tech Home Care: A Case Study. Researchers: P. Lehoux, R. Pineault, L. Richard, J. St-Arnaud, and H. Rosendal.

Publications Derived from this Study

Lehoux, P. 2004. Patients' perspectives on high-tech home care: A qualitative inquiry into the user-friendliness of four interventions. *BMC Health Services Research* 4 (28). http://www.biomedcentral.com/content/pdf/1472-6963-4-28.pdf.

Lehoux, P., J. Saint-Arnaud, and L. Richard. 2004. The use of technology at home: What patient manuals say and sell vs. what patients face and fear. *Sociology of Health & Illness* 26 (5): 617–644.

Lehoux, P., R. Pineault, L. Richard, J. Saint-Arnaud, S. Law, and H. Rosendal. 2003. High-tech home care delivered by Quebec primary care organizations: Are the sources of information about technology and relationships with hospitals of quality? *International Journal of Health Care Quality Assurance* 16(1): 37–46.

Lehoux, P., C. Charland, R. Pineault, L. Richard, and J. Saint-Arnaud. 2002. Technologies de pointe et soins à domicile: Où en sont les CLSC?" *Canadian Medical Association Journal* 166 (10): 1277–1278.

Lehoux, P., C. Charland, R. Pineault, L. Richard, and J. Saint-Arnaud. 2001a. Convivialité et cadre organisationnel des technologies utilisées à domicile." *Rapport 1: Résultats de l'enquête par questionnaire auprès des gestionnaires des programmes de soins à domicile des CLSC.* Report no. R01-07, GRIS, Université de Montréal. www.gris.umontreal.ca/publication2.asp?from-who=gris&no=5637

Lehoux, P., C. Charland, R. Pineault, L. Richard, and J. Saint-Arnaud. 2001b. Convivialité et cadre organisationnel des technologies utilisées à domicile. *Rapport 2: Analyse des entretiens menés auprès de gestionnaires et de professionels des programmes de soins à domicile des CLSC.* Report no. R01-13, GRIS, Université de Montréal. www.gris.umontreal.ca/publication2.asp?from-who=&no=7503

Satellite and Mobile Dialysis Units Study

This study was undertaken for the Quebec Ministry of Health and Social Services (Ministère de la Santé et de Services Sociaux [MSSS]), under a research contract. The goal was to assess the organizational and clinical outcomes of, and patients' perspectives on, the satellite and mobile dialysis units that had been implemented in two regions across the province. The satellite units were hosted in two local hospitals and supervised by nephrologists located in a regional hospital. The mobile unit was a bus adapted to host five dialysis stations. It traveled back and forth between a university-based teaching hospital and two sites within a 125-km radius. In both projects, nephrologists supervised from a distance via a videoconferencing system.

Assessment took place between January 2002 and March 2004. It relied on several sources of data: interviews with physicians, managers, and patients; two surveys with nurses—one examining their views and adaptation to change and one assessing their clinical knowledge; on-site observations; patient chart reviews focused on the compliance of clinical parameters with established guidelines; and longitudinal registers compiled by the project teams (i.e., patient cohort characteristics, technical incidents).

Interviews with Managers, Providers, and Patients   Semistructured interviews were conducted with managers (n=11; mostly nurses), physicians (n=7), and patients (n=8). Up to eight interviews were conducted by telephone, and interviews lasted between 30 minutes and 2.5 hours. All interviews were audiotaped with the consent of the interviewees. They were then transcribed in electronic format (approval was also obtained from each hospital's ethics committee).

Source of Funding   Research contract obtained after an open call for proposals by the MSSS (January 2002–January 2004). Title: Evaluation of Satellite and Mobile Dialysis Units. Researchers: P. Lehoux, C. Sicotte, R. Pineault, and J. Saint-Arnaud.

Publications Derived from this Study

Lehoux, P., B. Poland, G. Daudelin, D. Holmes, and G. Andrews. Under review. Emplacement and displacement of health technology: Making satellite and mobile dialysis units closer to patients? *Science, Technology and Human Values.*

Lehoux, P., G. Daudelin, R. Pineault, J. Saint-Arnaud, and C. Sicotte. 2004. *Evaluation des unités satellites et mobiles d'hémodialyse.* Report no. R04-02, GRIS, Université de Montréal. www.gris.umontreal.ca/publication2.asp?fromwho=&no=10450

Appendix B: Details of the Portfolio of the HTA Agencies Examined and Discussed in Chapter 1

Agency 1 had diversified its products to a limited extent, supported scientific publications, and specialized in health services assessment. This agency had a high percentage of contextualized documents addressing current practices and other outcomes. This characteristic was highly compatible with the aim of providing "information about utilization of healthcare services in the ... population. And this may be information in order to assess the equity or access to services, it may be information about the quality of care, or about the outcomes" (Researcher). All interviewees from this agency confirmed that even though the Ministry of Health "informs the agency agenda," most of its projects were investigator-initiated. Because several of these projects were eligible for funding through national and provincial research-funding bodies, this agency's portfolio was partly shaped by the funding criteria these bodies set and its investigators could maintain a high level of scientific autonomy.

Agency 2 had diversified its products, supported (albeit weakly) scientific publications, and had a balanced portfolio. Its stated mandate was to "explore ethical and social issues raised by the accelerating demand for technological interventions." This mandate suggested an interest in developing the "theoretical foundations for using large data sets to understand the determinants of health in population groups, and to derive better evidence-based approaches in healthcare" (Web site). These goals were compatible with the fact that 24% of its documents fit the "Essay and Research Tool" category. Even though we observed limited contextualization of findings, Agency 2 was explicit about its role in providing guidance for decision-makers: "Research findings are published in detailed reports, serving a principal objective of disseminating results in a form useful to decision-makers in a position to use them. By identifying and communicating how limited health care resources can be most effectively applied, [the agency] is able to assist the public sector in its policy development and planning efforts" (Web site). When deciding on technologies to assess, this agency considered input from several sources. The most important ones were prioritized because they raised significant, provincewide issues—"issues that have been raised from a number of different perspectives simultaneously" (Researcher). In other words, this agency's portfolio was shaped by an academic orientation to HTA and by recurring and convergent suggestions for assessments.

Agency 3, which specialized in assessing pharmacotherapies, also had diversified its products and supported (albeit weakly) scientific publications. Its drug assessment specialization was consistent with the fact that it was the agency that had the largest proportion (51%) of assessments that examined cost-effectiveness. This agency's priority-setting process was highly formalized and was significantly influenced by program-specific committees composed of representatives from various regions. An executive from this agency explained that a cumulative list of topics was built up throughout the year and then presented to members: "We had a list of almost 50 possible topics for them and some were clearly not appropriate and some were very appropriate. But we asked them to vote and, in the end, we got 10 that received multiple votes." Consequently, the agency's portfolio was the result of a structured process and reflects topics that matter to a wide set of stakeholders.

Agency 4 acted according to a broad mandate: "Support a community of researchers who generate knowledge that improves the health and quality of life of people ... throughout the world" (Web site). This agency had diversified its production to a limited extent, supported scientific publications and possessed a balanced portfolio. Its findings were contextualized as well, but with the goal of servicing its population, from decision-makers to members of the public. In the words of one researcher, "We don't select topics, we answer everything that comes to us. What differs is the level of analysis or the comprehensiveness of the assessment." This view was reinforced by the president of the organization of which this agency was a part, who stressed that the agency should never decline a request. As a result, according to the agency's head, only 5 to 10% of its projects were investigator-initiated. Overall, this agency's portfolio was oriented toward a public service pull rather than a scientific push.

Agency 5 had not diversified its products; however, it supported scientific publications and had a balanced portfolio. Its findings were contextualized and it frequently formulated recommendations. Input for priority-setting was sought from several sources, and criteria were used to decide which technologies to investigate. These criteria included burden of illness, number of individuals concerned, costs, and available evidence. While the agency believed requests formulated by the Ministry of Health or officials from the health care system should not be declined, response depth was based on available resources and the extent to which a request fit the criteria. Up to a third of this agency's projects were investigator-initiated. Thus, the final portfolio may have reflected an interest in the production of both scientific and user-oriented knowledge. This balanced approach helped HTA producers to maintain a certain level of scientific autonomy.

Agency 6 had diversified its products to a limited extent and specialized in health services assessment. Contextualizing its findings was important, and the agency frequently formulated recommendations. These activities were compatible with its mandate: to support the "development of strategic health policy by providing evidence on researchable issues" (Web site). Agency 6 had been engaged in an environmental scanning process that informed its priorities. This process facilitated frequent interactions between researchers and decision-makers. Because this process relied on bringing together the opinions of diverse stakeholders, one researcher noted that "it's difficult to say how much of that [i.e., the topics chosen] is us and how much of it them; there's an interplay there." In other words, agency representatives regarded the resulting portfolio as a response to both supply of and demand for HTA.

Notes

Introduction

1. According to Gillick (2004, 2201), "The framework that is best established for considering costs and values is cost-effectiveness analysis.... To be covered, a new procedure must be supported by scientific evidence that it offers patients a clinically meaningful benefit" and it should "demonstrate a cost-effectiveness ratio of not more than $50,000 to $100,000 per quality-adjusted life-year ($50,000 is a widely used benchmark reflecting the cost of dialysis in a patient with end-stage renal failure)." As Deber (1992) explains, although such reasoning seems logical, it cannot support a consistent form of rational decision-making in health care systems.
2. Some observers even see the future brightly: "We prefer to think of the next five years as an *era of unprecedented opportunity* for health care providers to meet the customer needs" (Coddington et al. 2000, xv).
3. A couple of decades ago, such a framing would have been met with some clear resistance: While financial ability is accepted as the means of distributing most goods, society has generally taken a different approach to medical care. There was public outrage in 1985 when the *Washington Post* reported that rich foreign nationals were receiving a disproportionate percentage of kidney transplants in the Washington, D.C., area. The foreign nationals' ability to pay more for a transplant than that provided by private insurance or public funds made them more valuable, and therefore more attractive, patients (Besharov and Dunsay Silver 1987, 519).
4. Coddington et al. (2000, 221) define "demand" as "the combination of a perceived need or desire for a product plus the ability to pay." This formula implies that health needs can be defined without examining them from a clinical perspective and without knowing whether or not specific products will fulfill those needs. It also suggests that the ability to pay is a legitimate component of health care utilization.
5. Coddington et al. (2000, xiv) also stress that "we sometimes forget that this is the revenue base and livelihood for seven hundred thousand physicians, over five million hospital employees, and over six million persons who work in other parts of health care (including physicians' offices, health plans, manufacturing and distribution of drugs and other health care products, association work, consulting, and so on)."

237

Chapter 1

1. This section partly draws on Lehoux and Blume (2000) and Lehoux (2002).

2. In recent decades, various studies have tried to elucidate the relationship between technology and costs. Chernew et al. (1998) reviewed this literature as well as studies on the impact of managed care on the adoption of new technologies in the United States. All eleven studies included in their review pertaining to the cost impacts of technology concluded that technology has contributed to a substantial increase in expenditures. For example, Newhouse (1992, 1993), adopting a "residual" approach that determines the total increase in health spending while neutralizing the effects of nontechnological factors such as inflation, population aging, and increases in personal income, concluded that technology was the main factor driving growth of expenditures in the period following World War II. Peden and Freeland (1995) estimated that since the 1960s, 70% of the increase in spending has been attributable to the development and distribution of medical technologies, an increase they claim was largely triggered by the deployment of health insurance (see Danzon and Pauly 2001). The studies cited by Chernew et al. and that adopted an "affirmative" approach that focused on the economic impact of a technology used for a specific health problem reached similar conclusions.

   It is clear that the choice of technology in an "affirmative" study will have a determining effect on its results. Weisbrod (1991) suggests that, for some pathologies, technology has been able to reduce costs substantially (e.g., the polio vaccine). In a special issue of *Health Affairs* (September/October 2001), a number of authors go so far as to say that the overall cost of technology development yields health gains that are significant enough to justify an increase in spending. For example, Cutler and McClellan (2001) observed that out of five clinical cases, four interventions (heart attacks, treatment of underweight babies, depression, and cataracts) have yielded benefits outweighing their costs; only one (breast cancer) showed costs equivalent to the benefits generated. To calculate these benefits, the authors estimated that a year of good health was valued at US$100,000 (if expenditures do not exceed that figure, an intervention is considered "cost-effective"). They also argue that people whose lives have been saved or whose health has been restored will make an economic contribution to society by (re)entering the labor market and spending their income. While they recognize the importance of reducing the use of technologies that yield marginal benefits, the authors fear that policies of technology cost containment, including managed care, will be detrimental to the productivity of health care systems over the long term by limiting innovation.

3. The work of two of these agencies would fit better under the broader label of health services research (HSR) than HTA. However, throughout the text I use HTA in order to facilitate reading.

4. Another, less common model is the hospital-based HTA unit that provides advice to a single hospital or a consortium of hospitals (e.g., the Comité d'Évaluation et de Diffusion des Innovations Technologiques [CEDIT] in France).

5. In this book I do not offer a detailed analysis of the methods of HTA, although I fully concur with Abraham (2002, 21), who aptly points out that social scientists may tend to neglect carefully examining *how* expertise and data are constituted. He stresses that "in addition to regulatory principles about *democratic* process and *political* procedures, there is also the matter of *methodological* principles."

   Pursuing this line of inquiry, Abraham provides a solid analysis of the regulatory weaknesses surrounding the decisions made in the United States regarding triazolam. In 1991, the British Medicines Control Agency suspended the license for this drug because, it was argued, its risks outweighed its benefits. Triazolam was banned in the United Kingdom, Norway, and Denmark, but remained on the market in the United States and many other countries. According to Abraham (27), in 1992 "the PDAC [the United States Food and Drug Administration's Psychopharmacological Drugs Advisory Committee] gave priority to anecdotal evidence about triazolam in use, when assessing efficacy, but to controlled clinical trial data, when assessing safety. In each instance the types of data which favored triazolam were given priority over those which threatened its viability."

6. Such an enlightenment function was instrumental in the emergence of national health insurance in Canada in the 1960s, which was facilitated by the fact that both researchers and policy-makers were arguing on behalf of the public's good:

This congruence in core values between researchers, their government audience, and the public therefore allowed the research information on inequitable access, inadequate private insurance coverage for the poor, and the high administrative cost of multiple private insurers to contribute to the design of a government-administered health insurance system. (Lomas 1990, 533)

7. This section draws heavily on Lehoux, Tailliez, Denis, and Hivon (2004).

8. The national-level agency receives funding from the provinces and the federal government because its mandate includes facilitating coordination across the country. Some agencies also receive additional funds from research-funding agencies (through open competition) and/or from specific research contracts with the federal Ministry of Health.

9. These finding are compatible with a recent study by Garcia-Altes et al. (2004). Examining the production of four agencies located in the United States (Veterans Administration Technology Assessment Program [VATAP]), United Kingdom (National Institute for Clinical Excellence [NICE]), Canada (Canadian Coordinating Office for Health Technology Assessment [CCOHTA]), and Spain (Agencia de Evaluación de Tecnologías Sanitárias [AETS]) between 1999 and 2001, these researchers found that those "organizations most commonly assessed drugs (58.7%) and devices (22.5%)" (301).

10. The findings covered here related to the scope of issues addressed in HTAs, and the nature of the conclusions reached coincide with the study by Garcia-Altes et al. (2004).

11. In Lehoux and Blume (2000), the results of a search on the 1999 International Society for Technology Assessment in Health Care (ISTAHC) CD-ROM database, which contains abstracts presented at the Annual Meetings (1994–1998) and all abstracts of papers published in the *International Journal* (1985–1999) were as follows: from a total of 2,906 records, 30 records contained "social" in their titles (1%), 5 contained "political" in their titles (0.2%), and 19 contained "ethical" in their titles (0.7%). A search of the abstracts was slightly more encouraging: 181 contained "social" (6%), 49 "political" (1.7%), and 80 "ethical" (2.8%).

12. This low level of negative conclusions converges to a certain extent with the observation of Garcia-Altes, et al. that "VATAP, NICE and AETS recommended the technology or recommended with conditions 33%, 51%, and 38% respectively," while "CCOHTA made general comments in 50% of cases and recommended against in 25%" (2004, 303).

13. In addition, building the foundations for and carving the paths of researchers' and users' individual careers nurture a different sense of time line and competence (and professional mobility). While researchers' careers are often grounded in consolidating expertise in a given area, those of civil servants seem to involve migrating from one sector to another.

14. This subsection and the following draw heavily on Hivon et al. (2005).

15. As one interviewee explained:

Yes, we do [use HTA reports]. We try . . . in addition to making sure our reports and our plans and our strategies are based on our good estimate of local needs and future requirements, we do want to make sure that our recommendations to the government are based on current and emerging best practice. So yes, so we do need to stay on top of health services research. So I'm quite familiar with [HTA agencies'] research, and so . . . just in terms of [HTA unit] specifically, as the reports come out, if they have relevance to work that we're doing, we would certainly analyze that and share that internally and see if it needs to be built into our reporting. (Decision-maker 1)

16. As noted earlier, HTA producers do not see the biomedical equipment industry as a potential user of their work. Representatives of the industry confirmed this nonrelationship:

Basically they say we're doing this assessment of this technology and we would like you to provide the data necessary. And that's it. There's no involvement in methodology or team approach or seeing drafts as when they're being done; at the end you do get to see a draft at some point, but with a very short time to respond back, but that's it. So you're basically contacted at the beginning for data, and then at the end. (Industry 3)

17. The range of opinions varied regarding the overall usability of HTA by patient associations. The following quotation both stresses the limited usefulness of HTA and one association's perception of not really being a target audience for that type of research:

Oh, I think [HTA reports] are of limited use. I mean some of their information is helpful, but most of it I think is more designed . . . because it's clinical, I mean that's what they are, the [Agency 1], I think that they're of more assistance to systemic improvement in health care as opposed to what we as a lay organization would be taking advantage of. I think we're not their primary target, it's so nice we had some interaction but it's not that significant. (Patient Association 3)

In addition, although some patient associations could use HTA instrumentally, it was observed that it can be integrated with various sources of information and knowledge, as one respondent explained:

Well, our national office is very good at getting the information about new technologies and new pharmaceutical innovations to us. As I said earlier, we also receive the [HTA unit] newsletters and they have excellent articles in there, so we follow up on some of those sometimes. And then the pharmaceutical companies, too. I find them to be very helpful if you have a question about their drug and research that might be ongoing on it. Or might have been completed. I find them a very good source. (Patient Association 4)

18. One respondent even stressed that an evidence-based approach was part of his organization's mission: "Our mandate is to foster the creation of an evidence-based culture for the provision of medical services and health services in the province" (Decision-maker 3).

19. These authors also argue that a "partnership among the many public and private organizations holding a stake in technology-related decisions is highly desirable" (375) and would enable setting priorities for assessment and pooling of a larger reservoir of financial and human resources.

20. Furthermore, as indicated earlier, HTAs can also end up with neutral conclusions or ambiguous recommendations. As one respondent explained, this may happen because the evidence base on which HTA usually relies is insufficiently developed and might not be consolidated in the near future:

You know, a common scenario from the health technology assessment unit is that there is information about the effectiveness and risks of a procedure, but not sufficient enough for conclusions to be reached, which doesn't leave us much further along [laughter] . . . most of the conclusions would be that there is insufficient evidence to warrant public expenditure on this technology. But that's not what we're usually interested in. We're interested in knowing whether or not it's sufficiently developed that a physician could employ it regardless of how it might get funded. (Physician Association 1)

21. As such, Abraham emphasizes: "Neither the precautionary principle nor the permissive principle is more scientifically valid in any straightforward technical sense" (2002, 28).

22. See also responses by Eccles (2004) and Littlejohns et al. (2004).

23. At http://www.cms.gov/coverage one can find a relatively clear definition (albeit not devoid of jargon and probably not easily accessible to everyone) of the clinical indications for which the use of a variety of technologies or procedures is cosidered beneficial, and therefore covered by Medicare and Medicaid.

Chapter 2

1. Although there is no consensus among social scientists about the best ways to integrate their knowledge in health care practices and policies, I am personally reluctant to embrace the utilitarian view, whereby the social sciences are seen as a reservoir of tools that can be selectively applied to fix health care problems. Keeping in mind the old debate around sociology *in* medicine versus sociology *of* medicine still can help one to understand the epistemological and normative challenges underlying interdisciplinary research. HTA is oriented toward policy and action—it asks for more guidance from social scientists about ways forward than most of them would agree to provide.

2. This section draws from a talk I gave in the "Technology" course taught in the Health Care, Technology and Place collaborative doctoral program at University of Toronto (January 8, 2004) and on a paper coauthored by mentors of that program (Poland et al. 2005).

3. According to the idiot-proof design imperative:

The product has to be made such that even an idiot can work it. So participants in design who abide by this norm work to shield the innards of their machinery from the user. They multiply internal redundancies, make it well nigh impossible for the user to get inside and poke around, then add "idiot lights" to inform and direct the operator to call the service department if something goes wrong. Setting impermeable interfaces with potential users is one way in which engineers try to extend their control over the functioning of their productions out into the marketplace. (Bucciarelli 1994, 124)

4. Joerges (1999) has analyzed Winner's bridge example as a case of Chinese whispers. See also Woolgar and Cooper (1999).

5. Figure 2.2 summarizes the core relationships between medical innovations and clinical expertise that I just explored. It reflects the fundamental dynamics that can be observed in Abbott's systems of professions. Abbott defined seven types of jurisdictional arrangements that may characterize how various competing groups maintain authority or partial authority over task domains. His detailed case studies have also shown how the history of professions is shaped by broader dynamics that influence the supply of professionals and the demand for their services (e.g., demographics, economy, culture).

6. Barley and Tolbert (1997, 108) used the term "script" with a different meaning: "The notion of a script usefully substitutes for Giddens' more abstract notion of modalities because scripts can be empirically identified, regardless of the type of actor or level of analysis in which a researcher is interested." They developed this notion for use when empirically investigating "institutions as being enacted through scripts."

Chapter 3

1. See, for example, an enlightening paper by Siu (2003) on users' creative responses to design. He describes how Hong Kong residents sometimes spontaneously hang out their quilts in public parks and recreational infrastructures. They believe that hanging quilts out in fresh, cold air kills the germs on them. Although the "need" for recreational infrastructures is not negated by such an unplanned use, it shows how other functions can be added to a flexible, versatile design.

2. According to Bucciarelli (1994, 72), the "uncertainty in the validation of a design scenario is what makes designing the challenge it is. *Uncertain* is perhaps not quite the right word to describe the participants' state of mind, for the authors of these stories display full confidence in their constructions. But it is impossible to carry out all the tests, to develop and pursue all the possible scenarios about the behavior of objects to fully verify a design."

3. Adopting a radically different approach, Haraway (1991), in introducing the notion of the "cyborg," made a major contribution to feminist analysis with her politicized and subversive conception (Oudshoorn and Pinch 2003) of the technology user as a human–technology hybrid whose (gendered) identity remains equivocal. Such an analysis could be applied to better understand how chronic care patients integrate high-tech home care equipment in their daily lives and reconstruct their identity.

4. According to Norman (1989, 189), the use of any device is learned more readily if the user has a good conceptual model: "This requires that the principles of operation be observable, that all actions be consistent with the conceptual model, and that the visible parts of the device reflect the current state of the device in a way consistent with that model." Hence, a designer must create a conceptual model that users can understand and that captures the important steps of the device's operation.

5. One of the dialysis units in which we conducted research had a wall-mounted gratitude plaque given by a patient who had successfully received a transplant. This plaque may have served as a concrete sign of the individual's hope for a better, positive future. In general, though, gloomy sickness, foreseeable death, and the impact of technology on patients are not easy topics for patients, clinicians, and researchers to articulate and discuss.

6. The term *user-friendly technology* is equivocal. On the one hand, it is widely used in the context of mundane social interactions where its meaning is rarely, if ever, contested. On the other, everyone is supposed to be a good judge of the level of user-friendliness of complex information systems or devices. It is even a selling point for a wide range of products, from coffee machines to global positioning system (GPS)-based car computers. While conducting a literature search on Medline, I identified a startling number of disparate things referred to as user-friendly, including diets, intrauterine devices, clinical practice guidelines, and nursing care.

7. Illich (1973, 11) adds, "I choose the term 'conviviality' to designate the opposite of industrial productivity. I intend it to mean autonomous and creative intercourse among persons,

and the intercourse of persons with their environment; and this in contrast with the conditioned response of persons to the demands made upon them by others, and by man-made environment." To illustrate his point, Illich offers the library as the "prototype of a convivial tool," stressing that "repositories for other learning tools can be organized on its model, expanding access to tapes, pictures, records, and very simple labs filled with the same scientific instruments with which most of the major breakthroughs of the last century were made" (1973, 65).

8. But it must be asked what "meaning and expectations" designers should build into technology. For Illich, the purpose of convivial tools is intimately linked to the fulfillment of his dream of a redesigned, convivial society, one that guarantees "for each member the most ample and free access to the tools of the community and limit this freedom only in favor of another member's equal freedom" (1973, 12).

9. This results in a paradoxical state of affairs because "the overriding ethos within the community of system designers has been to try to ensure that the system is user-friendly" (Wooffitt and MacDermid 1995, 126).

Chapter 4

1. Blumenthal et al. (1996) do stress, however, that it would be unwise for universities to depend too heavily on financial support from industry because such funding is not conducive to maintaining high levels of excellence in fundamental research (as opposed to applied research).

2. Angell also recommends setting up an independent national advisory panel to thoroughly study pharmaceutical industry practices.

3. The belief that manufacturers of devices and drugs had *already* gathered data on the costs and effectiveness of their products was also widespread among industry representatives. Several interviewees stressed that providing such data was a requirement for obtaining regulatory approval and market; as a result, they claimed that HTA was redundant.

4. Members of the medical administrative elite may also look for knowledge, but of a kind that would be more helpful in guiding the macro-allocation of resources (e.g., defining the number and distribution of physicians or more efficiently distributing resources across medical areas). One respondent from a college of physicians, for instance, stressed that he did not have any particular expectations concerning HTA: "We're often looking for data and information. . . . We need extremely precise data on the health care system and how it works. This is lacking" (Physician Association 2).

5. The health sector probably differs from others on this point. The mistrust of private-based research is generally more prominent in this sector because the pursuit of profit is widely seen as directly conflicting with the good of the patient. In the areas of telecommunications, electronics, or new materials, private research laboratories are more often regarded as highly competitive, more resourceful, and innovative.

6. This respondent's opinion on policy-making influence might also reflect his organization's mission—to raise funds for research. He did not position his association as one that provides information or services to patients or defends their interests, and therefore lobbying governments may be less important.

7. In their study of collaborative research experiences, Ross et al. (2003, 28) found three models of decision-maker involvement: "formal supporter"—"decision-makers were not actively involved in the research process"; "responsive audience"—"decision-makers were actively involved in the research process by responding to researcher approaches with ideas, information or tactical advice"; and "integral partner"—"decision-makers were actively involved in the research process as a significant partner in helping to shape the research process." According to these authors, all three models had a positive impact on the research process. They also observed that supporting interactions between researchers and decision-makers outside of the research process could leverage unforeseen rewards.

8. The timeliness argument was emphasized by a respondent who recommended that HTA agencies monitor and anticipate technological developments in order to enhance the timing of their assessments:

[It's key] to your survival as a professional organization to be able to see what's coming down the road and what the pressures will be, and some associations are doing that better than others. . . . you can develop the skill, but it's only as good, and as effective, as the environment you're working in. If you're working in a very erratic and unpredictable environment, it really doesn't matter how good your skills are. If you think things are going to fall into a certain sequence in the next twelve months, and they don't—because that's the way the environment works—that's the best you're going to be able to do. (Decision-maker 3)

9. As Martin notes, the word "meaning" connotes both intelligibility and values: "These dual connotations are connected, for it is in light of values that human beings make their lives intelligible. Meaning connects directly with motivation and commitment, with what people care about deeply in ways that evoke interest and energy, shape identities, and create pride or shame in work" (2002, 547).

Chapter 5

1. For instance, Cohen and Hanft (2004, 104) suggest that in order to avoid impeding the adoption of a beneficial, cost-effective technology, one must "improve the timeliness and rigor of technology evaluation methods and . . . develop mechanisms for disseminating evaluation findings at appropriate points in the diffusion process." This solution would indeed prove satisfactory if the time horizon were limited to five or ten years.

2. As Moran and Alexander (1997, 591) observe, the history of technological innovation in medicine is a history of "dazzling scientific research and engineering ingenuity." Nonetheless, "that dazzling history is due in large part to the investment of huge resources. The history of the assessment of that technology is, by contrast, an affair of very modest investment and correspondingly modest intellectual advance."

3. A similar observation could hold for the production of science in general. According to Fuller (2000, 148), in such production a "sense of continuity is reinforced by the idea that the primary aim of science is 'The Truth,' which, in turn, has tended to reduce normative questions about inquiry to disputes over the appropriate means to this already agreed-upon end. It is no accident that the philosophy of science has been primarily concerned with something called 'methodology' rather than 'axiology.'"

4. Through a mail survey of the adult population (n=1,187) in England and Wales on the subject of genetic technologies, Calnan et al. (2005, 1947) found "that those who are negative about new, innovative, health care technologies are also likely to have lower levels of trust and confidence in health care and health-care practitioners." In addition, they found "general public skepticism of many but not all new technologies, and that acceptance specifically depended to some extent on the technology's perceived utility value in terms of treating specific diseases" (1947). These findings may coincide with the emergence of a pragmatic stance toward the value of innovations.

5. Fuller (2000, 155) also believes that we should "take seriously the size and diversity of the activities and institutions devoted to the pursuit of knowledge."

6. Consumers are defined as "patients, carers, long-term users of services, organizations representing consumers' interests, members of the public who are the potential recipients of health promotion programs and groups asking for research because they believe they have been exposed to potentially harmful circumstances, products or services" (Royle and Oliver 2004, 494).

7. We need to be vigilant about using the consumerist perspective to define desirable health technologies. As Faulkner (1997, 202) aptly puts it, "If the existence of choice itself might affect health, then personal healthcare choices become part of the material from which some health technologies are manufactured."

8. One could argue that the decreasing proportion of public funding in the total research-funding envelope is due not to the private sector "invading" research, but brought about by decreasing support from public authorities, which are asking industry to increase their support of research. That is why data on absolute spending figures and their pattern over time are needed.

9. As Faulkner remarks, HTA may itself be seen as a rationalist technology that seeks to establish its own scientific authority:

The HTA movement, in its engagement of expert disciplines, its research alliances, its encompassing metaphors, its containment of uncertainty, its consultation of public voices, its bias-elimination methodologies, and its use of a rational aggregated voice speaking for the good of the public health, might be seen as part of a dialectical process involving decline in traditional medical authority and a reconstruction of a new framework of scientific authority. (1997, 203)

10. The assumption that these issues are too complex for the ordinary citizen to grasp, an attitude that is not unique to the health sector, may be invalid. As Fuller (2000, 148) comments, "The biggest obstacle facing Big Science's public accountability is not the public's lacking competence but its lacking a clear stake in the outcomes of research. To be sure, when the stakes are made clear—as in most cases surrounding biotechnology—the public is quite prepared to engage with highly complicated and technical issues."

11. For Bohman (1996, 229), disclosures are not disclosures of truth, but rather "are prior to truth, they concern what makes truth possible." Disclosures cannot be self-justifying or self-verifying; they require public reflection and deliberation.

12. Bohman asserts that three conditions are required for a deliberative democracy to flourish and to avoid the pitfalls associated with policy arenas in which experts and elite groups hold sway: "the discursive structures of informal and formal deliberations make it less likely that irrational and untenable arguments will decide outcomes"; "decision-making procedures are structured so as to allow revisions—of arguments, decisions, and even procedures—that either take up features of defeated positions or better their chances of being heard"; and "deliberative decision-making procedures are broadly inclusive, so that minorities may reasonably expect they will be able to affect future outcomes in ways they have not been able so far" (Bohman 1996, 100).

13. According to Sang (2004, 187), a new paradigm surfaces, one that "synthesizes the values of consumerism and citizenship, and which challenges public authorities, professions, and the public themselves to rethink their relationships, roles and responsibilities in relation to health-care delivery and service planning."

14. "This ideal of common citizenship does not demand that all citizens agree for the same reasons; it demands only that they continue to cooperate and to compromise in the same process of public deliberation. In deep conflicts, such continued cooperation and thus common citizenship is precisely what is at stake" (Bohman 1996, 89).

Conclusion

1. I nevertheless regard refusing to engage in collaborative research to be a legitimate position, because a number of researchers should devote their time entirely to producing knowledge and, therefore, to contributing to the overall scientific enterprise. I do not see why there should be just one position on the issue.

2. When discussing the significance of the emergence of a "risk society," Beck (2001, 343) argues that science becomes increasingly necessary in the governance of modern societies and, simultaneously, proves less and less sufficient.

3. According to Faulkner, many aspects of the HTA movement could form the basis of a proper sociological inquiry.

   [The national health technology assessment movement] raises issues to do with interests, values and inter-organisational relationships. It raises questions about the shaping of research agendas, healthcare policies, regulation of health technologies and, indeed, about the evolving patterns and methods of healthcare. . . . It also raises issues germane to some of the prime concerns of sociologies of medicine/healthcare and science/technology, including trust and contestability in medical authority, construction of healthcare risks, rhetorics of scientific projects and knowledge claims, relationships between the disciplines of medical and healthcare knowledge, and relationships between healthcare experiments, laboratories and technology tests. (Faulkner 1997, 184)

4. This requires first being aware of the institutional dynamics that steer knowledge production in certain directions, such as the ones Winner archly describes:

During the 80s many of those most delightfully detached and ironic about the Strategic Defense Initiative were also accepting paychecks to work on it. Similar attitudes are still with us, for example, in the playful hermeneutics that surround "virtual reality" and "interactive" media, while our populace is being manoeuvered toward new frameworks of manipulation and exploitation (1994, 109).

5. Against constructivists' generally evasive political stance, Winner recommends enforcing an "anticonstructivist" position. Elam gives a straightforward reply to this recommendation, in the form of a counter-proposition: "[Being anti anticonstructivist] does *not* mean 'sitting on the fence', because, as an intellectual attitude, it is well suited to combat the paranoia that leads to fences being raised in the first place" (1994, 102). An explicit reluctance to define and adhere to a party line, of blindly putting forward a sort of coherent ideology that pretends to be a universal application, is a judicious and mature intellectual attitude, but it is insufficient.

6. "Mais il faut penser le réseau en ce qu'il suscite, en certains endroits, la nécessité héroïque de n'être ni paresseux, ni conformiste, ni respectueux pour ne pas être dupe."

7. For Melzer there is a need to attain a "serene detachment" vis-à-vis the problem of technology: "We might begin to distance ourselves from technology . . . first, by attempting to overcome our forgetfulness of happiness and the human good; and second, by adopting, as part of this very attempt, a more humble attitude toward the past, especially the pretechnological past, both Eastern and Western" (Melzer 1993, 320).

8. Stengers offers an interesting comparison between irony and humor: A transcendental stance is adopted by the relativist who ironically grants him/herself a lucid, remote, and overmastering hindsight. This sharp demarcation from the Others enables critics to forge judgments that are aloof from the individuals and groups studied, and to remain highly confident of this Difference (Stengers 1993, 79). There is no commitment in time and space on the part of critics. On the other hand, humor is an immanent art, the ability to consider oneself a very product of the unfolding story that is actually being followed. Thus, irony and humor constitute different political projects. They create different arenas for debating with/ against scientists, engineers, the public, and policy-makers. According to Stengers, irony opposes power to power, whereas humor cultivates a shared perplexity and puts debaters on equal terms.

9. "The term *kairos* has a rich and varied history, but generally refers to the way a given context for communication both calls for and constrains one's speech. Thus, sensitive to *kairos*, a speaker or writer takes into account the contingencies of a given place and time, and considers the opportunities within this specific context for words to be effective and appropriate to that moment. As such, this concept is tightly linked to considerations of audience (the most significant variable in a communicative context) and to decorum (the principle of apt speech)." http//humanities.byu.edu/rhetoric/Encompassing%20Terms/kairos.htm (accessed April 20, 2005).

10. According to Brown and Webster, medical technologies "open up and so increase the diversity of existing socio-biological boundaries" (2004, 170).

11. Furthermore, recent technological developments such as genetic information banks have initiated a "move towards a *repositioning of choice and consent* beyond the conventional level of the individual, as patient or kin, to the institutional, collective level" (Brown and Webster 2004, 170).

12. According to Petre (2004, 477), "In high-performing engineering teams and companies, innovation happens deliberately, [because] teams have developed a number of systematic practices that support innovation and feed inspiration." Examining twelve firms operating in the United Kingdom and the United States, Petre observed that they tended to combine two modes for generating new products: "first-to-market, generating new ideas which they marketed to select clients" and "designing solutions for customer-identified problems" (479). Thus, new technologies are customized to address specific client needs, certain ones of which give rise to new technologies that are afterward applied in other contexts.

13. Needless to say, this paper triggered a spectrum of reactions. See, for instance, Goldstein (2001), Johnson (2000), Levin-Scherz (2001), and J. T. Smith (2000).

Bibliography

Abbott, A. 1988. *The system of professions: An essay on the division of expert labor.* Chicago: University of Chicago Press.

Abelson, J., P.-G. Forest, J. Eyles, P. Smith, E. Martin, and F.-P. Gauvin. 2003. Deliberations about deliberative methods: Issues in the design and evaluation of public participation processes. *Social Science and Medicine* 57 (2): 239–251.

Abraham, J. 2002. Drug safety and the safety of patients: The challenge to medicine and health from permissive expert risk assessments of triazolam (Halcion). *Health, Risk and Society* 4 (1): 19–29.

AETMIS (Agence d'Évaluation des Technologies et des Modes d'Intervention en Santé). 2002. *The efficacy and safety of electroconvulsive therapy: Issues in delivery and organization.* Montreal: AETMIS.

Akrich, M. 1994. Comment sortir de la dichotomie technique/société: Présentation des diverses sociologies de la technique. In *De la préhistoire aux missiles balistiques: De l'intelligence sociale des techniques,* ed. B. Latour and P. Lemonnier, 105–131. Paris: La Découverte.

Akrich, M. 1995. User representations: Practices, methods and sociology. In *Managing technology in society: The approach of constructive technology assessment,* ed. A. Rip, T. J. Misa, and J. Schot, 205–224. London: Pinter.

Akrich, M. and B. Latour. 1992. A summary of a convenient vocabulary for the semiotics of human and non-human assemblies. In *Shaping technology/building society: Studies in sociotechnical change,* ed. W. E. Bijker and J. Law, 259–264. Cambridge, MA: MIT Press.

Andrews, G. J. 2003. Locating a geography of nursing: Space, place and the progress of geographical thought. *Nursing Philosophy* 4: 231–248.

Angell, M. 2000. The pharmaceutical industry: To whom is it accountable? *New England Journal of Medicine* 342 (25): 1902–1904.

Armstrong, D. 1983. *Political anatomy of the body: Medical knowledge in Britain in the twentieth century.* Cambridge: Cambridge University Press.

Auditor General of Quebec. 2001. *Report to the National Assembly for 2000–2001,* official publication of the Quebec government. Highlights available in English: http://www.vgq.gouv.qc.ca/publications/rapp_2001_1/Highlights/Index.html

Australia, Productivity Commission. 2005. *The impact of advances in medical technology in Australia.* Melbourne: The Commission.

Baker C. F., C. J. Rudnisky, M. T. Tennant, P. Sanghera, B. J. Hinz, A. R. De Leon, and M. D. Greve. 2004. JPEG compression of stereoscopic digital images for the diagnosis of diabetic retinopathy via teleophthalmology. *Canadian Journal of Ophthalmolology* 39 (7): 746–754.

Baker, N. 1990. *The mezzanine.* New York: Vintage Books.

Banta, H. D. and B. R. Luce. 1993. *Health care technology and its assessment: An international perspective.* New York: Oxford University Press.

Banta, H. D., W. J. Oortwijn, and W. T. van Beekum. 1995. *The organization of health care technology assessment in the Netherlands.* The Hague: Rathenau Institute.

Banta, H. D., and S. Perry. 1997. A history of ISTAHC: A personal perspective on its first 10 years. *International Journal of Technology Assessment in Health Care* 13 (3): 430–453.

Barbot, J. 1998. Science, marché et compassion: L'intervention des associations de lutte contre le sida dans la circulation des nouvelles molécules. *Sciences Sociales et Santé* 16 (3): 67–93.

Barley, S. R., and P. S. Tolbert. 1997. Institutionalization and structuration: Studying the links between action and institution. *Organization Studies* 18 (1): 93–117.

Bartunek, J., J. Trullen, E. Bonet, and A. Sauquet. 2003. Sharing and expanding academic and practitioner knowledge in health care. *Health Services Research & Policy* 8 (2): 62–68.

Bastian, H. 1998. Speaking up for ourselves: The evolution of consumer advocacy in health care. *International Journal of Technology Assessment in Health Care* 14: 3–23.

Battista, R. N., H. D. Banta, E. Jonsson, M. Hodge, and Gelbland, H. 1994. Lessons from eight countries. *Health Policy* 30: 397–421.

Battista, R. N., J.-M. Lance, P. Lehoux, and G. Régnier. 1999. Health technology assessment and the regulation of medical devices and procedures in Quebec: Synergy, collusion or collision? *International Journal of Technology Assessment in Health Care* 15 (3): 593–601.

Beck, U. 1992. *La société du risque. Sur la voie d'une autre modernité.* Paris: Flammarion.

Berg, M. 1997. *Rationalizing medical work: Decision-support techniques and medical practices.* Cambridge, MA: MIT Press.

Berg, M., R. ter Meulen, and M. van den Burg. 2001. Guidelines for appropriate care: The importance of empirical normative analysis. *Health Care Analysis* 9: 77–99.

Berg, M., T. van der Grinten, and N. Klazinga. 2004. Technology assessment, priority setting, and appropriate care in Dutch health care. *International Journal of Technology Assessment in Health Care* 20 (1): 35–43.

Bero, L. A., and A. R. Jadad. 1997. How consumers and policymakers can use systematic reviews for decision-making. *Annals of Internal Medicine* 127: 37–42.

Bero, L. A., R. Grilli, J. M. Grimshaw, E. Harvey, A. D. Oxman, and M. A. Thomson. 1998. Closing the gap between research and practice: An overview of systematic reviews of interventions to promote the implementation of research findings. *British Medical Journal* 317 (7156): 465–468.

Besharov, D. J., and J. Dunsay Silver. 1987. Rationing access to advanced medical techniques. *Journal of Legal Medicine* 8 (4): 507–532.

Bijker, W. E. (1987). The social construction of Bakelite: Toward a theory of invention. In *The social construction of technological systems*, ed. W. E. Bijker, T. P. Hughes, and T. J. Pinch, 11–50. Cambridge, MA: MIT Press.

Blume, S. S. 1992. *Insight and industry: On the dynamics of technological change in medicine.* Cambridge, MA: MIT Press.

Blume, S. S. 1997. The rhetoric and counter-rhetoric of a "bionic technology." *Science, Technology and Human Values* 22 (1): 31–56.

Blumenthal, D., N. Causino, E. Campbell, and K. Seashore Louis. 1996. Relationships between academic institutions and industry in the life sciences: an industry survey. *New England Journal of Medicine* 334: 368–373.

Bohman, J. 1996. *Public deliberation: Pluralism, complexity, and democracy.* Cambridge, MA: MIT Press.

Bos, M., P. Carlsson, S. Kooij, L. Liaropoulos, L. Sampietro-Colom, J. Schilling, and the EUR-ASSESS Project, Technology Assessment and Insurance Coverage SubGroup. 1996. *Technology assessment and coverage policy: The case of invasive cardiology therapy in five European countries.* Barcelona: Catalan Agency for Health Technology Assessment and Research (CAHTA).

Brown, N., and A. Webster. 2004. *New medical technologies and society: Reordering life.* Cambridge: Polity Press.

Bucciarelli, L. L. 1994. *Designing engineers.* Cambridge, MA: MIT Press.

Burke, J., and R. Ornstein. 1997. *The axemaker's gift: Technology's capture and control of our minds and culture.* New York: Penguin Putnam.

Buxton, M., and S. Hanney. 1996. How can payback from health services research be assessed? *Journal of Health Services Research* 1 (1): 35–43.

Cabatoff, K. A. 1996. Getting on and off the policy agenda: A dualistic theory of program evaluation utilization. *Canadian Journal of Program Evaluation* 11: 35–60.

Callahan, D. 1990. *What kind of life: The limits of medical progress.* Washington, D.C.: Georgetown University Press.

Callon, M. 1986. Éléments pour une sociologie de la traduction: La domestication des coquilles Saint-Jacques et des marins-pêcheurs dans la baie de Saint-Brieuc. *L'Année Sociologique* 36: 169–208.

Callon, M. 1987. Society in the making: The study of technology as a tool for sociological analysis. In *The social construction of technological systems,* ed. W. E. Bijker, T. P. Hughes, and T. J. Pinch, 83–106. Cambridge, MA: MIT Press.

Calnan, M., D. Montaner, and R. Horne. 2005. How acceptable are innovative health-care technologies? A survey of public beliefs and attitudes in England and Wales. *Social Science and Medicine* 60: 1937–1948.

Campbell, J. L. 2002. Ideas, politics, and public policy. *Annual Review of Sociology* 28: 21–38.

Casey, S. 1998. *Set phasers on stun: And other true tales of design, technology, and human error.* Santa Barbara, CA: Aegean.

Champagne, F., L. Lemieux-Charles, and W. McGuire. 2004. Introduction: Toward a broader understanding of the use of knowledge and evidence in health care. In *Multidisciplinary perspectives on evidence-based decision-making in health care,* ed. L. Lemieux-Charles and F. Champagne, 3–17. Toronto: University of Toronto Press.

Chernew, M. E., R. A. Hirth, S. S. Sonnad, R. Ermann, and A. M. Fendrick. 1998. Managed care, medical technology, and health care cost growth: A review of the evidence. *Medical Care Research Review* 55 (3): 259–288; discussion 289–297.

Chervenak, F. K., and L. B. McCullough. 2001. The moral foundation of medical leadership: The professional virtues of the physician as fiduciary of the patient. *American Journal of Obstetrics and Gynecology* 18 (5): 875–880.

Christensen, C. M., R. Bohmer, and J. Kenagy. 2000. Will disruptive innovations cure health care? *Harvard Business Review* 78 (5): 102–112, 199.

Clarke, A. 1998. *Disciplining reproduction: Modernity, American life sciences, and "the problem of sex."* Chicago: University of Chicago Press.

Coburn, A. F. 1998. The role of health services research in developing state health policy. *Health Affairs* 17:139–151.

Cockburn, C. 1983. *Brothers: Male dominance and technological change.* London: Pluto Press.

Coddington, D. C., E. A. Fischer, K. D. Moore, and R. L. Clarke, eds. 2000. *Beyond managed care: How consumers and technology are changing the future of health care.* San Francisco: Jossey-Bass.

Cohen, A. B., and R. S. Hanft, with W. E. Encinosa, S. M. Spernak, S. A. Stewart, and C. C. White. 2004. *Technology in American health care: Policy directions for effective evaluation and management.* Ann Arbor: University of Michigan Press.

Collins, H., and M. Kush. 1998. *The shape of actions: What humans and machines can do.* Cambridge, MA: MIT Press.

Cooke, B., and U. Kothari, eds. 2001. *Participation: The New Tyranny?* London: Zed Books.

Cookson, R., and A. Maynard. 2000. Health technology assessment in Europe: Improving clarity and performance. *International Journal of Technology Assessment in Health Care* 16 (2): 639–650.

Coulter, A. 2004. Perspectives on health technology assessment: Response from the patient's perspective. *International Journal of Technology Assessment in Health Care* 20 (1): 92–96.

Couture, D. 1988. Technologies médicales et statut des corps professionnels dans la division du travail socio-sanitaire. *Sociologie et Sociétés* 20 (2): 77–88.

Cowan, R. S. 1983. *More work for mother: The ironies of household technology from the open hearth to the microwave.* New York: Basic Books.

Coyle, D., L. Davies, and M. F. Drummond. 1998. Trials and tribulations: Emerging issues in designing economic evaluations alongside clinical trials. *International Journal of Technology Assessment in Health Care* 14: 135–144.

Coyte, P., and W. Young. 1997. Applied home care research. *International Journal of Health Care Quality Assurance Incorporating Leadership in Health Services* 10 (1): i–iv.

Creditor, M. C., and J. B. Garrett. 1977. The information base for diffusion of technology: Computed tomography scanning. *New England Journal of Medicine* 297: 49–53.

Cross, N. 2004. Editorial. *Design Studies* 24: 425–426.

Cutler, D. M., and M. McClellan. 2001. Is technological change in medicine worth it? *Health Affairs* 20 (5): 11–29.

Daly, J., and E. Willis. 1989. Technological innovation and the labour process in health care. *Social Science and Medicine* 28 (11): 1149–1157.

Daniels, N., and J. E. Sabin. 1997. Limits to health care: Fair procedures, democratic deliberation and the legitimacy problem for insurers. *Philosophy and Public Affairs* 26 (4): 303–350.

Daniels, N., and J. E. Sabin. 1998. Ethics of accountability in managed care reform. *Health Affairs* 17: 50–64.

Danzon, P. M., and M. V. Pauly. 2001. Insurance and new technology: From hospital to drugstore. *Health Affairs* 20 (5): 86–100.

Davies, E., and P. Littlejohns. 2002. Views of directors of public health about NICE Appraisal Guidance: Results of a postal survey. *Journal of Public Health Medicine* 24: 319–325.

Deber, R. 1992. Translating technology assessment into policy. *International Journal of Technology Assessment in Health Care* 8 (1): 131–137.

Deber, R. 2003. Health care reforms: Lessons from Canada. *American Journal of Public Health* 93 (1): 20–24.

Denis, J.-L., P. Lehoux, and F. Champagne. 2004. Knowledge utilization in health care: From fine-tuning dissemination to contexualizing knowledge. In *Using knowledge and evidence in health care: Multidisiplinary perspectives*, ed. L. Lemieux-Charles and F. Champagne, 18–40. Toronto: University of Toronto Press.

Denis, J.-L., P. Lehoux, M. Hivon, and F. Champagne. 2003. Creating a new articulation between research and practice through policy? The views and experience of researchers and practitioners. *Journal of Health Services Research.* 8 (Suppl. 2): 44–51.

Dixon-Woods, M., S. Agarwal, B. Young, D. Jones, and A. Sutton. 2004. *Integrative approaches to qualitative and quantitative evidence.* London: National Health Service (NHS), Health Development Agency.

Dodier, N. 1995. *Les hommes et les machines: La conscience collective dans les sociétés technicisées.* Paris: Éditions Métailié.

Domenigehtti, G., R. Grilli, and A. Liberati. 1998. Promoting consumers' demand for evidence-based medicine. *International Journal of Technology Assessment in Health Care* 14: 97–105.

Dyer, S. 2004. Rationalising public participation in the health services: The case of research ethics committees. *Health and Place* 10: 339–348.

Eccles, M. 2004. NICE clinical guidelines: Health economics must engage with complexity of issues. Letter. *British Medical Journal* 329: 572.

Edquist, C., and B. Johnson. 1997. Institutions and organizations in systems of innovation. In *Systems of innovation: Technologies, institutions and organizations,* ed. C. Edquist, 41–63. London: Pinter.

Elam, M. 1994. Anti anticonstructivism or laying the fears of a Langdon Winner to rest. *Science, Technology & Human Values* 19 (1): 101–106.

Ellis, D. 2000. *Technology and the future of health care: Preparing for the next 30 years.* San Francisco: Jossey-Bass.

Elzinga, A. 2004. Book review: Making science and technology studies relevant for technology policy—Gains and losses? *Social Studies of Science* 34(6): 949–956.

Evans, R. 1984. *Strained mercy: The economics of Canadian health care.* Toronto: Butterworths.

Evans, R., M. L. Barer, and T. R. Marmor, eds. 1994. *Why are some people healthy and others not?: The determinants of health of the populations.* New York: A. de Gruyter.

Fagerhaugh, S., A. Strauss, B. Suczek, and C. Wiener. 1986. Chronic illness, medical technology, and clinical safety in the hospital. *Research in the Sociology of Health Care* 4: 237–270.

Faulkner, A. 1997. "Strange bedfellows" in the laboratory of the NHS? An analysis of the new science of health technology assessment in the United Kingdom. In *The Sociology of Medical Science and Technology,* ed. M. A. Elston, 183–207. Oxford: Blackwell.

Faulkner, A., I. Geesink, J. Kent, and D. Fitzpatrick. 2003. Human tissue engineered products: drugs or devices? Editorial. *British Medical Journal* 326: 1159–1160.

Finlay, J. F., B. Henderson, and D. Menon. 1994. Medical device regulation in Canada: Direction for change. *Health Policy* 28:185–195.

Foote, S. B. 1986. Coexistence, conflict, and cooperation: Public policies toward medical devices. *Journal of Health Politics, Policy and Law* 11 (3): 501–523.

Foray, D. 1997. Generation and distribution of technological knowledge: Incentives, norms, and institutions. In *Systems of Innovation: Technologies, Institutions, and Organizations*, ed. C. Edquist, 64–85. London: Pinter.

Fox, N. J., K. J. Ward, and A. J. O'Rourke. 2005. The "expert patient": Empowerment or medical dominance? The case of weight loss, pharmaceutical drugs and the Internet. *Social Science and Medicine* 60: 1299–1309.

Freidson, E. 1975. *Doctoring together: A study of professional social control.* New York: Elsevier.

Friedman, L., H. Cooper, J. Webb, A.Weinberg, and S. E. Plon. 2003. Primary care physicians' attitudes and practices regarding cancer genetics: A comparison of 2001 and 1996 survey results. *Journal of Cancer Education* 18 (2): 91–94.

Fuller, S. 1993. *Philosophy of science and its discontents*, 2nd ed. New York: Guilford Press.

Fuller, S. 2000. *The governance of science.* Buckingham, U.K.: Open University Press.

Galanti, G.-A. 1999. How to do ethnographic research. *Western Journal of Medicine* 171: 19–20.

Gallo, P. 2004. Integrating ethical enquiry and health technology assessment: Limits and opportunities for efficiency and equity. *Poiesis & Praxis* 2: 103–117.

Garcia-Altes, A., S. Ondategui-Parra, and P. J. Neuman. 2004. Cross-national comparison of technology assessment processes. *International Journal of Technology Assessment in Health Care* 20 (3): 300–310.

Garrety, K., and R. Badham. 2004. User-centered design and the normative politics of technology. *Science, Technology, & Human Values* 29 (2): 191–212.

Gauthier, P. 1999. Technological intervention and the malady of happiness. *Design Issues* 15 (2): 40–54.

Gelijns, A., and N. Rosenberg. 1994 The dynamics of technological change in medicine. *Health Affairs* 13 (3): 28–45.

Giacomini, M. 1999. The which-hunt: Assembling health technologies for assessment and rationing. *Journal of Health Politics, Policy, and Law* 24: 715–758.

Giacomini, M., F. Miller, and G. Browman. 2003. Confronting the "gray zones" of technology assessment: Evaluating genetic testing services for public insurance coverage in Canada. *International Journal of Technology Assessment in Health Care* 19 (2): 301–316.

Giacomini, M., J. Hurley, I. Gold, P. Smith, and J. Abelson. 2004. The policy analysis of "values talk": Lessons from Canadian health reform. *Health Policy* 67: 15–24.

Giacomini, M., D. J. Cook, D. L. Streiner, and S. S. Anand. 2000. Using practice guidelines to allocate medical technologies: An ethics framework. *International Journal of Technology Assessment in Health Care* 16 (4): 987–1002.

Gibbons, M., C. Limoges, H. Nowotny, P. Scott, S. Schwartzman, and M. Trow. 1994. *The new production of knowledge: The dynamics of science and research in contemporary societies.* London: Sage.

Giddens, A. 1984. *The constitution of society: Outline of the theory of structuration.* Berkeley: University of California Press.

Gillick, M. R. 2004. Medicare coverage for technological innovations: Time for new criteria? *New England Journal of Medicine* 350 (21): 2199–2203.

Goering, P., D. Butterill, N. Jacobson, and D. Sturtevant. 2003. Linkage and exchange at the organizational level: A model of collaboration between research and policy. *Health Services Research & Policy* 8 (2): 14–19.

Goffman, E. 1971. *The presentation of self in everyday life.* Harmondsworth, U.K.: Penguin.

Golden-Biddle, K., T. Reay, S. Petz, C. Witt, A. Casebeer, A. Pablo, and B. Hinings. 2003. Towards a communicative perspective of collaborating in research: The case of the researcher–decision-maker partnership. *Health Services Research & Policy* 8 (2): 20–25.

Goldstein, D. 2001. Disruptive innovations threaten revenues and profits. *Management Care Interface* 14 (4): 50–52.

Goodman, C. 1992. It's time to rethink health care technology assessment. *International Journal of Technology Assessment in Health Care* 8: 335–358.

Gortmaker, S. L., and P. H. Wise. 1997. The first injustice: Socioeconomic disparities, health services technology, and infant mortality. *Annual Review of Sociology* 23: 147–170.

Greenhalgh, T., G. Robert, F. MacFarlane, P. Bate, and O. Kyriakidou. 2004. Diffusion of innovations in service organizations: Systematic review and recommendations. *Milbank Quarterly* 82 (4): 581–629.

Greer, A. L. 1987. Rationing medical technology: Hospital decision making in the United States and England. *International Journal of Technology Assessment in Health Care* 3: 199–222.

Greer, A. L., J. S. Goodwin, J. L. Freeman, and Z. H. Wu. 2002. Bringing the patient back in: Guidelines, practice variations, and the social context of medical practice. *International Journal of Technology Assessment in Health Care* 18 (4): 747–761.

Grin, J. 2004. Health technology assessment between our health care system and our health. *Poiesis & Praxis* 2: 157–174.

Grint, K., and S. Woolgar. 1992. Computers, guns, and roses: What's social about being shot? *Science, Technology, & Human Values* 17 (3): 366–380.

Grunwald, A. 2004. The normative basis of (health) technology assessment and the role of ethical expertise. *Poiesis & Praxis* 2: 175–194.

Hailey, D. M. 1993. The influence of technology assessments by advisory bodies on health policy and practice. Health Policy, 25(3): 243–254.

Hailey, D. M., and B. L. Crowe. 1993. The influence of health technology assessment on the diffusion of MRI in Australia. *International Journal of Technology Assessment in Health Care* 9 (4): 522–529.

Halm, E. A., and A. Gelijns. 1991. An introduction to the changing economics of technological innovation in medicine. In *The changing economics of medical technology*, ed. A. Gelijns and E. A. Halm, 1–20. Washington, D.C.: National Academy Press.

Hammersley, M., and P. Atkinson. 1983. *Ethnography: Principles in practice.* London: Routledge.

Haraway, D. 1991. *Simians, cyborgs and women: The reinvention of nature.* New York: Routledge.

Hasman, A. 2003. Eliciting reasons: Empirical methods in priority setting. *Health Care Analysis* 11 (1): 41–58.

Heitman, E. 1996. The public's role in the evaluation of health care technology: The conflict over ECT. *International Journal of Technology Assessment in Health Care* 12 (4): 657–672.

Heitman, E. 1998. Ethical issues in technology assessment: Conceptual categories and procedural considerations. *International Journal of Technology Assessment in Health Care* 14 (3): 544–566.

Hirsch, P. 2005. Personal communication.

Hivon, M., P. Lehoux, J.-L. Denis, and S. Tailliez. 2005. The use of Health Technology Assessment (HTA) in decision-making: The co-responsibility of users and producers? *International Journal of Technology Assessment in Health Care* 21 (2): 268–275.

Hlatky, M. A. 2004. Evidence-based use of cardiac procedures and devices. *New England Journal of Medicine* 350 (21): 2126–2128.

Hogle, L. F. 2000. Réglementer les innovations utilisant des tissus humains: Hybrides et gouvernance. *Sciences Sociales et Santé* 18 (4): 53–73.

Ihde, D. 1990. *Technology and the lifeworld: From garden to earth.* Bloomington: Indiana University Press.

Illich, I. 1973. *Tools for conviviality.* New York: Harper & Row.

INHATA (International Agency for Health Technology Assessment). 1997. Newsletter. Stockholm: INAHTA.

Jacob, R., and M. McGregor. 1997. Assessing the impact of health technology assessment. *International Journal of Technology Assessment in Health Care* 13: 68–80.

Jasanoff, S. 1990. *The fifth branch: Science advisers as policymakers.* Cambridge, MA: Harvard University Press.

Joerges, B. 1999. Do politics have artifacts? *Social Studies of Science* 29 (3): 411–431.

Johnson, D. E. 2000. Will disruptive innovations cure health care? *Harvard Business Review* 78 (6): 197–198.

Johri, M., and P. Lehoux. 2003. The great escape? Health technology assessment as a means of cost control. *International Journal of Technology Assessment in Health Care* 19 (1): 179–193.

Kaiser, L. 2000. Foreword. In *Beyond managed care: How consumers and technology are changing the future of health care*, ed. D. C. Coddington, E. A. Fischer, K. D. Moore, and R. L. Clarke, ix–xii. San Francisco: Jossey-Bass.

Kaufman S. R. 2003. Hidden places, uncommon persons. *Social Science & Medicine* 56: 2249–2261.

Kaye, L. W., and J. Davitt. 1995. Importation of high technology services into the home. In *New developments in home care services for the elderly: Innovations in policy, program, and practice*, ed. L. W. Kay, 67–94. New York: Haworth Press.

Kearns, R. A. 1993. Place and health: Towards a reformed medical geography. *The Professional Geographer* 46: 67–72.

Kenen, R. G. 1996. The at-risk health status and technology: A diagnostic invitation and the "gift" of knowing. *Social Science and Medicine* 42 (11): 1545–1553.

Kent, J. 2003. Lay experts and the politics of breast implants. *Public Understanding of Science* 12: 403–421.

Kent, J., and A. Faulkner. 2002. Regulating human implant technologies in Europe: Understanding the new era in medical device regulation. *Health, Risk and Society* 4 (2): 189–209.

Kling, R. 1991. Computerization and social transformations. *Science, Technology, & Human Values* 16 (3): 342–367.

Kling, R. 1992a. Audiences, narratives, and human values in social studies of technology. *Science, Technology, & Human Values* 17 (3): 349–365.

Kling, R. 1992b. When gunfire shatters bone: Reducing sociotechnical systems to social relationships. *Science, Technology, & Human Values* 17 (3): 381–385.

Knorr Cetina, K. 1999. *Epistemic cultures: How the sciences make knowledge.* Cambridge, MA: Harvard University Press.

Koch, E. B. 1995. Why the development process should be part of medical technology assessment: Examples from the development of medical ultrasound. In *Managing technology in society: The approach of constructive technology assessment,* ed. A. Rip, T. J. Misa, and J. Schot, 231–260. London: Pinter.

Kuttner, R. 1998. Must good HMOs go bad? The commercialization of prepaid group health care. *New England Journal of Medicine* 338: 1558–1563.

LaCapra, R. 1997. Cultural studies, globalization, and neoliberalism. In *The politics of research,* ed. E. A. Kaplan and G. Levine, 69–89. New Brunswick, NJ: Rutgers University Press.

Latour, B. 1988. Mixing humans and nonhumans together: The sociology of a door-closer. *Social Problems* 35 (3): 298–310.

Latour, B. 1989. *La science en action.* Paris: Éditions La Découverte.

Latour, B. 1990. Postmodern? No, simply amodern! Steps towards an anthropology of science. *Studies in History and Philosophy of Science* 21 (1): 145–171.

Latour, B., and P. Lemonnier, eds.1994. *De la préhistoire aux missiles balistiques. De l'intelligence sociale des techniques.* Paris: Éditions La Découverte.

Laupacis, A. 2002. Inclusion of drugs in provincial drug benefit programs: Who is making these decisions, and are they the right ones? *Canadian Medical Association Journal* 166 (1): 44–47.

Laupacis, A., G. Anderson, and B. O'Brien. 2002. Drug policy: Making effective drugs available without bankrupting the healthcare system. *Healthcare Papers* 3 (1): 12–30.

Laupacis, A. and Evans, W. 2005. Diagnostic imaging in Canada. *Healthcare Papers* 6(1): 8–15.

Laupacis, A., D. Feeny, A. S. Detsky, and P. X. Tugwell. 1993. Tentative guidelines for using clinical and economic evaluations revisited. *Canadian Medical Association Journal* 148 (6): 927–929.

Lavis, J. N., S. E. Ross, J. E. Hurley, J. M. Hohenadel, G. L. Stoddart, C. A. Woodward, and J. Abelson. 2002. Examining the role of health services research in public policy-making. *The Milbank Quarterly* 80 (1): 125–154.

Lawton, J. 2003. Lay experiences of health and illness: Past research and future agendas. *Sociology of Health & Illness,* 25: 23–40.

Lehoux, P. 2000. Cohabitation des perspectives moderne et postmoderne dans la recherche en santé publique: Controverses et propositions. *Sciences Sociales et Santé* 18 (3): 37–75.

Lehoux, P. 2002. *Could new regulatory mechanisms be designed after a critical assessment of the value of health innovations?* Discussion Paper no. 37, Commission on the Future of Health Care in Canada.

Lehoux, P. 2004. Patients' perspectives on high-tech home care: A qualitative inquiry into the user-friendliness of four interventions. *BMC Health Services Research* 4 (28), http://www.biomedcentral.com/content/pdf/1472-6963-4-28.pdf.

Lehoux, P., and S. Blume. 2000. Technology assessment and the sociopolitics of health technologies. *Journal of Health Politics, Policy, and Law* 25 (6): 1083–1120.

Lehoux, P., C. Charland, R. Pineault, L. Richard, and J. Saint-Arnaud. 2002. Technologies de pointe et soins à domicile. Où en sont les CLSC? *Canadian Medical Association Journal* 166 (10): 1277–1278.

Lehoux, P., G. Daudelin, R. Pineault, J. St-Arnaud, and C. Sicotte. 2004. Évaluation des unités satellites et mobile d'hémodialyse. Report no. R04–02, GRIS, Université de Montréal.

Lehoux, P., J.-L. Denis, M. Hivon, and S. Tailliez. 2003. Dissemination and use of health technology assessment in Canada: The perception of providers, health care administrators, patients and industry. Report no. R03–01, GRIS, Université de Montréal.

Lehoux, P., J.-L. Denis, S. Tailliez, and M. Hivon. 2005. Disseminating health technology assessment: Identifying the visions guiding an evolving policy intervention in Canada. *Journal of Health Politics, Policy and Law*, 30 (4): 603–641.

Lehoux, P., J. Saint-Arnaud, and L. Richard. 2004. The use of technology at home: What patient manuals say and sell vs. what patients face and fear. *Sociology of Health & Illness*, 26 (5): 617–644.

Lehoux, P., C. Sicotte, and J.-L. Denis. 1999. Assessment of a computerized medical record system: Disclosing its scripts of use. *Evaluation and Program Planning* 22 (4): 439–453.

Lehoux, P., C. Sicotte, J.-L. Denis, M. Berg, and A. Lacroix. 2002. The theory of use behind telemedicine: How compatible with physicians' clinical routines? *Social Science & Medicine*, 54: 889–904.

Lehoux, P., C. Sicotte, J.-L. Denis, A. Lacroix, and M. Berg. 2000. Trust as a key component in the use of teleconsultation. *Annals of the Royal College of Physicians and Surgeons of Canada* 33 (8): 482–487.

Lehoux, P., S. Tailliez, J.-L. Denis, and M. Hivon. 2004. Redefining HTA in Canada: Diversification of products and contextualization of findings. *International Journal of Technology Assessment in Health Care* 20 (3): 325–336.

Lehtonen, T.-K. 2003. The domestication of new technologies as a set of trials. *Journal of Consumer Culture* 3 (3): 363–385.

Leslie, J. 1989. Women's time: A factor in the use of child survival technologies? *Health Policy and Planning* 4 (1): 1–16.

Levin-Scherz, J. 2001. Will disruptive innovations cure health care? *Harvard Business Review* 79 (2): 150–151.

Lewis, S., P. Baird, R. G. Evans, W. A. Ghali, C. J. Wright, E. Gibson, and F. Baylis. 2001. Dancing with the porcupine: Rules governing the university-industry relationship. *Canadian Medical Association Journal* 165 (6): 783–785.

Leys, M. 2003. Health technology assessment: The contribution of qualitative research. *International Journal of Technology Assessment in Health Care* 19 (2): 319–329.

Light, D. W., R. Castellblanch, P. Arredondo, and D. Socolar. 2003. No exit and the organization of voice in biotechnology and pharmaceuticals. *Journal of Health Politics, Policy and Law*, 28 (2–3): 473–507.

Littlejohns, P., G. Leng, T. Culyer, and M. Drummond. 2004. NICE clinical guidelines: Maybe health economists should participate in guideline development. Letter. *British Medical Journal* 329: 571.

Lock, M., A. Young, and A. Cambrosio, eds. 2000. *Living and working with new medical technologies.* Cambridge: Cambridge University Press.

Lomas, J. 1990. Finding audiences, changing beliefs: The structure of research use in Canadian health policy. *Journal of Health Politics, Policy, and Law* 15 (3): 525–542.

Lomas, J. 1993. Making clinical policy explicit. *International Journal of Technology Assessment in Health Care* 9 (1): 11–25.

Lomas, J. 2004. Postscript: Understanding evidence-based decision-making or why keyboards are irrational? In *Multidisciplinary perspectives on evidence-based decision-making in health care,* ed. L. Lemieux-Charles and F. Champagne, 281–290. Toronto: University of Toronto Press.

Longman dictionary of the English language. 1984. Harlow, U.K.: Longman.

Lowton, K., and J. Gabe. 2003. Life on a slippery slope: Perceptions of health in adults with cystic fibrosis. *Sociology of Health & Illness* 25 (4): 289–319.

Luck, R. 2003. Dialogue in participatory design. *Design Studies* 24: 523–535.

Lun, K. C. 1995. New user interfaces. *International Journal of Biomedical Computing* 39:147–150.

MacKenzie, D., and J. Wacjman, eds. 1985. *The social shaping of technology: How the refrigerator got its hum.* Milton Keynes, U.K.: Open University Press.

Malpani, A., A. Malpani, and D. Modi. 2002. Preimplantation sex selection for family balancing in India. *Human Reproduction* 17 (1): 11–12.

Marmor, T. R., and J. Blustein. 1994. Cutting waste by making rules: Promises, pitfalls and realistic prospects. In *Understanding health care reform*, ed. T. R. Marmor, 86–106. New Haven, Conn.: Yale University Press.

Marteau, T. M., and C. Lerman. 2001. Genetic risk and behavioural change. *British Medical Journal* 322 (7293): 1056–1059.

Martin, D. K., M. Giacomini, and P. A. Singer. 2002. Fairness, accountability for reasonableness, and the views of priority setting decision-makers. *Health Policy* 61: 279–290.

Martin, M. W. 2002. Personal meaning and ethics in engineering. *Science and Engineering Ethics* 8: 545–560.

Mather, C. 2004. The pipeline and the porcupine: Alternate metaphors of the physician-industry relationship. *Social Science and Medicine* 60: 1323–1334.

Mather, C., U. Fleising, and L. Taylor. 2004. Translating knowledge from bench to bedside: The controversial social life of t-PA. *Risk Management: An International Journal* 6 (2): 49–60.

May, C., M. Mort, T. Williams, F. Mair, and L. Gask. 2003. Health technology assessment in its local contexts: Studies of telehealthcare. *Social Science and Medicine* 57 (4): 697–710.

McGregor, M. 1992. Can our health services be saved by technology evaluation? The Quebec experience. *Clinical Investigative Medicine* 17 (4): 334–342.

McKeever, P., and P. Coyte. 1999. *Place in health care: Sites, roles, rights and responsibilities.* Report prepared under the auspices of an SSHRC/CHSRF Health Institute Design Grant.

McKeever, P. 2001. Home care in Canada: Housing matters. *Canadian Journal of Nursing Research* 33 (2): 3–4.

McKeever, P., J. Angus, K.-L. Miller, and D. Reid. 2003. "It's more of a production": Accomplishing mothering using a mobility device. *Disability & Society* 18 (2): 179–197.

McKinlay, J. 1981. From "promising report" to "standard procedure": Seven stages in the career of a medical innovation. *Milbank Memorial Fund Quarterly: Health and Society* 59 (3): 374–411.

Mechanic, D. 2002. Socio-cultural implications of changing organizational technologies in the provision of care. *Social Science and Medicine* 54 (3): 459–467.

Melzer, A. M. 1993. The problem with the "problem of technology." In *Technology in the western political tradition*, ed. A. M. Melzer, J. Weinberger, and M. R. Zinman, 287–322. Ithaca, N.Y.: Cornell University Press.

Menkes, D. B., M. P. Davison, S. A. Costello, and C. Jaye. 2005. Stereotactic radiosurgery: The patient's experience. *Social Science and Medicine* 60: 2561–2573.

Menon D., and L. A. Topfer. 2000. Health technology assessment in Canada: A decade in review. *International Journal of Technology Assessment in Health Care* 16: 896–902.

Merleau-Ponty, M. 1969. *Phénoménologie de la perception.* Paris: Gallimard.

Merleau-Ponty, M. 1962. *Phenomenology of perception*, trans. Colin Smith. New York: The Humanities Press.

Mitchell, L. M., and A. Cambrosio. 1997. The invisible topography of power: Electromagnetic fields, bodies and the environment. *Social Studies of Science* 27 (2): 221–271.

Mol, A. 2000. What diagnostic devices do: The case of blood sugar measurement. *Theoretical Medicine and Bioethics* 21: 9–22.

Mol, A.-M. 2002. *The body multiple: Ontology in medical practice.* Durham, N.C.: Duke University Press.

Mol, A.-M., and J. Law. 1994. Regions, networks, and fluids: Anaemia and social topology. *Social Studies of Science* 24 (4): 641–671.

Molewijk, A. C., A. M. Stiggelbout, W. Otten, H. M. Dupuis, and J. Kievit. 2004. Implicit normativity in evidence-based medicine: A plea for integrated empirical ethics research. *Health Care Analysis* 11 (1): 69–92.

Moran, M., and E. Alexander. 1997. Technology, American democracy and health care. *British Journal of Political Sciences* 27: 573–594.

Moreira, T. 2005. Diversity in guidelines: The role of repertoires of evaluation. *Social Science and Medicine* 60: 1975–1985.

Morgall, J. M. 1993. *Technology assessment: A feminist perspective.* Philadelphia: Temple University Press.

Mort, M., C. May, and T. Williams. 2003. Remote doctors and absent patients: Acting at a distance in telemedicine? *Science, Technology and Human Values* 28: 274–295.

Murphy, E., R. Dingwall, D. Greatbatch, S. Parker, and P. Watson. 1998. Qualitative research methods in health technology assessment: A review of the literature. *Health Technology Assessment* 2 (16), http://www.ncchta.org/fullmono/mon216.pdf.

Murray, S. A., E. Grant, A. Grant, and M. Kendall. 2003. Dying in developed and developing countries: Lessons from two qualitative interview studies of patients and their carers. *British Medical Journal* 326: 368.

Mykhalovskiy, E., and L. Weir. 2004. The problem of evidence-based medicine: Directions for social science. *Social Science and Medicine* 59 (5): 1059–1069.

Nélisse, C. 1996. La trousse médico-légale: Technologie sociale et protocolorisation de l'intervention. *Sociologie et Sociétés* 28 (2): 157–171.

Neves, M. P. 2004. Cultural context and consent: An anthropological view. *Medicine, Health Care and Philosophy* 7: 93–98.

Newhouse, J. P. 1992. Medical care costs: How much welfare loss? *Journal of Economic Perspectives* 6: 3–21.

Newhouse, J. P. 1993. An iconoclastic view of health cost containment. *Health Affairs* 15: 152–171.

Neyland, D. 2004. Closed-circuits of interactions? The mobilization of images and accountability through high-street CCTV. *Information, Communication and Society* 7 (2): 252–271.

Neyland, D. 2005. Personal communication.

Nieusma, D. 2004. Alternative design scholarship: Working toward appropriate design. *Design Issues* 20 (3): 13–24.

Nord, E. 1999. *Cost-value analysis in health care: Making sense out of QALYs.* Cambridge, Cambridge University Press.

Norman, D. 1989. *The design of everyday things.* Toronto: Doubleday.

Oliver S., L. Clarke-Jones, R. Rees, R. Milne, P. Buchanan, G. Gyte, A. Oakley, and K. Stein. 2004. Involving consumers in research and development agenda setting for the NHS: Developing an evidence-based approach. *Health Technology Assessment* 8 (15), http://www.ncchta.org/fullmono/mon815.pdf.

Oortwijn, W., R. Reuzel, and M.Decker. 2004. Introduction. *Poiesis &Praxis*, 2: 97–102.

Oudshoorn, N., and T. Pinch. 2003. *How users matter: The co-construction of users and technologies.* Cambridge, MA: MIT Press.

Pacey, A. 1999. *Meaning in technology.* Cambridge, MA: MIT Press.

Paravic, J., B. Brajenovic-Milic, D. Tislaric, M. Kapovic, A. Botica, V. Jurcan, and S. Milotti. 1999. Maternal serum screening for Down syndrome: A survey of pregnant women's views. *Community Genetics* 2 (2–3): 109–112.

Parent, K., and M. Anderson. 2000. Developing a home care system by design. *Healthcare Papers* 11 (4): 46–52.

Pasveer, B. 1989. Knowledge of shadows: The introduction of x-ray images in medicine. *Sociology of Health & Illness* 11 (4): 360–381.

Peden, E. A., and M. S. Freeland.1995. A historical analysis of medical spending growth, 1960–1963. *Health Affairs* 14: 235–247.

Pelz, D. C. 1978. Some expanded perspectives on the use of social science in public policy. In *Major social issues: A multidisciplinary view*, ed. J. M. Yinger and S. J. Cutler, 346–357. New York: Free Press.

Peters, B. E. 2000. Hospitals and the forces of change. In *Technology and the future of health care: Preparing for the next 30 years*, ed. D. Ellis, 193–208. San Francisco: Jossey-Bass.

Petre, M. 2004. How expert engineering teams use disciplines of innovation. *Design Studies* 25: 477–493.

Pierret, J. 2003. The illness experience: State of knowledge and perspective for research. *Sociology of Health & Illness* 25: 4–22.

Pinch, T. J., and W. E. Bijker. 1987. The social construction of facts and artifacts or how the sociology of science and the sociology of technology might benefit from each other. In *The social construction of technological systems*, ed. W. E. Bijker, T. P. Hughes, and T. J. Pinch, 11–50. Cambridge, MA: MIT Press.

Pinch, T. and T. Pinch. 1988. Reservations about reflexivity and new literary forms or why let the devil have all the good tunes? In *Knowledge and reflexivity: New frontiers in the sociology of knowledge*, ed. S. Woolgar, 178–197. London: Sage.

Pippin, K., and G. R. Fernie. 1997. Designing devices that are acceptable to the frail elderly: A new understanding based upon how older people perceive a walker. *Technology & Disability* 7: 93–102.

Pivik, J., E. Rode, and C. Ward. 2004. A consumer involvement model for health technology assessment in Canada. *Health Policy* 69: 253–268.

Poland, B., P. Lehoux, D. Holmes, and G. Andrews. 2005. How place matters: Unpacking technology and power relations in health and social care. *Health and Social Care in the Community* 13 (2): 170–180.

Prasad, P. 1993. Symbolic processes in the implementation of technological change: A symbolic interactionist study of work computerization. *Academy of Management Journal* 36 (6): 1400–1429.

Prout, A. 1996. Actor-network theory, technology and medical sociology: An illustrative analysis of the metered dose inhaler. *Sociology of Health and Illness* 18 (2): 198–219.

Reese W. L. 1980. *Dictionary of philosophy and religion*. Atlantic Highlands, N.J.: Humanities Press.

Reiter-Theil, S. 2004. Does empirical research make bioethics more relevant? The "embedded researcher" as a methodological approach. *Medicine, Health Care and Philosophy* 7: 17–29.

Remennick, L. I., and R. A. Shtarkshall. 1997. Technology versus responsibility: Immigrant physicians from the former Soviet Union reflect on Israeli health care. *Journal of Health and Social Behavior* 38: 191–202.

Reuzel, R., W. Oortwijn, M. Decker, C. Clausen, P. Gallo, J. Grin, A. Grunwald, L. Hennen, G. van der Wilt, and Y. Yoshinaka. 2004. Ethics and HTA: Some lessons and challenges for the future. *Poiesis & Praxis* 2: 247–256.

Rip, A., T. J. Misa, and J. Schot, eds. 1995. *Managing technology in society: The approach of constructive technology assessment*. London: Pinter.

Robins, R., and S. Metcalfe. 2004. Integrating genetics as practices of primary care. *Social Science & Medicine* 59: 223–233.

Rocher, G. 1990. Y a-t-il des normes d'allocation des équipements couteux en milieu hospitalier? *Revue de Droit de l'Université de Sherbrooke* 20: 219–229.

Ross, S. E., J. N. Lavis, C. Rodriguez, J. M. Woodside, and J.-L. Denis. 2003. Partnership experiences: Involving decision-makers in the research process. *Journal of Health Services Research and Policy* 8 (Suppl. 2): 26–34.

Rouse, J. 1991. Philosophy of science and the persistent narratives of modernity. *Studies in History and Philosophy of Science* 22 (1): 141–162.

Royle, J., and S. Oliver. 2004. Consumer involvement in the health technology assessment program. *International Journal of Technology Assessment in Health Care* 20 (4): 493–497.

Sanders, C. A. 1995. Industry's efforts: Devices and pharmaceuticals. *Annals of Thoracic Surgery* 60: 1537–1540.

Sang, B. 2004. Choice, participation and accountability: Assessing the potential impact of legislation promoting patient and public involvement in health in the UK. *Health Expectations* 7: 187–190.

Savage, J. 2000. Ethnography and health care. *British Medical Journal* 321: 1400–1402.

Savoie, I., A. Kazanjian, and F. Brunger. 1999. Women, the media, and heart disease. *International Journal of Technology Assessment in Health Care* 15 (4): 729–737.

Scott, S., L. Prior, F. Wood, and J. Gray. 2005. Repositioning the patient: The implications of being "at risk." *Social Science and Medicine* 60: 1869–1879.

Serres, M. 1991. *Le tiers-instruit*. Paris: Gallimard.

Serres, M. 2001. *Hominescence*. Paris: Pommier.

Shemer, J., and T. Schersten, eds. 1995. *Technology assessment in health care: From theory to practice*. Jerusalem: Gefen.

Shostak, S. 2003. Locating gene-environment interaction: At the intersections of genetics and public health. *Social Science and Medicine* 56: 2327–2342.

Sicotte, C., J.-L. Denis, P. Lehoux, and F. Champagne. 1998. The computer-based patient record: Challenges towards timeless and spaceless medical practice. *Journal of Medical Systems* 22 (4): 237–256.

Sinding, C. 2003. Disarmed complaints: Unpacking satisfaction with end-of-life care. *Social Science & Medicine* 57: 1375–1385.

Siu, K. W. M. 2003. Users' creative responses and designers' roles. *Design Issues* 19 (2): 64–73.

Smith, J. T. 2000. Will disruptive innovations cure health care? *Harvard Business Review* 78 (6): 198.

Smith, K. 1997. Economic infrastructures and innovation systems. In *Systems of innovation: Technologies, institutions and organizations*, ed. C. Edquist, 86–105. London: Pinter.

Stengers, I. 1993. *L'invention des sciences modernes*. Paris: Éditions La Découverte.

Sullivan, M. 2003. The new subjective medicine: Taking the patient's point of view on health care and health. *Social Science & Medicine* 56: 1595–1604.

Tatum, J. S. 2004. The challenge of responsible design. *Design Issues* 20 (3): 66–80.

Tenery, R. M. 2000. Interactions between physicians and the health care technology industry. *Journal of the American Medical Association* 283 (3): 391–393.

Tenner, E. 1996. *Why things bite back: Technology and the revenge of unintended consequences*. New York: Vintage Books.

Timmermans, S., and M. Berg. 2003. The practice of medical technology. *Sociology of Health and Illness* 25: 97–114.

Tunis, S. 2004. Why Medicare has not established criteria for coverage decisions. *New England Journal of Medicine* 350 (21): 2196–2198.

Udow, M., and K. L. Seitz. 2000. A payer's perspective on the future. In *Technology and the future of health care: Preparing for the next 30 years*, ed. D. Ellis, 209–230. San Francisco: Jossey-Bass.

U.S. Congress, Office of Technology Assessment. 1985. *Medicare's prospective payment system: Strategies for evaluating cost, quality, and medical technology*. Washington, D.C.: Government Printing Office.

van der Scheer, L., and G. Widdershoven. 2004a. A response to Levitt and Molewijk. *Medicine, Health Care and Philosophy* 7: 89–91.

van der Scheer, L., and G. Widdershoven. 2004b. Integrated empirical ethics: Loss of normativity? *Medicine, Health Care and Philosophy* 7: 71–79.

van der Wilt, G. J. 2004. Health technology assessment: Trying to bring empirical and ethical inquiry together. *Poiesis & Praxis* 2: 195–206.

Vicente, K. 2003. *The human factor: Revolutionizing the way people live with technology*. New York: Taylor & Francis.

Vos, R., and D. L. Willems. 2000. Technology in medicine: Ontology, epistemology, ethics and social philosophy at the crossroads. *Theoretical Medicine and Bioethics* 21: 1–7.

Wailoo, A., J. Roberts, J. Brazier, and C. McCabe. 2004. Efficiency, equity, and NICE clinical guidelines. *British Medical Journal* 328: 536–537.

Webster, A. 2004a. Health technology assessment: A sociological commentary on reflexive innovation. *International Journal of Technology Assessment in Health Care* 20 (1): 61–66.

Webster, A. 2004b. Healthy innovation: An international workshop held at the University of Manchester, July 8–10, 2004, http://www.york.ac.uk/res/iht/events/healthyinnov/healthyinnov2004.htm (accessed January 27, 2005).

Weisbrod, B. A. 1991. The health care quadrilemma: An essay of technological change, insurance, quality of care, and cost containment. *Journal of Economic Literature* 29: 523–552.

Weiss, C., ed. 1977. *Using social research in public policy making*. Toronto: Lexington Books.

Weiss, C. H. 1991. Policy research: Data, ideas, or arguments? In *Social sciences and modern states: National experiences and theoretical crossroads*, ed. P. Wagner, C. H. Weiss, B. Wittrock, and H. Wollman, 307–332. Cambridge: Cambridge University Press.

Wensing, M., and G. Elwyn. 2003. Methods for incorporating patients' views in health care. *British Medical Journal* 326: 877–879.

Wiktorowicz, M., and R. Deber. 1997. Regulating biotechnology: a rational-political model of policy development. *Health Policy* 40 (3): 115–138.

Williams, R., and D. Edge. 1996. The social shaping of technology. *Research Policy* 25: 865–899.

Williams, T., C. May, F. Mair, M. Mort, and L. Gask. 2003. Normative models of health technology assessment and the social production of evidence about telehealth care. *Health Policy* 64 (1): 39–54.

Williams-Jones, B., and J. E. Graham. 2003. Actor-network theory: A tool to support ethical analysis of commercial genetic testing. *New Genetics and Society* 22 (3): 271–296.

Winner, L. 1980. Do artifacts have politics? *Daedalus* 109 (1): 121–135.

Winner, L. 1994. Reply to Mark Elam. *Science, Technology, & Human Values* 19 (1): 107–109.

Witz, A. 1992. *Professions and patriarchy.* London: Routledge.

Wooffitt, R., and C. MacDermid. 1995. Wizards and social control. In *The social and interactional dimensions of human-computer interfaces*, ed. P. J. Thomas, 126–141. Cambridge: Cambridge University Press.

Woolgar, S. 1988. Reflexivity is the ethnographer of the text. In *Knowledge and reflexivity: New frontiers in the sociology of knowledge*, ed. S. Woolgar, 14–35. London: Sage.

Woolgar, S. 1991. Configuring the user: The case of usability trials. In *A sociology of monsters: Essays on power, technology and domination*, ed. J. Law, 58–97. London: Routledge.

Woolgar, S., and M. Ashmore. 1988. The next step: An introduction to the reflexive project. In *Knowledge and reflexivity: New frontiers in the sociology of knowledge*, ed. S. Woolgar, 1–11. London: Sage.

Woolgar, S., and G. Cooper. 1999. Do artefacts have ambivalence? Moses' bridges, Winner's bridges and other urban legends in S&TS. *Social Studies of Science* 29 (3): 433–449.

Wyer, M., ed. 2001. *Women, science, and technology: A reader in feminist science studies.* New York: Routledge.

Zimmern, R., and C. Cook. 2000. *Genetics and health: Policy issues for genetic science and their implications for health and health services.* London: The Nuffield Trust.

Permissions

Chapter 1. Health Technology Assessment: Promises and pitfalls

Figure 1.1 The Institutionalization of HTA-based Change in Health Care Systems

> Originally published in *Journal of Health Politics, Policy, and Law* (2005). Permission to reprint obtained from Duke University Press.

Table 1.1 Number of HTA Documents Published by Six Canadian HTA Agencies (1995–2001)

> Originally published in *International Journal of Technology Assessment in Health Care* (2004). Permission to reprint obtained from Cambridge University Press.

Table 1.2 Types of Documents Published by Six Canadian HTA Agencies (1995–2001)

> Originally published in *International Journal of Technology Assessment in Health Care* (2004). Permission to reprint obtained from Cambridge University Press.

Table 1.3 Types of Technology Assessed by Six Canadian HTA Agencies (1995–2001)

> Originally published in *International Journal of Technology Assessment in Health Care* (2004). Permission to reprint obtained from Cambridge University Press.

Table 1.4 Issues Addressed by Six Canadian HTA Agencies (1995–2001)

Originally published in *International Journal of Technology Assessment in Health Care* (2004). Permission to reprint obtained from Cambridge University Press.

Table 1.5 Examples of Negative, Neutral, and Positive Conclusions

Originally published in *International Journal of Technology Assessment in Health Care* (2004). Permission to reprint obtained from Cambridge University Press.

Table 1.6 Summary of the Portfolio Characteristics of the Six Canadian HTA Agencies

Originally published in *International Journal of Technology Assessment in Health Care* (2004). Permission to reprint obtained from Cambridge University Press.

Table 1.9 The Various Forms of HTA Use by Three Types of User

Originally published in *International Journal of Technology Assessment in Health Care* (2005). Permission to reprint obtained from Cambridge University Press.

Table 1.10 Limitations in the Use of HTA

Originally published in *International Journal of Technology Assessment in Health Care* (2005). Permission to reprint obtained from Cambridge University Press.

Table 1.11 Five Categories of Technology and Their Associated Ethical Issues

Originally published in *International Journal of Technology Assessment in Health Care* (2003). Permission to reprint obtained from Cambridge University.

Chapter 3. What Do Humans Want and for Whom?

Figure 3.2 Technical and Human Dimensions That Shape User-friendliness of Health Technology

Originally published in *BMC Health Services Research* (2004). Permission to reprint obtained from BioMed Central.

Table 3.1 Accountability for Reasonableness and Fairness According to Decision-makers

Originally published in *Health Policy* (2002). Permission to reprint obtained from Elsevier.

Chapter 5. An Alternative Framework

Table 5.2 Strengthening HTA and Research on Health Technology

Originally published in *Journal of Health Politics, Policy, and Law* (2000). Permission to reprint obtained from Duke University Press.

Appendices

Box A.1 Sampling Criteria for Interviews and Survey Respondents

Originally published in *International Journal of Technology Assessment in Health Care* (2005). Permission to reprint obtained from Cambridge University Press.

Table A.1 Structure and Resources of the Six Agencies (2001–2002)

Originally published in *Journal of Health Politics, Policy, and Law* (2000). Permission to reprint obtained from Duke University Press.

Index